Clinical Cases in Neurology

Clinical Cases in Neurology

Editor: Foster Jones

AMERICAN
MEDICAL PUBLISHERS
www.americanmedicalpublishers.com

AMERICAN
MEDICAL PUBLISHERS
www.americanmedicalpublishers.com

Cataloging-in-Publication Data

Clinical cases in neurology / edited by Foster Jones.
p. cm.
Includes bibliographical references and index.
ISBN 979-8-88740-631-2
1. Neurology. 2. Nervous system--Diseases. I. Jones, Foster.
RC346 .C55 2023
616.8--dc23

American Medical Publishers,
41 Flatbush Avenue,
1st Floor, New York,
NY 11217, USA

ISBN 979-8-88740-631-2 (Hardback)

Contents

Preface

Neurology refers to a medical specialty that focuses on the diagnosis, treatment and management of diseases and disorders that affect the nervous system, which comprises the brain, spinal cord, nerves, and muscles. Some common diseases and conditions which are treated under this field are stroke, epilepsy and multiple sclerosis. Stroke occurs when the blood supply to the brain is disrupted, leading to brain cell damage. Epilepsy is a neurological disorder characterized by recurrent seizures. Multiple sclerosis refers to an autoimmune disease that affects the central nervous system, leading to inflammation and damage to the protective covering of nerve fibers. This book unravels the recent studies in the field of neurology. From theories to research to practical applications, clinical cases related to all contemporary topics of relevance to this field have been included herein. The book will serve as a reference to a broad spectrum of readers.

This book is the end result of constructive efforts and intensive research done by experts in this field. The aim of this book is to enlighten the readers with recent information in this area of research. The information provided in this profound book would serve as a valuable reference to students and researchers in this field.

At the end, I would like to thank all the authors for devoting their precious time and providing their valuable contribution to this book. I would also like to express my gratitude to my fellow colleagues who encouraged me throughout the process.

Editor

1

Compressive Dorsal Myelopathy Secondary to Extramedullary Hematopoiesis in a Thalassemic Patient

Ismail Ibrahim Ismail,[1] **Fathi Massoud**,[1] **K. J. Alexander**,[1] **and Jasem Youssef Al-Hashel**[1,2]

[1]*Department of Neurology, Ibn Sina Hospital, Kuwait*
[2]*Department of Medicine, Faculty of Medicine, Health Sciences Centre, Kuwait University, Kuwait*

Correspondence should be addressed to Ismail Ibrahim Ismail; dr.ismail.ibrahim2012@gmail.com

Academic Editor: Andreas K. Demetriades

Background. Extramedullary hematopoiesis (EMH) is one of the rare causes of spinal cord compression (SCC). It results from noncancerous proliferation of hematopoietic tissue outside the bone marrow as a compensatory mechanism for ineffective erythropoiesis. It occurs in the paraspinal area in 11–15% of thalassemic patients in intermediate and severe cases causing a paraspinal compressive mass. We present a rare case of spinal EMH with thoracic cord compression in a 22-year-old female with beta thalassemia who presented with paraparesis and we provide a review of literature. *Case Report.* A 22-year-old female patient with a known history of beta thalassemia presented with subacute onset of weakness and numbness of both lower limbs with a sensory level at T6. Magnetic resonance imaging (MRI) of the dorsal spine showed cord compression secondary to paraspinal EMH from T2 to T9 with most prominent compression over T5. She was managed with blood transfusion and low-dose radiotherapy. *Conclusion.* Although rare, EMH should be suspected in thalassemic patients presenting with paraplegia. Treatment with blood transfusions is usually effective. Other options include radiotherapy, surgery, hydroxyurea or a combination of these modalities.

1. Introduction

Thalassemia is an autosomal recessive blood disease which leads to a chronic anemic state. It is classified into α-thalassemia and β-thalassemia according to which chain of the hemoglobin molecule is affected. Non-transfusion-dependent thalassemia (NTDT) is a state that does not require regular blood transfusion, contrary to transfusion-dependent thalassemia (TDT) that is usually treated with repeated blood transfusions and iron chelation. The clinical phenotype and severity of β-thalassemia can manifest as major, minor, or intermedia. Bone marrow transplantation is curative and despite being expensive, it is usually offered to thalassemic patients in Kuwait [1].

EMH is a well-documented complication of conditions associated with ineffective hematopoiesis resulting in a chronic anemic state. The noncancerous proliferation of hematopoietic tissue outside the bone marrow causes expansion into nearby normal tissues. Paraspinal EMH affects 11–15% of thalassemic patients and is usually asymptomatic in the majority of them [2].

We report a rare case of spinal EMH with dorsal cord compression and myelopathy in a 22-year-old female with beta thalassemia who presented with paraparesis and we provide a review of literature.

2. Case Report

A 22-year-old Kuwaiti female with a past history of non-transfusion dependent beta-thalassemia who do not receive any current active treatment presented with a two months history of subacute onset of gait difficulty secondary to weakness and stiffness of both lower limbs with recurrent falls. Her condition was associated with back pain, mainly in the thoracic region and bilateral numbness of the lower part of her body up to the level of the costal margin. She had no sphincteric affection, no

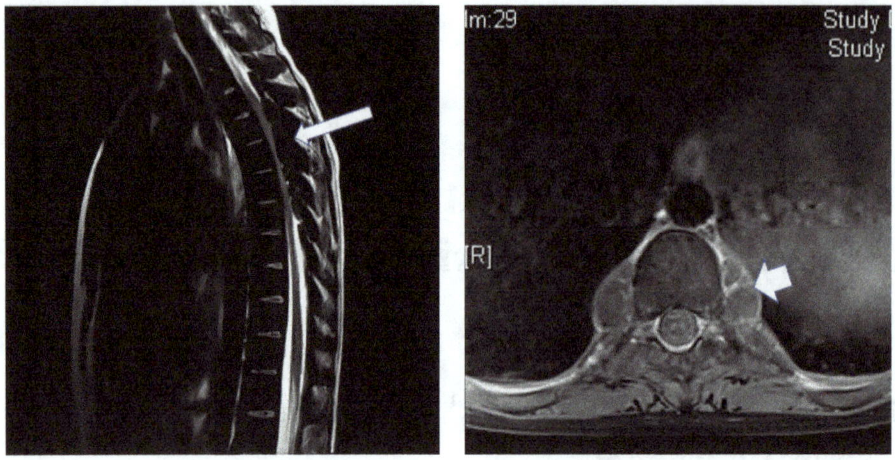

(a) (b)

Figure 1: MRI of the dorsal spine: (a) sagittal T2-weighted, (b) axial T1-weighted images with contrast showing posterior epidural multilobulated extramedullary hematopoietic mass from T2 to T9 (arrows) with the largest at T5 causing the most prominent cord compression and showing no contrast enhancement.

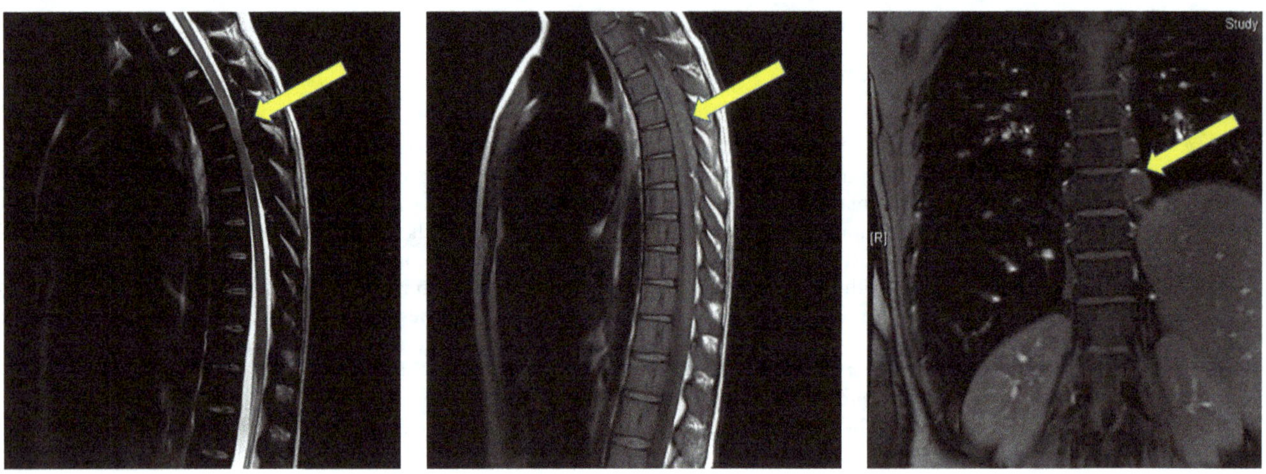

(a) (b) (c)

Figure 2: Follow up MRI of the spine after blood transfusion: (a) sagittal T2-weighted, (b) sagittal T1-weighted, (c) coronal T1-weighted images showing interval reduction in cord compression.

history of trauma or fever and no history of previous similar condition.

Neurological examination showed a fully conscious and oriented patient with normal speech, higher mental functions and cranial nerves. Motor examination was normal in both upper limbs. Lower limbs examination showed spastic paraparesis with hypertonia, power of grade 4+/5, hyperreflexia (3+) and bilateral extensor plantar response. Sensory examination showed a sensory level at T6 with poor joint position and movement sensation. She had no cerebellar signs while her gait was spastic.

Laboratory investigations were as follows: hemoglobin (Hb): 66 g/L, Hematocrit (Hct): 0.198, mean corpuscular volume (MCV): 63.2 and mean corpuscular hemoglobin (MCH): 22.2. Iron level was 25.7 umol/L, transferrin: 1.4 g/L, ferritin: 39 ng/mL and saturation: 74%. Serum electrolytes, renal function, liver function, coagulation profile, vasculitic work-up and thyroid function were normal.

MRI of the brain was normal. MRI of the spine showed multi-lobulated soft tissue masses at the posterior epidural spaces of the thoracic spine from T2 to T9, with the most prominent cord compression at T5 level. These masses are isointense to bone marrow and show no significant enhancement suggestive of extramedullary hematopoiesis (Figure 1).

She was evaluated by hematologist and she received blood transfusion in the form of one unit of packed red blood cells. Hemoglobin level increased from 6.6 to 9.1 g/L. She showed partial clinical improvement after transfusion. Follow up MRI the following day showed reduction in cord compression (Figure 2).

She was further evaluated by neurosurgery who refrained from surgical management due to initial improvement and Oncologist advised for adjuvant low dose radiotherapy to prevent recurrence. She was also put on scheduled blood transfusions and she remained clinically and radiologically stable on follow up visits for one year with improved strength in both lower limbs (G 5/5), 2+ reflexes and down-going plantar response bilaterally.

3. Discussion

EMH has been observed in numerous hematological disorders, including thalassemia, sickle cell anemia, hereditary spherocytosis and idiopathic thrombocytopenic purpura. It occurs as a response to chronic anemia states as a homeostatic mechanism via the production of erythropoietin [3].

The carrier rates of β-thalassemia in the Arab countries range from 1% to 11% of the population [4]. In Kuwait, it is estimated that the number of thalassemic patients are more than 475 cases [5, 6]. Galanello et al. estimated the percentage of β-thalassemia carriers in Kuwait to be 3% of population [7].

The association between EMH and NTDT is well-recognized and Gatto et al. was the first to report SCC in these patients in 1954 [8]. The incidence of EMH in thalassemia vary in literature between 0.8% in thalassemia major and up to 20% in thalassemia intermedia. EMH is particularly common in NTDT patients (20%) and rare in TDT (<1%) due to underlying bone marrow suppression from repeated transfusions [9, 10].

It affects the paraspinal region in 11–15% of the cases followed by the liver, spleen, and lymph nodes [11]. The most frequent location of paraspinal EMH is thoracic and it is usually asymptomatic and incidentally discovered on imaging in the majority of cases with only 20% presenting with SCC and significant disability [12]. The reason why there is a predilection for thoracic cord region is unclear, however, some authors believe that stem cells could have leaked into the thoracic epidural space from the expanding bone marrow [13].

Paraspinal EMH is more common in males with a M:F ratio ranging from 2.5 : 1 to 5 : 1 and occurs mainly in chronic cases in the third and fourth decades of life. The clinical manifestations depend on the site and size of the mass and include: back and lower limb pain, paresthesia, paraplegia, paraparesis and sphincteric dysfunction [14].

The gold standard for diagnosis is MRI as it can show clearly the site and extent of EMH and can differentiate between active and inactive lesions. Active lesions contain blood while inactive lesions contain fat and iron deposits. Active recent lesions show intermediate signal intensity in T1 and T2 weighted images while inactive lesions show high signal intensity in both T1 and T2 weighted images if it contains fatty tissue or low signal intensity if it contains iron deposition. Gadolinium enhancement varies in literature between no/minimal enhancement to marked enhancement [15]. In our patient, the lesion was isointense to bone marrow with no contrast enhancement.

Treatment of paraspinal EMH should be individualized, in the absence of large randomized controlled trials and evidence-based guidelines in literature. Management modalities include repeated blood transfusions with iron chelation, radiotherapy, surgical decompression, hydroxyurea, or a combination therapy depending on the size of the mass, severity of symptoms and clinical status [16, 17].

In patients presenting with acute cord syndrome, surgical interreference is warranted. An open approach with laminectomies and multi-level decompression is known to be effective. An alternative approach is minimally invasive incisions along the posterior midline with each incision being used to reach four adjacent levels [18].

In our patient, a conservative approach with a combination of blood transfusion and radiotherapy was performed. The mass regressed in size after one unit of blood transfusion due to elevation of hemoglobin level to 9.1 g/dl. This was followed by low-dose radiation (20 Gy in 10 fractions) as adjunctive therapy as hematopoietic tissue is extremely radiosensitive. In literature, up to 50% of patients shows neurological improvement within 3–7 days of radiotherapy.

4. Conclusion

Paraspinal EMH must be suspected in any thalassemic patient presenting with paraplegia. MRI is the modality of choice in diagnosis and evaluation of SCC secondary to EMH. Early diagnosis and management can prevent irreversible neurological damage.

References

[1] D. J. Weatherall, "The Thalassemias," in *Williams Hematology*, B. Beutler, M. A. Lichtman, B. S. Coller, T. J. Kipps, and S. Seligsohn, Eds., pp. 562–564, McGraw-Hill, New York, 6th edition, 2001.

[2] U. Ghieda, M. Elshimy, and A. H. El Beltagi, "Progressive spinal cord compression due to epidural extramedullary hematopoiesis in thalassemia intermedia," *The Neuroradiology Journal*, vol. 26, no. 1, pp. 111–117, 2013.

[3] K. Yamamoto, Y. Miwa, S. Abe-Suzuki et al., "Extramedullary hematopoiesis: elucidating the function of the hematopoietic stem cell niche," *Molecular Medicine Reports*, vol. 13, no. 1, pp. 587–591, 2016.

[4] Hanan A. Hamamy and Nasir A. S. Al-Allawi, "Epidemiological profile of common haemoglobinopathies in Arab countries," *Journal of Community Genetics*, vol. 4, no. 2, pp. 147–167, 2013.

[5] L. Al-Fuzae, K. C. Aboolbacker, and Q. Al-Saleh, "β-Thalassaemia major in Kuwait," *Journal of Tropical Pediatrics*, vol. 44, no. 5, pp. 311–312, 1998.

[6] M. Burseli, "Kuwait records 475 cases of Thalassemia," *Arab Times*, vol. 18, p. 6, 2013.

[7] R. Galanello, A. Eleftheriou, J. Traeger-Synedinos, J. Old, M. Petrou, and M. Angastiniotis, *Prevention of Thalassaemia and Other Haemoglobin Disorders*, vol. 1, Thalassaemia International Federation Publications, Nicosia, 2003.

[8] I. Gatto, V. Terrana, and L. Biondi, "Compression of the spinal cord due to proliferation of bone marrow in epidural space in a splenectomized person with Cooley's disease," *Haematologica*, vol. 38, no. 1, pp. 61–76, 1954.

[9] M. Angastiniotis and B. Modell, "Global epidemiology of hemoglobin disorders," *Annals of the New York Academy of Sciences*, vol. 850, no. 1, pp. 251–269, 1998.

[10] A. Taher, H. Ismaeel, and M. D. Cappellini, "Thalassaemia intermedia: revisited," *Blood Cells, Molecules, and Diseases*, vol. 37, pp. 12–20, 2006.

[11] D. Sohawon, K. K. Lau, T. Lau, and D. K. Bowden, "Extramedullary haematopoiesis: a pictorial review of its typical and atypical locations," *Journal of Medical Imaging and Radiation Oncology*, vol. 56, no. 5, pp. 538–544, 2012.

[12] R. Haidar, H. Mhaidli, and A. T. Taher, "Paraspinal extramedullary hematopoiesis in patients with thalassemia intermedia," *European Spine Journal*, vol. 19, no. 6, pp. 871–878, 2010.

[13] S. K. Lau, C. K. Chan, and Y. Y. Chow, "Cord compression due to extramedullary hemopoiesis in a patient with thalassemia," *Spine*, vol. 19, no. 21, pp. 2467–2470, 1994.

[14] S. a Salehi, T. Koski, and S. l Ondra, "Spinal cord compression in beta-thalassemia: case report and review of the literature," *Spinal Cord*, vol. 42, no. 2, pp. 117–123, 2004.

[15] A. D. Gouliamos, G. A. Plataniotis, E. S. Michalopoulos, L. J. Vlahos, and C. G. Papavasiliou, "Magnetic resonance imaging spinal cord compression in thalassaemia before and after radiation treatment," *Clinical Radiology*, vol. 50, no. 7, pp. 504–505, 1995.

[16] B. Moncef and J. Hafedh, "Management of spinal cord compression caused by extramedullary hematopoiesis in beta-thalassemia," *Internal Medicine*, vol. 47, no. 12, pp. 1125–1128, 2008.

[17] S. S. Bukhari, M. Junaid, and M. U. Rashid, "Thalassemia, extramedullary hematopoiesis, and spinal cord compression: a case report," *Surgical Neurology International*, vol. 7, no. 6, p. 148, 2016.

[18] Z. A. Smith, C. D. Lawton, A. P. Wong et al., "Minimally invasive thoracic decompression for multi-level thoracic pathologies," *Journal of Clinical Neuroscience*, vol. 21, no. 3, pp. 467–472, 2014.

2

CPEO and Mitochondrial Myopathy in a Patient with *DGUOK* Compound Heterozygous Pathogenetic Variant and mtDNA Multiple Deletions

V. Montano,[1] C. Simoncini,[1] Cassi L. Calì,[2] A. Legati,[3] G. Siciliano,[1] and M. Mancuso[1]

[1]*Department of Clinical and Experimental Medicine, Neurological Clinic, University of Pisa, Pisa, Italy*
[2]*Department of Hand Surgery and Reconstructive Microsurgery, University of Pisa, Pisa, Italy*
[3]*Unit of Medical Genetics and Neurogenetics, Fondazione IRCCS Istituto Neurologico "C. Besta", Milan, Italy*

Correspondence should be addressed to M. Mancuso; mancusomichelangelo@gmail.com

Academic Editor: Chin-Chang Huang

The classic features of deoxyguanosine kinase (*DGUOK*) deficiency are infantile onset hepatic failure with nystagmus and hypotonia; mitochondrial DNA studies on affected tissue reveal mitochondrial DNA depletion. Later, it has been shown that the mutations in the same gene may present with adult-onset mitochondrial myopathy and mitochondrial DNA multiple deletions in skeletal muscle. Here we report the case of a 42-year-old Italian woman presenting with a chronic progressive external ophthalmoplegia and myopathy with mtDNA multiple deletions and the compound heterozygous c.462T>A (p.Asn154Lys) and c.707+2T>G pathogenic variants in *DGUOK*.

1. Introduction

Mitochondrial diseases are multisystem disorders caused by mutation in mitochondrial DNA (mtDNA) or in nuclear DNA (nDNA). Many proteins encoded by nDNA control the replication of mtDNA and the pull of the mtDNA nucleotides necessary for replication; the deficit of these proteins causes mtDNA depletion or multiple deletions or both [1]. The deoxyguanosine kinase (dGK), encoded by *DGUOK* gene (chromosome 2p13, MIM 601465), is an enzyme that catalyzes the phosphorylation of purine deoxyribonucleosides into the corresponding nucleotides; it is necessary for the maintenance of mitochondrial deoxyribonucleoside triphosphate (dNTP) pools and its deficiency results in impaired synthesis of mitochondrial dNTPs, the building blocks for mtDNA, leading to decreased mtDNA amount and mtDNA depletion. The phenotypes associated with the mutation of those gene are most frequently mtDNA depletion syndrome 3 (hepatocerebral type, phenotype MIM number 251880), noncirrhotic portal hypertension (MIM number 617068), and, less frequently, chronic progressive external ophthalmoplegia (cPEO) with mtDNA deletions (MIM number 617070) [2–4].

Here we describe a case of cPEO and myopathy with mtDNA multiple deletions and the compound heterozygous c.462T>A (p.Asn154Lys) and c.707+2T>G pathogenic variants in *DGUOK* gene.

2. Case Report

A 42-year-old Italian woman arrived to our attention for a two-year history of eyelid ptosis, ophthalmoparesis, dysphagia, exercise intolerance, and myalgia. She presented mild hyperCKemia (243U/L). Patient's parents were not consanguineous. She had no family history of neurological disorder. In the past, she has suffered of anxiety disorder. Neurological examination showed mild proximal weakness of lower and upper limbs, weakness of facial muscles, bilateral eyelid ptosis, and ophthalmoparesis. Forearm ischaemic test revealed basal hyperlactacidemia (25 mg/dL, reference value: 4,5-19,8 mg/dl), increased production, and delay in the recovery of lactate. Electromyography showed a myopathic pattern. Echocardiogram was normal but the ergospirometric test showed a functional limitation; spirometry was normal but maximal inspiratory pressure (MIP) and maximal expiratory pressure (MEP) were reduced (MIP=4,1

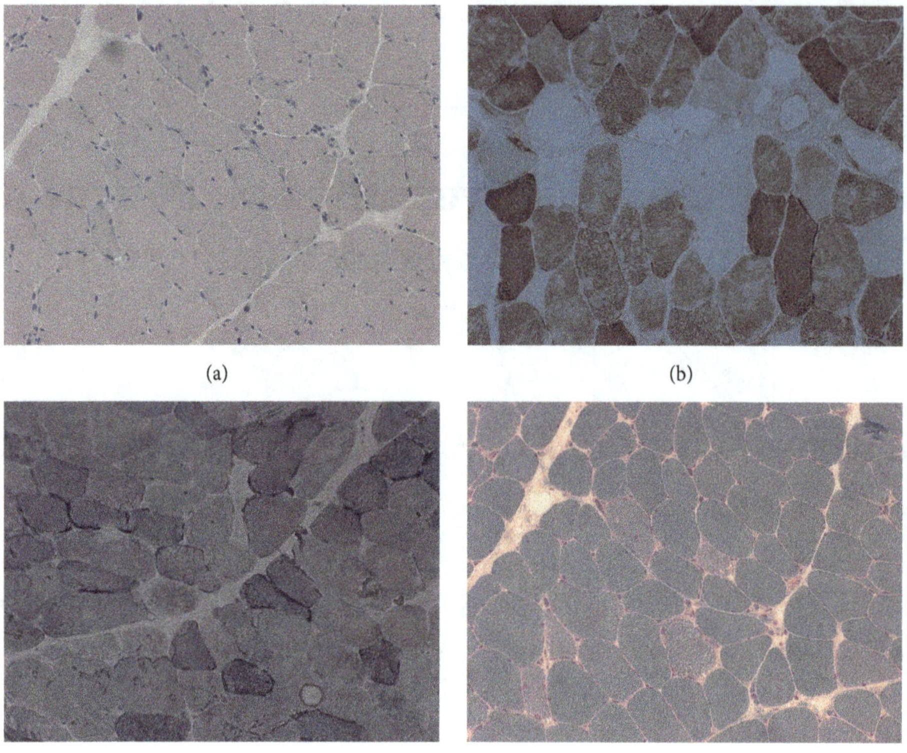

Figure 1: Muscle biopsy: (a) hematoxylin eosin; (b) staining for cytochrome oxidase; (c) succinate dehydrogenase (SDH) staining; (d) Gömöri trichrome stain.

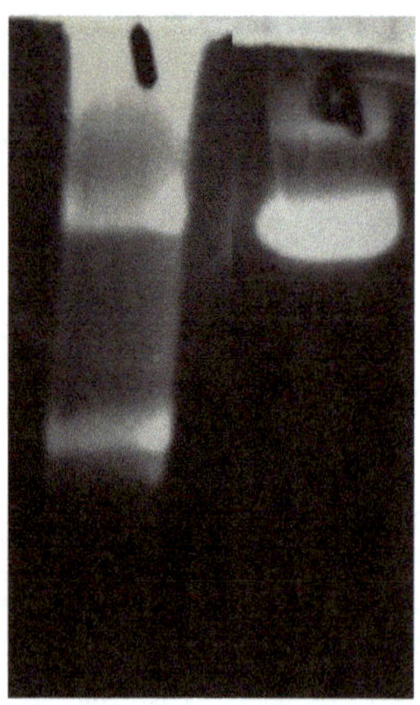

Figure 2: Long-PCR analysis of mitochondrial DNA in muscle tissue: on the left, the test performed on our patient, which shows multiple deletions of mtDNA, and, on the right, a normal control.

kPA, n.v. >7,61, MEP 5,17 kPA, n.v. >10,2). Muscle biopsy revealed ragged red and ragged blue fibers and COX negative fibers (Figure 1). Sequencing of the entire mtDNA from muscle was normal. Long-PCR analysis, in muscle tissue, showed mtDNA multiple deletions (Figure 2), and next-generation sequencing (NGS) analysis detected two *DGOUK* compound heterozygous mutations: the known pathogenetic variant c.462T>A (p.Asn154Lys) and a new variant of the donor splice site of intron 5 c.707+2T>G, predicted to alter the splicing on Human Splicing Finder (http://www.umd.be/HSF3/HSF.shtml) and thus considered pathogenetic. While we could not test their parents, two asymptomatic siblings harbored the c.707+2T>G pathogenetic variant. Since we could not test the parents, it is possible to assume that the two variants were inherited in an autosomal recessive manner in the patient; however, it is equally possible one arose de novo.

3. Discussion

Mitochondrial disorders are the largest group of inherited metabolic disorders and the commonest adult forms of inherited neurological disorders that arise as a result of dysfunction of the mitochondrial respiratory chain and, consequently, deficient energy production [5]. mtDNA encodes for part of its machinery, while most of the mitochondrial proteins are encoded by the nDNA. Accordingly, mitochondrial disorders can be due to mutation of genes encoded by either nuclear DNA or mtDNA. A number of nuclear-encoded factors control mtDNA replication and the maintenance of qualitative and quantitative mtDNA integrity. The impaired cross-talk between the two genomes gives rise to so-called nuclear-mitochondrial intergenomic communication disorders, which result in loss or instability of the mitochondrial genome and impaired maintenance of qualitative and quantitative mtDNA integrity: multiple deletions, depletion, or combinations of the two in critical tissues are "hallmarks" of disease conditions arising from altered communication between these two genomes [6]. The mtDNA depletion syndromes are usually clinically classified as myopathic (*TK2* [thymidine kinase 2] mutation), encephalomyopathic (mutation in *SUCLA2* [Succinate-Coa Ligase, Adp-Forming, Beta Subunit], *SUCLG1* [Succinate-Coa Ligase, Alpha Subunit] and *RRM2B* [Ribonucleotide Reductase M2 B Subunit]), hepatocerebral (due to mutation in DGUOK, *MPV17* [Mitochondrial Inner Membrane Protein], *POLG* [DNA Polymerase Subunit Gamma] and *TWNK* [Twinkle mtDNA Helicase]), or neurogastrointestinal (mutations in TYMP [Thymidine Phosphorylase]) [7, 8].

The other hallmarks of mtDNA instability are mtDNA multiple deletions, which have been shown to accumulate even in the aging of postmitotic tissue [9, 10]. Multiple deletions due to nuclear gene mutation in *POLG1, POLG2, C10Orf2, SLC25A4, RRM2B, OPA1,* and many others may present with clinical phenotypes ranging from chronic external ophthalmoplegia to multisystem involvement including ataxia, parkinsonism, sensory axonal neuropathy, and optic atrophy [11–13].

The deoxyguanosine kinase (dGK), encoded by *DGUOK* gene, plays an important role in maintaining of mitochondrial deoxyribonucleoside triphosphate (dNTP) pools; its deficiency results in impaired synthesis of mitochondrial dNTPs.

DGUOK mutations were firstly associated with mtDNA depletion syndrome by Mandel et al. in 2001 [2]. Classical features associated with *DGUOK* deficiency are lactic acidosis, hypoglycemia, hepatic disease leading to liver failure and neurologic dysfunction with developmental regression, and typical rotary nystagmus or opsoclonus [14]. In 2012, Ronchi et [3] al. identified with NGS sequencing five patients with multiple deletions and autosomal recessive mutations in the *DGUOK* gene, with heterogeneous neuromuscular presentations ranging from PEO with limb girdle weakness to lower motor neuron disease with bulbar symptoms; interestingly, extra muscle involvement was reported (cataract and sensorineural deafness) and only two of the five patients presented hepatic involvement [3]. Buchaklian in the same year reported a patient with mitochondrial myopathy, mtDNA depletion, and a novel *DGUOK* mutation. Vilarinho in 2016 identified with whole exome sequencing the p.Asn46Ser *DGUOK* missense mutation in childhood or infancy onset portal hypertension of indeterminate etiology [15]; multisystem involvement with CPEO, mitochondrial myopathy, parkinsonism, and mtDNA deletions has recently been described by Caporali [16].

Our patient harbored the well-known pathogenic c.462T>A (p.Asn154Lys) pathogenic variant, already described as pathogenic [3, 8, 14], and a new variant not reported in the available databases (HGMD and ClinVar), predicted to be pathogenic altering the wild-type donor site.

We believe that the *DGUOK* mutations are pathogenic for the following reasons: (i) the phenotype of our patient is suggestive of a mitochondrial disease; (ii) all genes causing nuclear-mitochondrial intergenomic communication disorders have been screened in our patient, together with the entire mtDNA, with no mutations detected besides the ones in *DGUOK;* (iii) we have detected mtDNA multiple deletions, which are commonly observed as a consequence of *DGUOK* mutations.

Our report expands the *DGUOK* mutations causing mitochondrial myopathy and reinforces the concept that *DGUOK* mutations should be screened in adulthood patients with mitochondrial myopathy.

Acknowledgments

This work was partially supported by Telethon Grant (GUP09004) and Telethon-MITOCON Grant (GSP16001).

References

[1] S. DiMauro and E. A. Schon, "Mitochondrial respiratory-chain diseases," *The New England Journal of Medicine*, vol. 348, no. 26, pp. 2656–2668, 2003.

[2] H. Mandel, R. Szargel, V. Labay et al., "The deoxyguanosine kinase gene is mutated in individuals with depleted hepatocerebral mitochondrial DNA," *Nature Genetics*, vol. 29, no. 3, pp. 337–341, 2001.

[3] D. Ronchi, C. Garone, A. Bordoni et al., "Next-generation sequencing reveals DGUOK mutations in adult patients with mitochondrial DNA multiple deletions," *Brain*, vol. 135, no. 11, pp. 3404–3415, 2012.

[4] S. Vilarinho, S. Sari, G. Yilmaz et al., "Recurrent recessive mutation in deoxyguanosine kinase causes idiopathic noncirrhotic portal hypertension," *Hepatology*, vol. 63, no. 6, pp. 1977–1986, 2016.

[5] G. S. Gorman, A. M. Schaefer, Y. Ng et al., "Prevalence of nuclear and mitochondrial DNA mutations related to adult mitochondrial disease," *Annals of Neurology*, vol. 77, no. 5, pp. 753–759, 2015.

[6] A. W. El-Hattab and F. Scaglia, "Mitochondrial DNA depletion syndromes: review and updates of genetic basis, manifestations, and therapeutic options," *Neurotherapeutics*, vol. 10, no. 2, pp. 186–198, 2013.

[7] C. Nogueira, L. S. Almeida, C. Nesti et al., "Syndromes associated with mitochondrial DNA depletion," *Italian Journal of Pediatrics*, vol. 40, no. 1, p. 34, 2014.

[8] A. Spinazzola, F. Invernizzi, F. Carrara et al., "Clinical and molecular features of mitochondrial DNA depletion syndromes," *Journal of Inherited Metabolic Disease*, vol. 32, no. 2, pp. 143–158, 2009.

[9] K. J. Krishnan, A. K. Reeve, D. C. Samuels et al., "What causes mitochondrial DNA deletions in human cells?" *Nature Genetics*, vol. 40, no. 3, pp. 275–279, 2008.

[10] P. Yu-Wai-Man and P. F. Chinnery, "Dysfunctional mitochondrial maintenance: what breaks the circle of life?" *Brain*, vol. 135, no. 1, pp. 9–11, 2012, Comment on: The MFN2 gene is responsible for mitochondrial DNA instability and optic atrophy 'plus' phenotype. [Brain. 2012].

[11] P. Amati-Bonneau, M. L. Valentino, P. Reynier et al., "OPA1 mutations induce mitochondrial DNA instability and optic atrophy 'plus' phenotypes," *Brain*, vol. 131, pp. 338–351, 2008.

[12] G. Hudson, P. Amati-Bonneau, E. L. Blakely et al., "Mutation of OPA1 causes dominant optic atrophy with external ophthalmoplegia, ataxia, deafness and multiple mitochondrial DNA deletions: a novel disorder of mtDNA maintenance," *Brain*, vol. 131, no. 2, pp. 329–337, 2008.

[13] C. Rouzier, S. Bannwarth, A. Chaussenot et al., "The MFN2 gene is responsible for mitochondrial DNA instability and optic atrophy 'plus' phenotype," *Brain*, vol. 135, no. 1, pp. 23–34, 2012.

[14] D. P. Dimmock, Q. Zhang, C. Dionisi-Vici et al., "Clinical and molecular features of mitochondrial DNA depletion due to mutations in deoxyguanosine kinase," *Human Mutation*, vol. 29, no. 2, pp. 330-331, 2008.

[15] A. H. Buchaklian, D. Helbling, S. M. Ware, and D. P. Dimmock, "Recessive deoxyguanosine kinase deficiency causes juvenile onset mitochondrial myopathy," *Molecular Genetics and Metabolism*, vol. 107, no. 1-2, pp. 92–94, 2012.

[16] L. Caporali, L. Bello, F. Tagliavini et al., "DGUOK recessive mutations in patients with CPEO, mitochondrial myopathy, parkinsonism and mtDNA deletions," *Brain*, vol. 141, no. 1, p. e3, 2018.

3

Rare Case of Spinal Neurosarcoidosis with Concomitant Epidural Lipomatosis

Nesreen Jaafar,[1] Maria Khoueiry,[1] Samia J. Khoury,[2] and Achraf Makki[1]

[1]*Department of Neurology, American University of Beirut Medical Center, Beirut, Lebanon*
[2]*Nehme and Therese Tohme Multiple Sclerosis Center, American University of Beirut Medical Center, Beirut, Lebanon*

Correspondence should be addressed to Achraf Makki; am132@aub.edu.lb

Academic Editor: Samuel T. Gontkovsky

Introduction. Spinal neurosarcoidosis is a rare disease that can manifest as myelopathy, radiculopathy, or cauda equine syndrome. Spinal epidural lipomatosis is also a rare condition resulting from overgrowth of epidural fat tissue causing compressive myelopathy. To our knowledge, there are no reports linking epidural lipomatosis and spinal neurosarcoidosis. *Case Report.* We describe a case of progressive myelitis in the presence of concomitant spinal neurosarcoidosis and epidural lipomatosis which was a challenging diagnosis with complete response to treatment after addressing both diseases. Both etiologies are inflammatory in nature and share similar expression of inflammatory factors such as TNF-α and IL-1β. *Conclusion.* The common inflammatory process involved in these two diseases might explain a pathophysiological interconnection between both diseases that may underlie their concomitant development in our patient. If these two diseases are interconnected, in their pathophysiological mechanism remains a hypothesis that will need further investigation.

1. Introduction

Sarcoidosis is a multisystem chronic disease that commonly presents with pulmonary manifestations [1]. Neurosarcoidosis is less common accounting for 5–16% of all sarcoidosis cases [2]. Spinal cord involvement is yet a very rare entity occurring at less than 1% of sarcoidosis patients [3], and because of its insidious, progressive, and nonspecific symptoms, it is usually a challenging diagnosis. Spinal neurosarcoidosis can present as transverse myelitis, myelopathy, cauda equine syndrome, radiculopathy, syringomyelia, or cord atrophy [4]. Myelitis from neurosarcoidosis was found to be an ultraextensive longitudinal myelitis, involving more than three consecutive vertebral body lengths [5]. Here, we present a case of spinal neurosarcoidosis initially presenting as epidural lipomatosis with cord compression. To our knowledge, there are no reports linking epidural lipomatosis and spinal neurosarcoidosis.

2. Case Presentation

A 43-year-old Lebanese man residing in Saudi Arabia presented to our medical center with bilateral lower extremity weakness, severe burning electric such as sensation in both lower extremities, and erectile dysfunction that was preceded by lower back pain. He is sexually active and overweight with no significant past medical history except for a treated sexually transmitted gonorrhea infection. He has no family history of relevant neurologic disease.

The symptoms progressed over one month with worsening neuropathic pain in both lower extremities, paresthesia starting at the umbilicus and radiating down to the medial thighs, inability to walk long distances due to lower extremities weakness and claudication, erectile dysfunction, dribbling and slow urine stream, and constipation. He underwent extensive workup in Saudi Arabia that showed a longitudinal transverse myelitis. Cerebrospinal fluid (CSF) studies showed mildly elevated protein (0.56 g/L), normal sugar (55 mg/dl), absent pleocytosis, and no oligoclonal bands. Magnetic resonance imaging (MRI) of the brain and cervical spine was negative, while MRI of the dorsal spine showed a high T2 signal extending from T4 to T9 vertebrae with enhancement at the T7-T8 level. According to his CSF and MRI results, he was diagnosed with inflammatory myelitis of unclear etiology. He received intravenous pulse steroids twice with no improvement, followed by a tapering dose of oral steroids without any improvement or stabilization of symptoms; so, he presented for further work up.

His physical exam was notable for a sensory level at T10 with allodynia in both lower extremities, very mild weakness in hip flexion on the right (4+/5), and an antalgic gait.

MRI of the dorsal spine was repeated at our institution (Figure 1) showing the same longitudinally extensive dorsal lesion with diffuse cord edema and enhancement. The MRI also showed thickened epidural fat tissue encircling and effacing the CSF at these levels. This was followed by a computed tomography (CT) myelography (Figure 2) that showed near complete obstruction of CSF flow extending from T4 to T9 vertebrae. Autoimmune panel including antinuclear antibody, anti-Sjögren's syndrome-related antigen A autoantibodies, anti-Sjögren's syndrome-related antigen B autoantibodies, and antineutrophil cytoplasmic antibodies was negative. Infectious workup, including Brucella titers, human T-lymphotrophic virus serology, Toxocara antibodies, human immunodeficiency virus, and syphilis serology, was also negative. Antiaquaporin antibodies and antimyelin oligodendrocyte glycoprotein antibodies were negative too. Angiotensin converter enzyme, cobalamin, copper, and calcium levels were normal in blood.

With these MRI findings and negative autoimmune, infectious, demyelinating, and metabolic workup, the diagnosis of epidural lipomatosis causing compressive myelitis was raised, and neurosurgical evaluation recommended T4–T10 laminectomy for decompression and epidural fat removal (Figure 3).

After surgery, the patient reported a precipitous and significant improvement of his back pain, medial thighs burning sensation, and lower extremity weakness and claudication but persistent paresthesia, neuropathic pain, and erectile dysfunction.

Four months later, during follow-up in the clinic, the patient reported persistence of his erectile dysfunction, with some remnant neuropathic pain, with normal motor function. A follow-up MRI spine (Figure 4) showed resolution of the epidural lipomatosis with resolution of the mass effect on the spinal cord and decrease in the extent of the lesion (from T6 to T9) with a decrease in the enhancement. However, mediastinal and hilar lymph nodes seemed to be enlarged on this MRI; so, a CT chest (Figure 5) was performed and confirmed this finding. This was followed by bronchoscopy and mediastinal lymph node biopsy that showed noncaseating granulomas. The diagnosis of pulmonary sarcoidosis was made and that raised the possibility of spinal neurosarcoidosis as the etiology of his residual neurologic symptoms and continued enhancement on the spinal imaging.

Since the patient has tried two courses of steroids in the early stages of his myelitis with no improvement, we started him on mycophenolate mofetil (Cellcept) 1000 mg twice daily as treatment for his sarcoidosis.

Follow-up after two months of starting mycophenolate mofetil, he reported resolution of his erectile dysfunction, but persistent numbness and paresthesia mainly around the genital area. MRI of the dorsal spine showed decrease in the extent of the lesion to T7-T8 vertebrae with persistent enhancement anteriorly at this level (Figure 6). When comparing the enhancing lesion from initial MRI to the one after surgery and the one after treatment with mycophenolate mofetil, one can appreciate the marked decrease in the extent of enhancement (Figure 7). This decrease in enhancement is consistent with an inflammatory myelitis that can be a manifestation of neurosarcoidosis on top of spinal epidural lipomatosis. The gold standard diagnostic test to confirm spinal neurosarcoidosis, on the other hand, is a spinal cord biopsy, which we thought is too invasive to pursue in our patient. Given his improvement after treatment with mycophenolate mofetil and surgery, we considered a presumed diagnosis of spinal neurosarcoidosis with concomitant epidural lipomatosis that might have been exacerbated after steroid use.

3. Discussion

We report a case of spinal neurosarcoidosis with concomitant epidural lipomatosis presenting with longitudinally extensive myelitis that improved partially after surgical decompression and improved further after immunotherapy with mycophenolate mofetil. Due to the diversity in clinical presentations, rarity, and absence of the noninvasive confirmatory test, the diagnosis of spinal neurosarcoidosis is usually delayed especially when it is the first manifestation of sarcoidosis. This would be more challenging in a case such as ours in which there is concomitant pathology such as epidural lipomatosis that is also relatively rare and might explain this myelitis. Whether the resolution in the lesion was related to decrease in venous congestion after surgical repair of epidural lipomatosis only or is a combination of both responses to mycophenolate mofetil and surgery remains a possibility, given similar reported cases of epidural lipomatosis that improve after surgery [6].

Based on the clinical presentation and progression of symptoms, diagnostic considerations might include demyelinating diseases (e.g., multiple sclerosis and neuromyelitis optica), rheumatologic diseases (e.g., vasculitis, systemic lupus erythematosus, Sjogren syndrome, and Behcet's disease), infectious etiologies (e.g., brucellosis, Lyme disease, and tuberculosis), and neoplastic syndromes (e.g., leptomeningeal carcinomatosis) [7].

Spinal neurosarcoidosis can manifest as an acute/subacute process with cord lesions located in the dorsal more commonly than in the cervical spine [5]. Extraneural biopsy with the finding of noncaseating granulomas especially in the lungs is very helpful in the diagnosis [5]. Serum and CSF ACE levels are less sensitive and of limited value in the diagnosis of neurosarcoidosis, but elevated protein in the

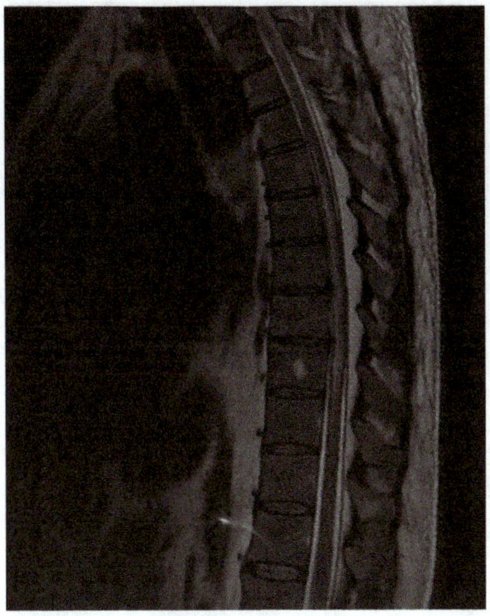

(a)

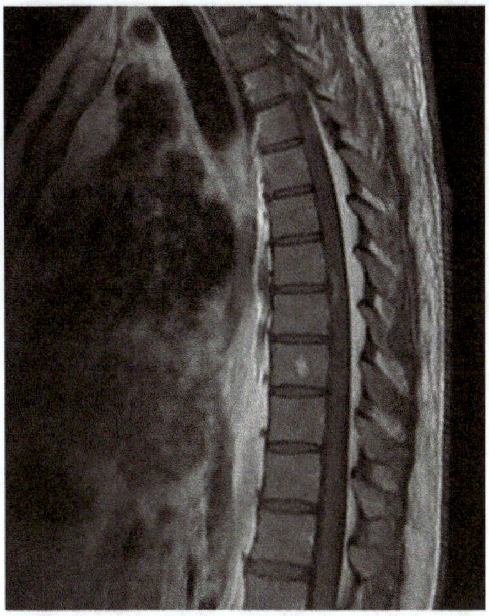

(b)

FIGURE 1: (a) Sagittal T2 MRI of dorsal spine showing high T2 signal with cord edema from T4 to T9 levels with thickened epidural fat tissue posteriorly. (b) Sagittal T1 MRI with gadolinium of dorsal spine showing an enhancing lesion at T7-T8 level.

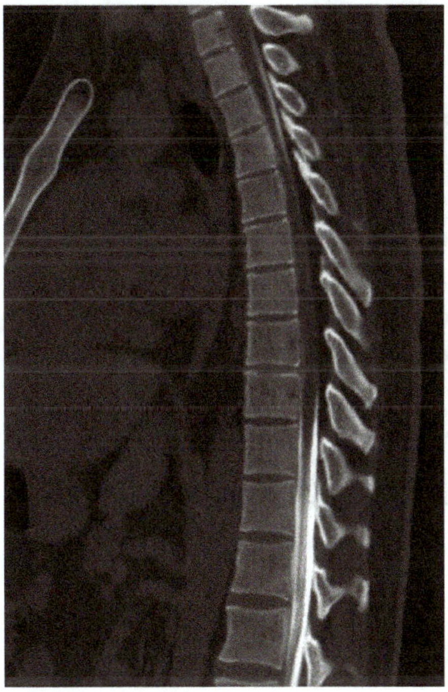

FIGURE 2: CT myelogram showing obstruction of CSF flow extending from T4 to T9 vertebrae.

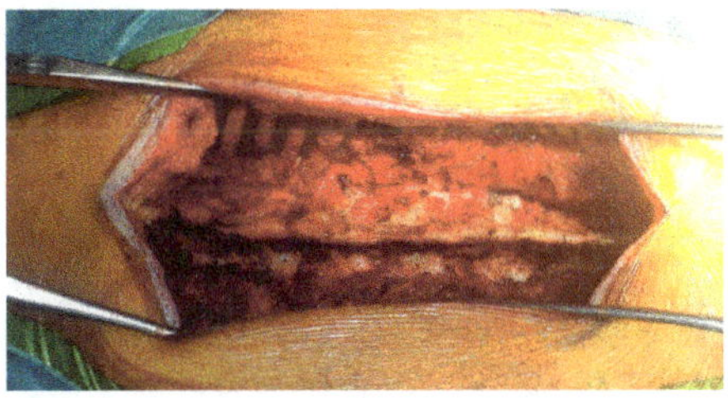

FIGURE 3: Intraoperative image showing the thickened epidural fat before excision.

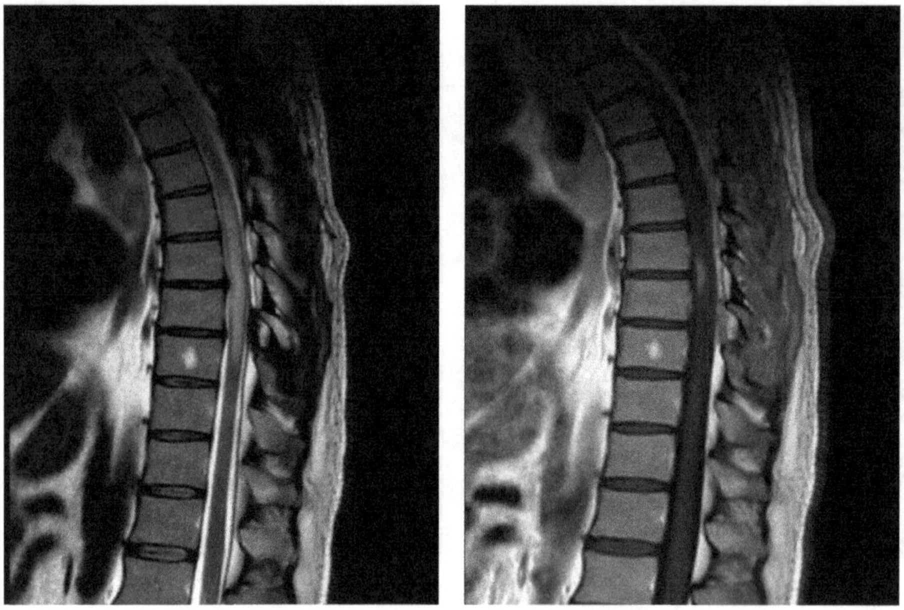

(a) (b)

Figure 4: (a) Sagittal T2 MRI showing resolution of the epidural lipomatosis with resolution of the mass effect on the spinal cord and decrease in the extent of the lesion (from T6 to T9). (b) Sagittal T1 MRI with gadolinium showing mild decrease in the size of enhancing lesion.

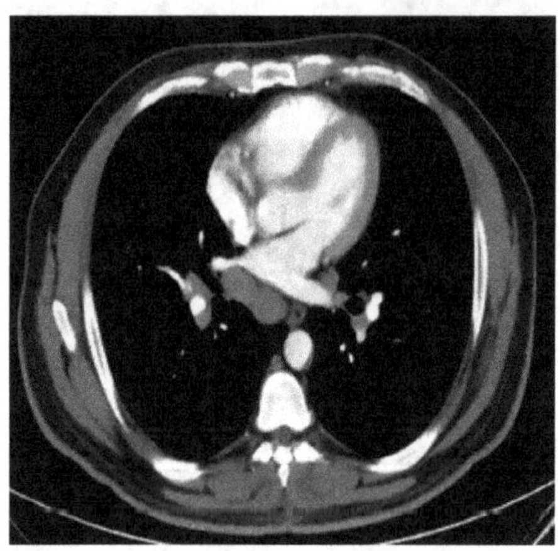

Figure 5: CT chest showing bilateral mediastinal and hilar adenopathy.

CSF is usually helpful [5]. The pathophysiology of sarcoidosis remains unknown; however, studies have shown elevated levels of tumor necrosis factor-α, interleukin-1β, and interleukin-6 secreted by alveolar macrophages in sarcoidosis patients when compared to alveolar macrophages of controls [8, 9]. Accordingly, steroids and cytotoxic drugs such as methotrexate, azathioprine, mycophenolate mofetil, and cyclophosphamide are used to alter the granulomatous inflammatory process and are the mainstay treatment in sarcoidosis [10]. Regarding the treatment of spinal neurosarcoidosis, it is largely based on experience in the absence of evidence based guidelines [4]. However, regardless of the treatment used, the recovery of the neurologic deficit depends on the severity of symptoms at initial presentation [11].

Spinal epidural lipomatosis is also a rare condition resulting from overgrowth of epidural fat tissue causing compressive myelopathy [12]. The main etiology of epidural lipomatosis is endogenous steroids overproduction or exogenous use of long-term steroids [12]. Nevertheless, idiopathic epidural lipomatosis and epidural lipomatosis in obese patients with an unclear etiology have been reported. A potential causal relationship between chronic inflammation and the development of epidural lipomatosis was suggested by studies that found higher expression levels of transcripts of TNF-α and interleukin-1β in adipocytes of patients with spinal epidural lipomatosis compared to healthy controls [13].

In our case, we describe a progressive myelitis in the presence of preexisting lipomatosis that worsened after the

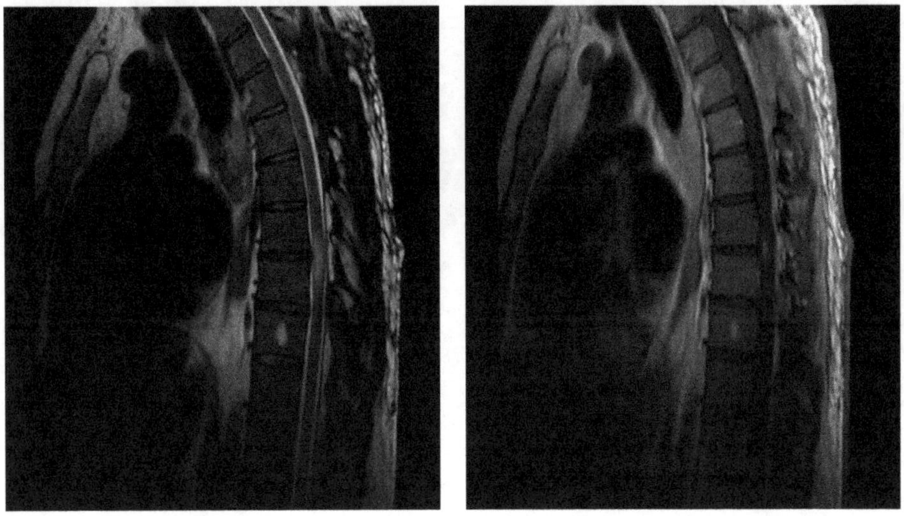

(a) (b)

FIGURE 6: (a) Sagittal T2 MRI of whole spine after 2 months of treatment with mycophenolate mofetil showing decrease in T2 signal involving T7-T8. (b) Sagittal T1 MRI with gadolinium after 2 months of treatment showing further decrease in extent of enhancing lesion.

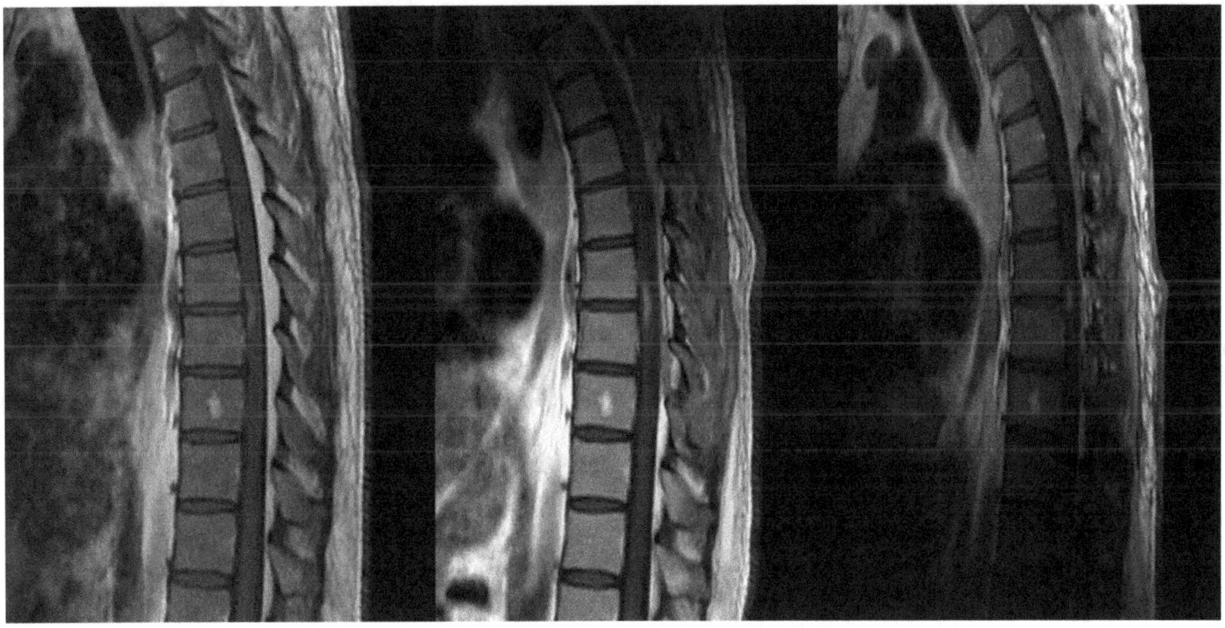

FIGURE 7: Sagittal T1 MRI with gadolinium showing the decrease in extent of enhancing lesion from initial MRI, after surgery, and after treatment.

administration of exogenous steroids with compressive myelopathy and obstruction of CSF flow that is typical of epidural lipomatosis. However, the partial response after decompression by surgical removal of the lipomatosis and the presence of hilar and mediastinal enlarged lymph nodes with pathology showing noncaseating granuloma pointed to the diagnosis of neurosarcoidosis on top of the epidural lipomatosis. Furthermore, the resolution of symptoms and decrease in the extent of the enhancing lesion on MRI after starting mycophenolate mofetil can be explained by the concomitant presence of inflammatory myelitis in association with compressive myelitis.

Sarcoidosis (a chronic inflammatory disease) and epidural lipomatosis (a consequence of chronic inflammation) share similar expression of inflammatory factors such as TNF-α and IL-1β and could have interconnected pathophysiological mechanisms that may underlie the concomitant development of both diseases in our patient. However, this hypothetical relationship between these two entities will need further investigations.

References

[1] M. C. Iannuzzi, B. A. Rybicki, and A. S. Teirstein, "Sarcoidosis," *New England Journal of Medicine*, vol. 357, no. 21, pp. 2153–2165, 2007.

[2] B. J. Stern, A. Krumholz, C. Johns, P. Scott, and J. Nissim, "Sarcoidosis and its neurological manifestations," *Archives of Neurology*, vol. 42, no. 9, pp. 909-917, 1985.

[3] D. A. Bradley, E. E. Lower, and R. P. Baughman, "Diagnosis and management of spinal cord sarcoidosis," *Sarcoidosis, Vasculitis, and Diffuse Lung Diseases: Official Journal of WASOG*, vol. 23, no. 1, pp. 58–65, 2006.

[4] A. M. Scott, J. Yinh, T. McAlindon, and R. Kalish, "Two cases of sarcoidosis presenting as longitudinally extensive transverse myelitis," *Clinical Rheumatology*, vol. 37, no. 10, pp. 2899–2905, 2018.

[5] L. Wang and Y. Li, "Longitudinal ultra-extensive transverse myelitis as a manifestation of neurosarcoidosis," *Journal of the Neurological Sciences*, vol. 355, no. 1-2, pp. 64–67, 2015.

[6] I. Lotan, R. W. Charlson, G. M. Fatterpekar et al., "Progressive myelopathy associated with spinal epidural lipomatosis in three non-obese patients with type 1 diabetes mellitus," *Journal of the Neurological Sciences*, vol. 411, 2020.

[7] J. P. Zajicek, N. J. Scolding, O. Foster et al., "Central nervous system sarcoidosis diagnosis and management," *QJM: An International Journal of Medicine*, vol. 92, no. 2, pp. 103–117, 1999.

[8] P. R. Bachwich, J. P. Lynch, J. Larrick, M. Spengler, and S. L. Kunkel, "Tumor necrosis factor production by human sarcoid alveolar macrophages," *American Journal of Pathology Volume*, vol. 125, no. 3, pp. 421-425, 1986.

[9] S. Martin, J. Petersen, M. Oldigs et al., "Increased secretion of tumor necrosis factor-alpha, interleukin-1 -beta, and interleukin-6 by alveolar macrophages from patients with sarcoidosis," *Journal of Allergy and Clinical Immunology*, vol. 91, 1993.

[10] D. Valeyre, A. Prasse, H. Nunes, Y. Uzunhan, P.-Y. Brillet, and J. Müller-Quernheim, "Sarcoidosis," *The Lancet*, vol. 383, no. 9923, pp. 1155–1167, 2014.

[11] C.-A. Durel, R. Marignier, D. Maucort-Boulch et al., "Clinical features and prognostic factors of spinal cord sarcoidosis: a multicenter observational study of 20 biopsy-proven patients," *Journal of Neurology*, vol. 263, no. 5, pp. 981–990, 2016.

[12] D. Al-Khawaja, K. Seex, and G. D. Eslick, "Spinal epidural lipomatosis - a brief review," *Journal of Clinical Neuroscience*, vol. 15, no. 12, pp. 1323–1326, 2008.

[13] N. Fujita, N. Hosogane, and T. Hikata, "Potential involvement of obesity-associated chronic inflammation in the pathogenesis of idiopathic spinal epidural lipomatosis," vol. 41, no. 23, pp. E1402–E1407, 2016.

4

Mitochondrial Neurogastrointestinal Encephalomyopathy: Novel Pathogenic Mutation in Thymidine Phosphorylase Gene in a Patient from Cape Verde Islands

Catarina Falcão de Campos ,[1,2] Miguel Oliveira Santos,[1,2] Rafael Roque,[3] Isabel Conceição,[1,2] and Mamede de Carvalho[1,2]

[1]*Department of Neurology, Department of Neurosciences and Mental Health, Hospital de Santa Maria, Centro Hospitalar Universitário Lisboa Norte, Lisbon, Portugal*
[2]*Instituto de Medicina Molecular and Instituto de Fisiologia, Faculdade de Medicina, Universidade de Lisboa, Lisbon, Portugal*
[3]*Neuropathology Unit, Department of Neurosciences and Mental Health, Hospital de Santa Maria, Centro Hospitalar Universitário Lisboa Norte, Lisbon, Portugal*

Correspondence should be addressed to Catarina Falcão de Campos; catarinahfcampos@gmail.com

Academic Editor: Norman S. Litofsky

Mitochondrial Neurogastrointestinal Encephalomyopathy (MNGIE) is a rare autosomal recessive disorder caused by mutations in the gene encoding the Thymidine Phosphorylase (TP). It is clinically characterized by severe gastrointestinal dysmotility, cachexia, palpebral ptosis, ophthalmoparesis, sensorimotor polyneuropathy and leukoencephalopathy. The diagnosis is established by the presence of typical clinical and neuroimaging features, positive family history, and abnormal genetic test. A 19-year-old Cape Verdean patient with a history since childhood of recurrent episodes of nausea, vomiting, diarrhoea and painful abdominal distension associated with progressive motor disability with difficulty in climbing stairs and running and clumsiness with her hands. The diagnostic workup was suggestive of MNGIE. Genetic screening of the *TYMP* gene identified a novel mutation (c. 1283 G>A). Patients with MNGIE have significant comorbidity and mortality, and they are frequently misdiagnosed. A better acknowledgment of this disorder is essential to permit an earlier diagnosis and to improve disease management.

1. Introduction

Mitochondrial disorders (MDs) are a complex group of neuromuscular diseases in which the main features derive from mitochondrial dysfunction. Their prevalence has been difficult to establish and it is not yet known, mainly due to its clinical and genetic heterogeneity. Recent studies suggest that MDs are more frequent than previously considered, with an estimated prevalence of 1/4300 [1]. MDs heterogeneity can be explained by the fact that mitochondria metabolism requires two genomes: mitochondrial DNA (mtDNA) and nuclear DNA (nDNA), with a maternal and Mendelian inheritance, respectively [2].

Mitochondrial Neurogastrointestinal Encephalomyopathy (MNGIE) is a rare autosomal recessive disorder, and is considered as a classic example of MD secondary to a defect in the intergenomic communication [3]. Its prevalence is unknown; fewer than 100 cases have been reported. MNGIE is caused by loss of function mutations in *TYMP* gene, a nuclear gene encoding thymidine phosphorylase (TP), located on chromosome 22 [4]. TP initiates the catabolism of the pyrimidine nucleosides thymidine (dThd) and deoxyuridine (dUrd) by catalyzing the phosphorolysis of both nucleosides to deoxyribose phosphate and the corresponding bases, namely thymine and uracil [5]. In MNGIE patients, TP activity is very low resulting in systemic accumulation of dThd and dUrd, mitochondrial nucleotide pool imbalances with secondary depletion, multiple deletions and point mutations of mtDNA [6]. There is also evidence that TP activity is critical for angiogenic activity, which may further contribute to the pathophysiological mechanism of MNGIE [5].

MNGIE is clinically characterized by ptosis, external ophthalmoplegia, severe gastrointestinal dysmotility, cachexia, sensorimotor polyneuropathy and leukoencephalopathy. This disorder typically has an onset before the age of 30 years, associated with a severe prognosis and high mortality rate between the ages of 20 and 40 years [7]. Recently, allogeneic haematopoietic stem cell transplantation (HSCT) and orthotopic liver transplantation (OLT) have been proposed as a disease-modifying treatment [8, 9].

We report a young woman from Cape Verde origin, with a clinical diagnosis of MNGIE and a novel homozygous mutation in association with a frequent synonymous polymorphism in the *TYMP* gene.

2. Case Report

A 19-year-old female born and living in Cape Verde islands was admitted with a history of recurrent episodes of nausea and vomiting, gastric regurgitation, diarrhoea and painful abdominal distension, since 5 years of age. Those episodes became more frequent and severe in late adolescence resulting in a significant weight loss (≈15 kg) over the previous year. In association, she complained of slowly progressive gait impairment, difficulty in climbing stairs and inability to run. She referred poor gymnastic classes performance in school. She also mentioned progressive weakness of upper limbs with functional impact in combing her hair, writing and using cutlery. There was no history of cognitive impairment and academic achievement was good. She rejected pain, sensory or other dysautonomic symptoms. She was the second daughter of a consanguineous marriage. Her older sister had a similar clinical picture with gastrointestinal complaints; she received the diagnosis of superior mesenteric artery syndrome.

She developed cachexia (Body Mass Index of 10.9). On neurological examination, she had mild bilateral symmetric ptosis with no ocular paresis, generalized muscle weakness and atrophy, more pronounced in lower extremities and in distal segments, absent tendon reflexes, decreased nociception below knees, reduced vibration and position sense in toes and fingers, and required bilateral support to walk.

Routine laboratory studies were unremarkable, including creatine kinase and thyroid hormone levels. Plasma lactate level was above normal range (2.83 mM/L, normal 0.5–1). CSF analysis disclosed 2.5-fold increased protein content with normal number of cells; lactate level was also increased (2.7 mmol/L, normal 0.88–1.4).

Upper gastrointestinal endoscopy showed gastric aperistalsis associated with major dilation and ulcerative esophagitis. A nasojejunal feeding tube was required for enteral feeding.

Nerve conduction studies revealed marked demyelinating sensorimotor polyneuropathy (Table 1) and needle electromyography showed a superimposed myopathic pattern in proximal muscles.

Patient's muscle biopsy of the deltoid muscle disclosed unspecific myopathic changes such as type I fibre predominance and increased variation in fiber size with small, angular muscle fibres and round hypertrophic fibers. No signs of mitochondrial dysfunction (ragged red fibers, Cox-negative fibers and increased oxidative staining on SDH) were seen (Figure 1).

Table 1: Patient's nerve conduction studies (NCS).

Motor NCS	Latency (ms)	Amplitude (mV)	Velocity (m/s)	F-Wave
Median		5.4	**28.4** (NV>50)	Absent
Wrist	4.9			
Elbow	12.3			
Ulnar		4	**24.4** (NV>50)	Absent
Wrist	4.1			
Elbow	12.7			
Peroneal		0.4	**15.4** (NV>40)	Absent
Ankle	4.8			
Fibula (below)	11.3			
Sensory NCS	**Latency (ms)**	**Amplitude (μV)**	**Velocity (m/s)**	
Median		Absent		
Ulnar		Absent		
Radial		Absent		
Sural		Absent		

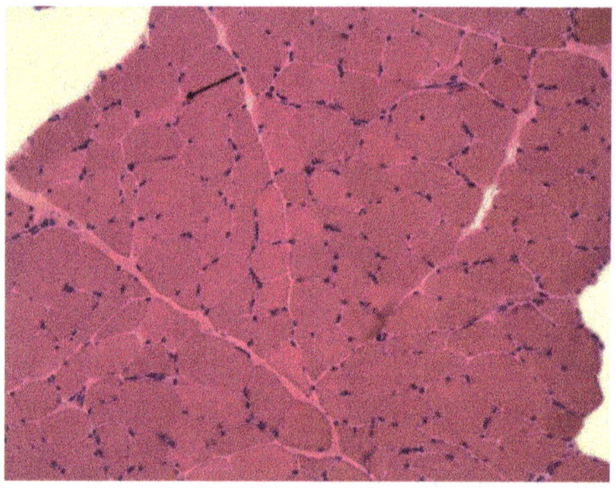

Figure 1: Muscle biopsy H&E ×10. It is observed increased variation in fiber size, with round hypertrophic fibres (*) associated with angular atrophic fibres (arrow). No mitochondrial changes were detected.

Brain MRI revealed unspecific symmetric and confluent T2-hyperintensity images in the deep white matter (Figure 2).

The presence of severe gastrointestinal dysmotility associated with a demyelinating sensorimotor polyneuropathy and myopathic changes suggested a mitochondrial disorder, specifically MNGIE. Genetic screening of the TYMP gene identified two homozygous contiguous mutations (c. 1283G>A, c.1284 T>A), affecting the same codon (GGT>GAA), causing together cause the amino acid change p.Gly428Asp. Prediction tools of pathogenicity (Polyphen, SIFT, Provean, SNP&GO) agreed with the damaging role of this genetic change. Unfortunately, DNA samples from family members were not available to perform segregation study.

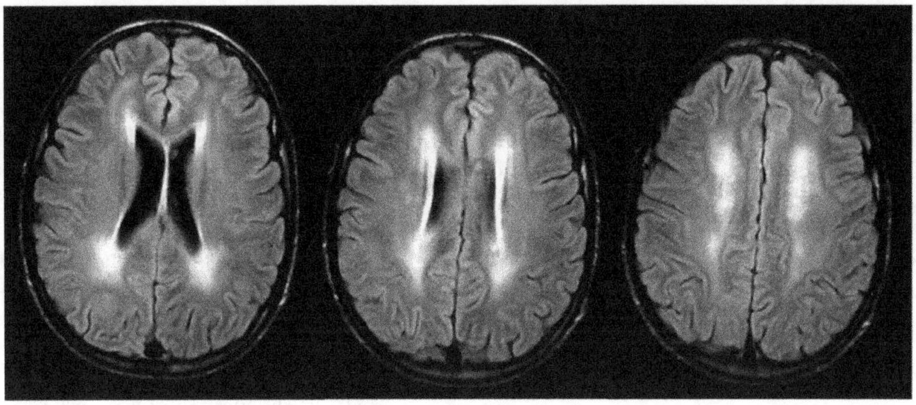

FIGURE 2: Brain MRI. Axial FLAIR images show symmetric and confluent increase signal intensity in deep white matter.

The patient died three months after admission from medical complications associated with poor absorption and profound cachexia.

3. Discussion

We report a 19-year-old Cape Verdean woman with typical clinical features of MNGIE syndrome in whom we identified a novel homozygous *TYMP* gene mutation.

The gastrointestinal symptoms were the most prominent manifestation resulting in gastric atony, poor absorption and cachexia. Her older sister, living in Cape Verde islands, had milder but similar gastrointestinal symptoms. She was diagnosed as "superior mesenteric artery syndrome", which is a common misdiagnosis in patients with MNGIE in the early course of the disease [7]. Their parents were asymptomatic but consanguineous, indicating an autosomal recessive transmission.

Patient poor functional ability was probably related to the presence of a marked demyelinating polyneuropathy. Indeed some cases of MNGIE syndrome have been misdiagnosed as chronic demyelinating inflammatory neuropathy [10]. It is hypothesized that the pathogenic mtDNA accumulates in the peripheral nerve, causing segmental and focal defects [10]. However, proximal weakness and ptosis were probably associated with the muscle fibres dysfunction observed in mitochondrial myopathies.

The main laboratory findings in these patients are plasma lactic acidosis and high CSF protein, as seen in our patient [7]. Muscle biopsy typically shows morphological and biochemical findings suggestive of mitochondrial abnormalities, such as the presence of ragged red fibers and Cox-deficient fibers. In our case, the muscle biopsy was not helpful. To our knowledge, there are few described MNGIE cases with normal muscle biopsy [7]. Therefore, a normal muscle biopsy does not exclude a MNGIE syndrome, in particular in young subjects. As reported elsewhere, our patient had symmetrical confluent T2-hyperintensity in the deep white matter. However, these changes do not impair cognition [11].

The genetic screening confirmed the diagnosis. Two homozygous contiguous mutations (c. 1283G>A, c.1284T>A), affecting the same codon (GGT>GAA) were identified. To our knowledge, the first mutation has never been described in literature. The second is a frequent synonymous polymorphism. However, both mutations together caused the amino acid change p.Gly428Glu [12]. Although we were not able to perform TP activity and dThd and dUrd serum levels measurement and family segregation study in order to confirm its pathogenicity, bioinformatics genetic analysis (Polyphen, SIFT, Provean, SNP&GO) suggested a pathogenic role for this genetic change. Also, the associated typical patient's phenotype, compatible with MNGIE syndrome, further supported its pathogenicity.

Different therapeutic strategies have been proposed for patients with MNGIE syndrome. Some attempts were made to reduce the toxic accumulation of the nucleoside levels (dThd and dUrd) with dialysis and platelets transfusion, since platelets are rich with TP. However, both these approaches are not feasible as long-term therapies because there is an accumulation of the nucleosides [13, 14]. Halter and his colleagues showed that allogeneic HSCT could be an effective disease-modifying treatment. However, it was associated with a non-negligible mortality [8]. Additionally, OLT has been proposed as a new treatment in patients with MNGIE since the liver may be a tissue source of TP. OLT was successfully performed in two patients with early normalization of nucleosides levels with no serious adverse events [9]. Whether this finding is associated with a long-term quality of life improvement and increased survival remains to be elucidated. However, both these treatments may be considered in carefully selected patients, before severe organ damage occurs, making crucial an early diagnosis of MNGIE in these patients. Unfortunately, our patient was admitted in a late stage of the disease, dying few months later. More recently, treatment with adeno-associated virus vector containing the *TYMP* coding sequencing targeting the liver showed a persistent reversion of biochemical abnormalities in murine models without adverse effects. This observation indicates that in the future gene therapy may also be a feasible and efficient therapeutic strategy for MNGIE patients [15].

To date, more than 50 mutations have been reported. Here, we report a novel mutation (c. 1283G>A) in a patient with severe gastrointestinal dysmotility and polyneuropathy phenotype.

Disclosure

We acknowledge that this manuscript has been previously presented in the 3rd Congress of the European Academy of Neurology—Amsterdam 2017 which abstract is available in C. Campos, M. Oliveira Santos, R. Roque, I. Conceição, M. Carvalho. Mitochondrial Neurogastrointestinal Encephalomyopathy: Novel pathogenic mutation in Thymidine Phosphorylase gene in a patient from Cape Verde. 2017 European Journal of Neurology, 24 (Suppl. 1), 445–678.

Acknowledgments

We would like to thank Valerio Carelli, Leonardo Caporali and Chiara la Morgia from IRCCS Institute of Neurological Sciences of Bologna for providing the genetic screening of *TYMP* gene.

References

[1] G. S. Gorman, A. M. Schaefer, Y. Ng et al., "Prevalence of nuclear and mitochondrial DNA mutations related to adult mitochondrial disease," *Annals of Neurology*, vol. 77, no. 5, pp. 753–759, 2015.

[2] M. Hirano, Y. Nishigaki, and R. Marti, "Mitochondrial neurogastrointestinal encephalomyopathy: a disease of two genomes," *The Neurologist*, vol. 10, no. 1, pp. 8–17, 2004.

[3] I. Nishino, A. Spinazzola, and M. Hirano, "MNGIE: from nuclear DNA to mitochondrial DNA," *Neuromuscular Disorders*, vol. 11, pp. 7–10, 2001.

[4] I. Nishino, A. Spinazzola, and M. Hirano, "Thymidine phosphorylase gene mutations in MNGIE, a human mitochondrial disorder," *Science*, vol. 283, no. 5402, pp. 689–692, 1999.

[5] N. Brown and R. Bicknell, "Thymidine phosphorylase, 2-desoxy-D-ribose and angiogenesis," *Biochemical Journal*, vol. 334, pp. 1–8, 1998.

[6] A. Slama, C. Lacroix, L. A. Plante-Bordeneuve et al., "Thymidine phosphorylase gene mutations in patients with mitochondrial neurogastrointestinal encephalomyopathy syndrome," *Molecular Genetics and Metabolism*, vol. 84, no. 4, pp. 326–331, 2005.

[7] C. Garone, S. Tadesse, and M. Hirano, "Clinical and genetic spectrum of mitochondrial neurogastrointestinal encephalomyopathy," *Brain*, vol. 134, pp. 3326–3332, 2011.

[8] J. Halter, W. Michael, M. Schupbach et al., "Allogeneic haematopoietic stem cell transplantation for mitochondrial neurogastrointestinal encephalomyopathy," *Brain*, vol. 138, pp. 2847–2858, 2015.

[9] R. D'Angelo, R. Rinaldi, L. Pironi et al., "Liver transplant reverses biochemical imbalance in mitochondrial neurogastrointestinal encephalomyopathy," *Mitochondrion*, vol. 34, pp. 101–102, 2017.

[10] R. S. Bedlack, T. Vu, S. Hammans et al., "MNGIE neuropathy: five cases mimicking chronic inflammatory demyelinating polyneuropathy," *Muscle & Nerve*, vol. 29, no. 3, pp. 364–368, 2004.

[11] W. S. Millar, A. Lignelli, and M. Hirano, "MRI of five patients with mitochondrial neurogastrointestinal encephalomyopathy," *AJR American Journal of Roentgenology*, vol. 182, pp. 1537–1541, 2004.

[12] M. Hirano, "Mitochondrial Neurogastrointestinal Encephalopathy Disease," in *GeneReviews® [Internet]*, M. P. Adam, H. H. Ardinger, and R. A. Pagon, Eds., University of Washington Seattle, Seattle (WA), 2005, 1993–2019.

[13] M. C. Lara, B. Weiss, I. Illa, L. Massuet, A. L. Andreu, and M. L. Valentino, "Infusion of platelets transiently reduces nucleoside overload in MNGIE," *Neurology*, vol. 67, pp. 1461–3, 2006.

[14] A. Spinazzola, R. Marti, I. Nishino et al., "Altered thymidine metabolism due to defects of thymidine phosphorylase," *Journal of Biological Chemistry*, vol. 277, pp. 4128–4133, 2002.

[15] J. Torres-Torronteras, R. Cabrera-Pérez, F. Vila-Julià et al., "Long-term sustained effect of liver-targeted adeno-associated virus gene therapy for mitochondrial neurogastrointestinal encephalomyopathy," *Human Gene Therapy*, vol. 29, pp. 708–718, 2018.

5

Successful Clipping of a Giant Anterior Inferior Cerebellar Artery Aneurysm with Combined Transpetrosal Approach

The-Hao Nguyen,[1] Van-Thanh-Cong Pham,[1] Quynh-Trang Pham,[1] Hao Nguyen Si Anh,[2] Phong Tran Nhu,[3] and Hoang-Long Vo[2]

[1]*Department of Neurosurgery, Bach Mai Hospital, Hanoi, Vietnam*
[2]*Institute for Preventive Medicine and Public Health, Hanoi Medical University, Hanoi, Vietnam*
[3]*Public Health Department, Nursing Faculty, Dai Nam University, Hanoi, Vietnam*

Correspondence should be addressed to Hoang-Long Vo; vohoanglonghmu@gmail.com

Academic Editor: Samuel T. Gontkovsky

Background. The anterior inferior cerebellar artery (AICA) aneurysms are rare lesions whose treatment can be challenging. There are only a few previous reports of surgical treatment for such lesions. *Objectives*. We present a case of a basilar-AICA aneurysm undergoing surgery with the combined transpetrosal approach. *Case Description*. A 58-year-old female patient presented clinical signs including headache, diplopia, and right hemiparesis. The radiological imaging showed a basilar-AICA aneurysm measuring 25×19 mm. The patient was operated via left combined transpetrosal approach. The outcome was graded mRankin 1. Follow-up computerized tomographic angiography showed no aneurysmal residual and total preservation of basilar artery. *Discussions*. Surgical indication's purposes were aneurysmal elimination and reduction of mass effect. Combined transpetrosal approach: proximal segment control and enough space for clipping manipulation. Clipping techniques: Temporary clip for aneurysmal collapsing, "orienting clip". *Conclusion*. Giant basilar-AICA aneurysm is very rare lesion. Combined transpetrosal approach is appropriate for surgical clipping. Good surgical outcome is achieved with complete elimination of aneurysm.

1. Introduction

The aneurysms located near the verterbrobasilar junction or the anterior inferior cerebellar artery (AICA) aneurysms are uncommon lesions, accounting for only about 1% of all intracerebral aneurysms. There are important structures in this region concerning middle and lower clivus such as the pontine and the cranial nerves. Surgical approach to this region is still a challenge for neurosurgeons. Samii (1992) named the clivus as "no man's land" [1]. In 1948, Schwartz performed the first surgically treated case of AICA aneurysm clipping [2]. Until 2005, one of the biggest series of AICA aneurysm clipping was reported by Gonzalez with 34 cases. Subtemporal approach described by Drake (1978) was quite successful except for some cases with the vein of Labbé infarct. This approach requires the temporal lobe retraction, but it is still hard to control the lower part of basilar artery [3]. Kawase (1985) reported two cases of AICA aneurysm clipping via anterior petrosectomy without any complications; however, he acknowledged that he had difficulty controlling the proximal artery [4]. In 1996, Kawase reported another series of 14 cases experiencing midbasilar artery aneurysms clipping with anterior petrosectomy, posterior petrosectomy, and far-lateral approach [5]. Lawton (1997) applied modified orbitozygomatic and far-lateral approaches to treat 28 patients with large and giant midbasilar artery aneurysms. Then this surgical treatment outcome was recorded to be 75% patients with good outcome and 11% of those were having permanent treatment-associated neurological deficits [6]. Nowadays, with modern microsurgical instruments and better anatomical understanding, it is easier for neurosurgeons to treat the lesions of this region. The combined transpetrosal approach for the tumoral lesions is quite common; however, it is still controversial for aneurysmal clipping (Figure 1). We present

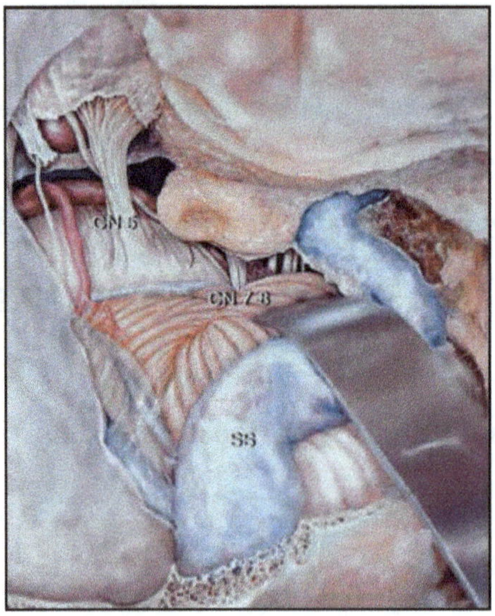

Figure 1: Combined transpetrosal approach schema.

a case of giant AICA aneurysm successfully clipped via combined transpetrosal approach, and evaluate the possibility, the advantages, and the inconveniences of this approach, along with sharing our experiences on used approach.

2. Case Presentation

2.1. Clinical and Imaging Features. A 58-year-old woman with medical history of hypertension presented with onset of headache, diplopia, and right sided weakness within 2 weeks. She was admitted to the Department of Neurosurgery (Bach Mai hospital) on 12 February 2018. Here, a cerebral computed tomography (CT) was performed, showing a hyperdense mass in the brainstem. CT angiography (CTA) revealed that a partially thrombosed aneurysm measuring 25 × 19 mm was located at the vertebrobasilar junction (AICA arises), causing mass effect on the pons (Figure 2). The radiologists found that endovascular treatment was a challenge for this aneurysm because of its wide neck and its compression on the brainstem. Our patient underwent the surgery on 28 February 2018 with combined transpetrosal approach.

2.2. Operation. The patient was in the supine position with the head turned right 80° and extended 30° (Figure 3). C-shaped incision was made from mastoid process to hairline on the left side (Figure 4). Temporal muscle was dissected to expose the temporobasal region as well as zygomatic root, and the lateral suboccipital region as well as the complete mastoid (Figures 5 and 6). The posterior petrosectomy was performed with high speed drill under the microscope to expose the atrium while preserving the semicircular canals, unroofing the sigmoid sinus, and a part of tranverse sinus until the presigmoid dura was exposed. A subtemporal craniotomy was performed for the exposure of Kawase triangle. The anterior part of the petrous bone was totally drilled until the posterior fossa dura and the inferior petrosal sinus were exposed. When the temporobasal dura was opened, the cerebrospinal fluid (CSF) was drained for the brain relaxation. Through the Kawase triangle opening, the posterior fossa dura was incised with two cuts crossing the superior petrosal sinus at anterior one-third and the cerebellar tentorium to its border. Transverse and sigmoid sinuses were retracted posteriorly, then the presigmoid dura was opened close to the inferior border of the superior petrosal sinus. The arachnoid was opened to expose the vertebrobasilar junction, the aneuryms, and the middle part of the basilar artery. One temporary clip was put on the proximal basilar artery through the posterior petrosal opening. The aneurysm wall was torn during the first clip application. Finally, the aneurysm was clipped with two long Yasargil clips through Kawase triangle opening. Dura closure was performed with the free flap of the temporal fascia, the abdominal fat tissue, and the biological glue.

3. Results

The patient was extubated after 48 hours. Despite without motor deficit, CSF leak through the external auditory canal and facial paralysis (House-Brackmann Grade III) were observed. The management for the CSF leak was with lumbar drainage within 10 days. At three-month follow-up, the patient had full recovery of facial nerve palsy, and was able to walk normally. CTA showed that the aneurysm was totally occluded with no sign of basilar artery stenosis (Figures 7–11).

4. Discussion

4.1. Surgical Indication. In this endovascular era, surgical indication for the complex aneurysms becomes less and less. In 2004, the biggest series of operated AICA aneurysms were firstly reported by Gonzalez [7]. A Xialin' literature review (2016) through Pubmed reported 47 cases of anterior inferior cerebellar aneurysms (in 30 previous reports), in which 21 cases were treated surgically [8]. We did not find any other large series of AICA aneurysms operated in the literature. Most previous authors made case reports for only endovascular treatment of AICA aneurysms. For example, Kawase (1996) reported 14 cases of vertebrobasilar aneurysms, in which there were only 2 cases of AICA aneurysms [5]. In another publication, six cases of operated AICA aneurysms were reported by XinLi (2012) [9]. According to Gonzalez (2004), the endovascular coiling should be indicated for treating residual aneurysms after surgery, proximal aneurysms located anterior to the arteriovenous malformations, and high-grade patients with small aneurysms with an adequate dome-to-neck ratio. However, endovascular coiling has not been indicated for the large and giant aneurysms resulting in compression of the brainstem.

We did not choose the coiling treatment because of the mass effect on the brainstem. The radiologists performed the flow diversion for this case but they did not succeed. Finally, we decided the surgical clipping for giant AICA aneurysm using combined petrosectomy approach with two purposes: (i) eliminating the aneurysm, and (ii) relieving the mass effect on the brainstem.

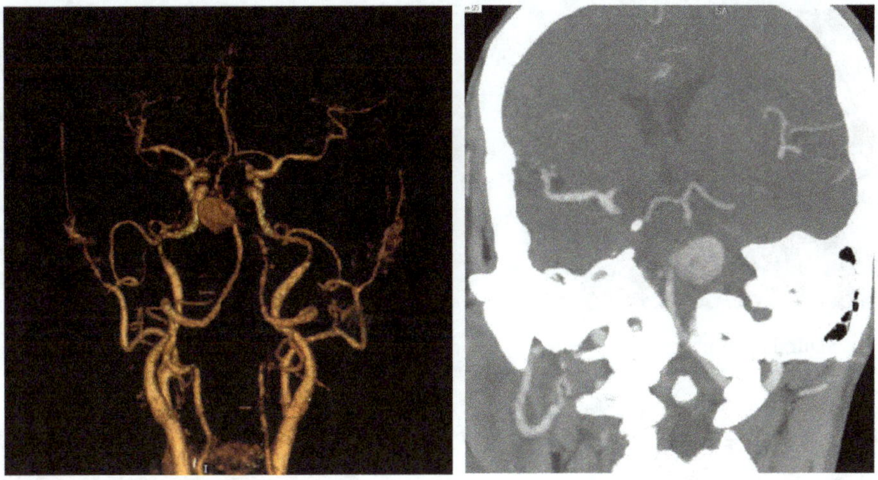

FIGURE 2: Pre-op CTA.

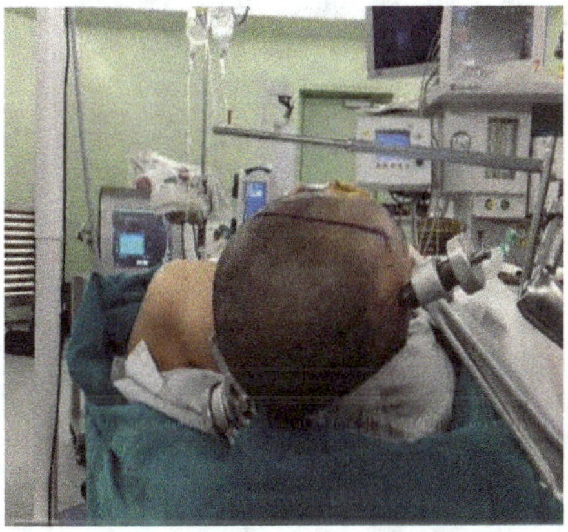

FIGURE 3: Head position.

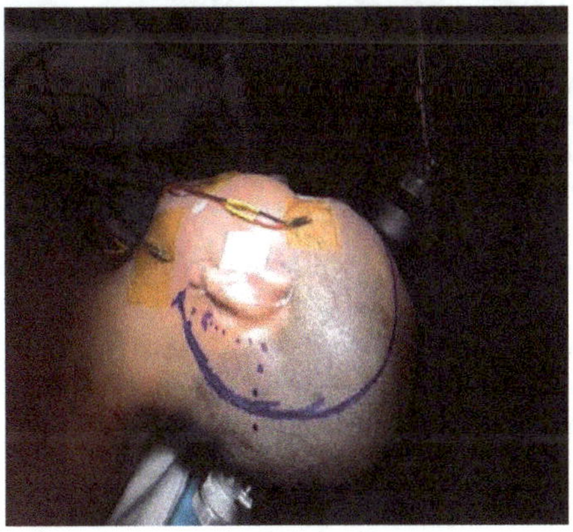

FIGURE 4: C-shaped incision.

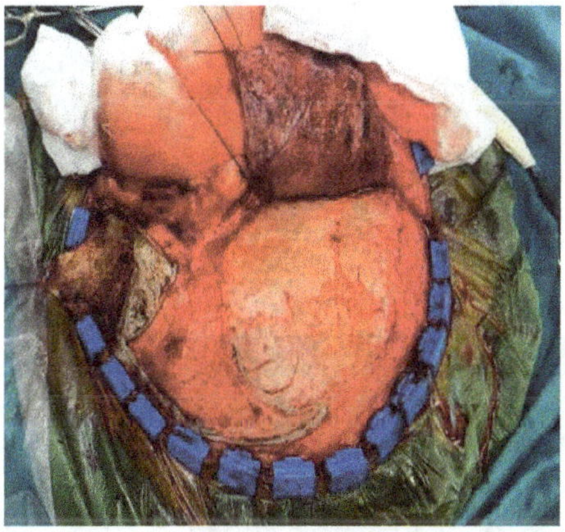

FIGURE 5: Temporal muscle dissection.

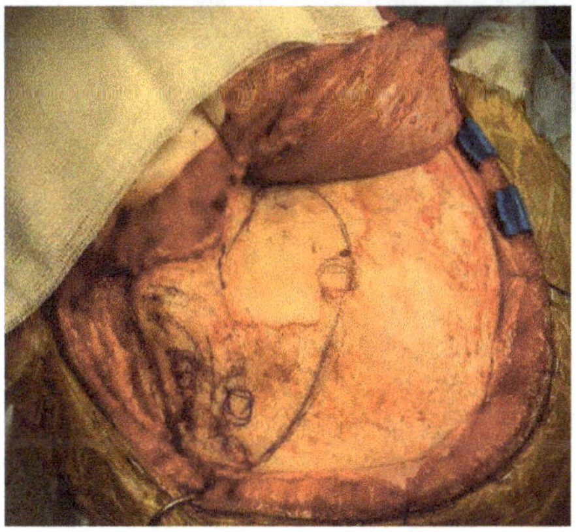

FIGURE 6: Mastoid drilling.

4.2. Combined Transpetrosal Approach. Gonzalez (2004) performed hypothermic cardiac standstill in 9 patients with large and giant aneurysms. This surgical technique softens the aneurysmal sac, therefore, proximal control is no longer necessary [7]. At our hospital, we did not have the possibility for the cardiac standstill, so the approach for our patient must be large enough for both clipping and proximal control. The anterior petrosectomy is enough to clip AICA aneurysm. Inferior limit of anterior approach is internal auditory canal. AICA aneurysm surgery requires more space, especially for the proximal control. The posterior petrosectomy responded to this requirement.

In our case, the limitation of the combined transpetrosal approach was that its operating time was longer than others such as pterional, subtemporal, or pure Kawasé approach. It took us 5 hours 20 minutes for this approach, in which 3 hours

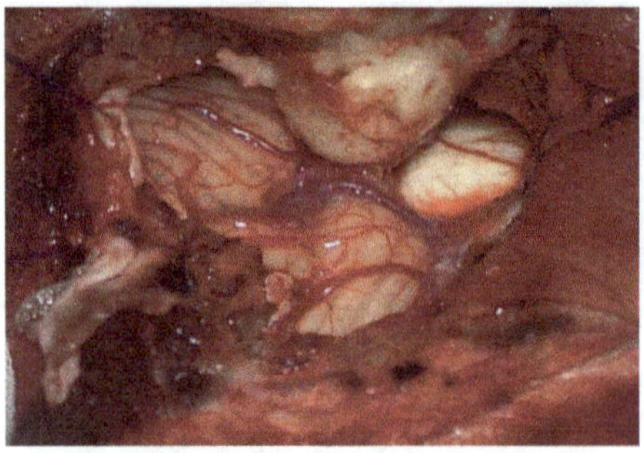

FIGURE 7: Dural opening.

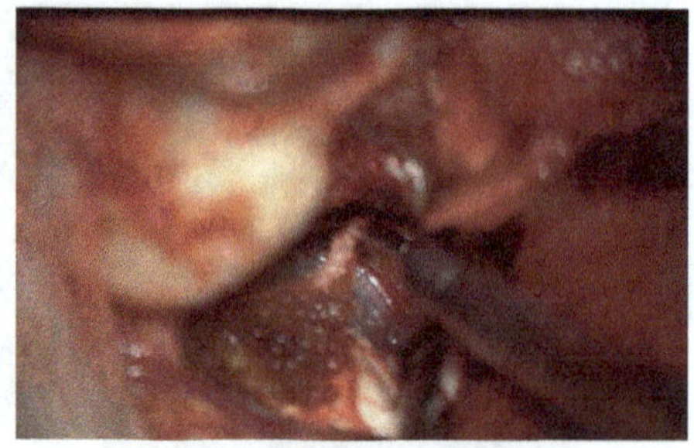

FIGURE 9: Applying clip.

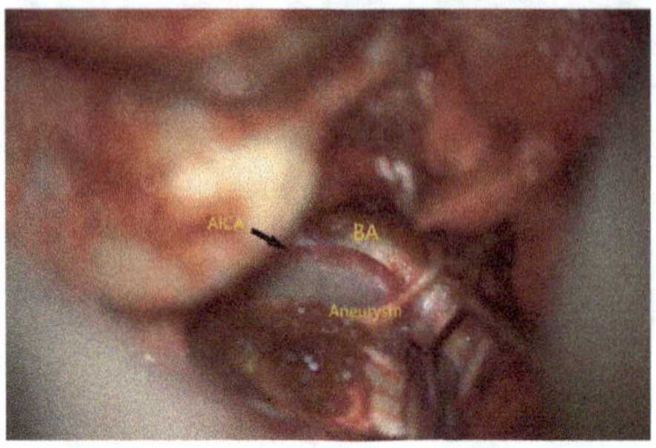

FIGURE 8: Aneurysm exposure.

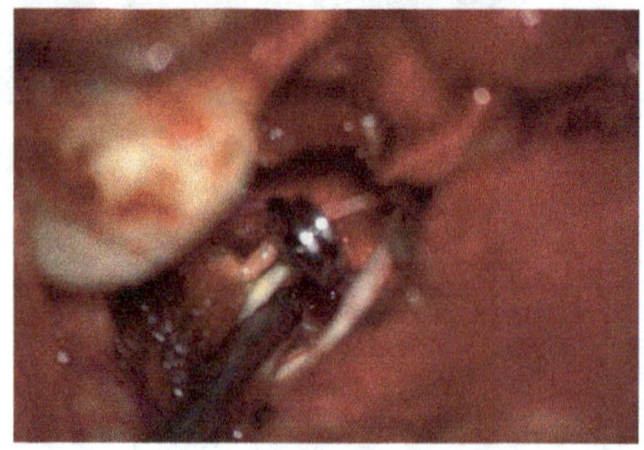

FIGURE 10: Clip applied.

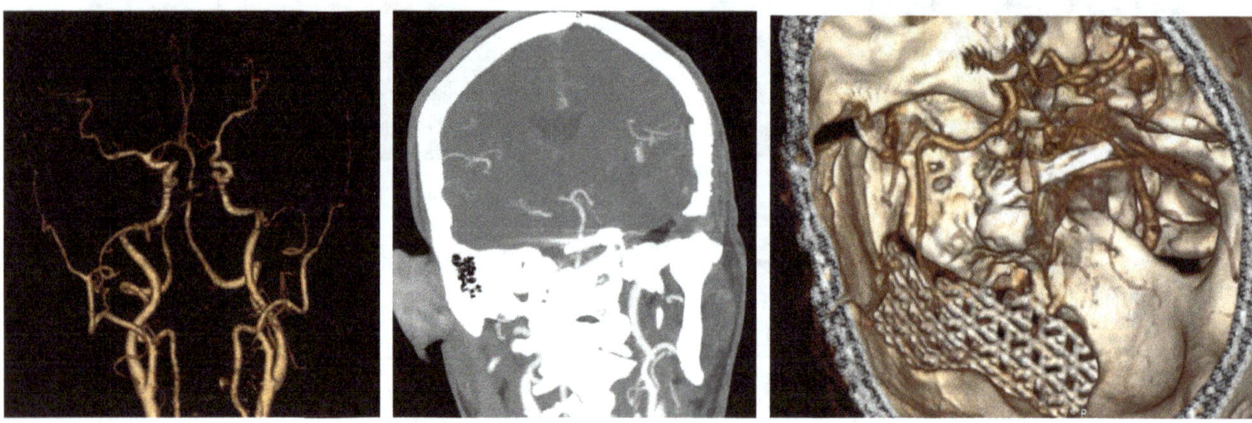

FIGURE 11: Post-op CTA.

15 minutes is for the posterior petrosectomy. This long time for the posterior petrosectomy was recorded because some steps such as unroofing of the sigmoid sinus or skeletonizing the semicircular canal must be taken meticulously. However, we have not found any comment about the operating time concerning skullbase approaches in the literature.

Kawase was the first surgeon who used anterior petrosectomy for midbasilar aneurysm clipping. However, he realized that it was difficult to control the proximal artery [4]. Later, anterior petrosectomy was used for the tumoral lesions. Inferior limit of anterior approach was internal auditory canal. Aneurysm clipping required more space, especially for the proximal control in the large and giant aneurysms. Posterior petrosectomy responded to this requirement.

4.3. Clipping Technique. Based on general techniques, we put temporary clips on 2 vertebral arteries through the posterior petrosal opening in order to soften the giant aneurysm. The temporary clipping time was about 6 min. Calcification of aneurysmal wall, intraluminal thrombus can make this step challenging.

We had no difficulties in clipping this aneurysm because its projection was anterior-posterior and superior-inferior. Therefore, the clips could be put on the neck directly through the drilled Kawase triangle. However, because of the wide neck and thin wall, the aneurysm wall was torn during the first clip application. Fortunately, this first clip was put far from the real neck, hence, with the second clip, the laceration was completely closed. Lawton (2011) described the technique of "orientation". He put the first long clip not too close to the aneurysmal neck, just to orientate the following clips [6, 8].

In this case, the anterior petrosectomy is sufficient enough for clip application. However, if the aneurysm is more complex or the projection is superiorly/anteriorly, maybe there will not be enough space for the manipulation. An extended approach to zygomatic bone may be necessary to gain more space for the surgeon.

4.4. Surgical Results. Giant AICA aneurysm was totally occluded. The mRankin was 1 after 3 months. In the earlier reports, good surgical outcome for the basilar aneurysms was about 80%, but no study was big enough to evaluate the surgical outcome of midbasilar aneurysm [5, 6], Mass effect disappeared after 3 months. This is also an advantage of clipping in comparison with endovascular treatments according to other authors' reports [8, 10].

5. Conclusion

Giant AICA aneurysm is a very rare lesion. Based on our experience in this case, we propose that combined transpetrosal approach is appropriate for surgical clipping. A good surgical outcome is achieved with the complete elimination of aneurysm.

Consent

Written informed consent was obtained from the patient for publication of this case report and accompanying images.

Acknowledgments

All authors want to sincerely thank the patient and her families. All members working at Department of Neurosurgery (Bach Mai Hospital) during the treatment time are gratefully acknowledged.

References

[1] M. Samii and E. Knosp, *Approaches to the Clivus: Approaches to No Man's Land*, Springer Science & Business Media, 1992.

[2] H. G. Schwartz, "Arterial aneurysm of the posterior Fossa," *Journal of Neurosurgery*, vol. 5, no. 3, pp. 312–316, 1948.

[3] C. Drake, "Treatment of Aneurysms of the Posterior Cranial Fossa," *Microsurgical Approach to Cerebro-Spinal Lesions*, Karger Publisherspp. 122–194, 1978.

[4] T. Kawase, S. Toya, R. Shiobara, and T. Mine, "Transpetrosal approach for aneurysms of the lower basilar artery," *Journal of Neurosurgery*, vol. 63, no. 6, pp. 857–861, 1985.

[5] T. Kawase, H. Bertalanffy, M. Otani, R. Shiobara, and S. Toya, "Surgical approaches for vertebro-basilar trunk aneurysms located in the midline," *Acta Neurochirurgica*, vol. 138, no. 4, pp. 402–410, 1996.

[6] M. T. Lawton, C. P. Daspit, and R. F. Spetzler, "Technical aspects and recent trends in the management of large and giant midbasilar artery aneurysms," *Neurosurgery*, vol. 41, no. 3, pp. 513–521, 1997.

[7] L. F. Gonzalez, M. J. Alexander, C. G. McDougall, and R. F. Spetzler, "Anteroinferior cerebellar artery aneurysms surgical approaches and outcomes-a review of 34 cases," *Neurosurgery*, vol. 55, no. 5, pp. 1025–1035, 2004.

[8] X. Lv, H. Ge, H. He, C. Jiang, and Y. Li, "Anterior inferior cerebellar artery aneurysms segments and results of surgical and endovascular managements," *Interventional Neuroradiology*, vol. 22, no. 6, pp. 643–648, 2016.

[9] X. Li, D. Zhang, and J. Zhao, "Anterior inferior cerebellar artery aneurysms: six cases and a review of the literature," *Neurosurgical Review*, vol. 35, no. 1, pp. 111–119, 2012.

[10] L. F. Gonzalez, M. J. Alexander, C. G. McDougall, and R. F. Spetzler, "Anteroinferior cerebellar artery aneurysms: surgical approaches and outcomes—a review of 34 cases," *Neurosurgery*, vol. 55, no. 5, pp. 1025–1035, 2004.

6

A First Case Report of Subependymoma in *PTPN11* Mutation-Associated Noonan Syndrome

Boonchai Boonyawat,[1] Mongkon Charoenpitakchai,[2] and Piradee Suwanpakdee [3]

[1]*Division of Genetics, Department of Pediatrics, Phramongkutklao Hospital and Phramongkutklao College of Medicine, Bangkok, Thailand*
[2]*Department of Pathology, Phramongkutklao Hospital and Phramongkutklao College of Medicine, Bangkok, Thailand*
[3]*Division of Neurology, Department of Pediatrics, Phramongkutklao Hospital and Phramongkutklao College of Medicine, Bangkok, Thailand*

Correspondence should be addressed to Piradee Suwanpakdee; piradee@pedpmk.org

Academic Editor: Mathias Toft

Noonan syndrome (NS) is an autosomal dominant disorder in some cases caused by *PTPN11* mutations. Since somatic mutations in *PTPN11* are seen in several tumor types, NS which causes germline *PTPN11* mutations are also increase the risk of hematologic malignancies and brain solid tumors. However, the report of brain tumors in Noonan syndrome remains rather rare. Here, we report the first case of an 11-year-old Thai boy with Noonan syndrome who presented with symptoms related to hydrocephalus secondary to subependymoma in the fourth ventricle, and *PTPN11* mutation was identified in this patient.

1. Introduction

Noonan syndrome (NS, OMIM 163950) is an autosomal dominant multiple congenital anomaly syndrome, which was first described by Jacqueline Noonan in 1968 [1]. The estimated prevalence is between 1 : 1,000 and 1 : 2,500 live births [2]. NS is characterized by short stature, distinctive facial dysmorphism, congenital heart defects, and a variable degree of developmental delay. Heterozygous activating mutations of the protein-tyrosine phosphatase, nonreceptor-type 11 genes (*PTPN11*, OMIM 176876) is the main cause of NS, which was elucidated by Tartaglia et al. in 2001 [3, 4]. The *PTPN11* gene encodes the nonreceptor protein tyrosine phosphatase (PTP) SHP-2 which is one of the proteins in the RAS-MAPK signaling pathway involved in the process of cell growth and differentiation.

Somatic mutations of *PTPN11* have been identified as the main cause of juvenile myelomonocytic leukemia (JMML) and in a small percentage of myelodysplastic syndrome (MDS) and acute myeloid leukemia (AML) [5]. Similarly, solid tumors have also been associated with somatic *PTPN11* mutations [6]. Thus, individuals with NS are also increased risk of cancer, in particular, hematologic malignancies and, less frequently, solid tumors including central nervous system (CNS) tumors [7]. Among CNS tumors, previous studies reported the low-grade glial and glioneural tumors, primarily dysembryoplastic neuroepithelial tumors (DNET) and low-grade gliomas [8, 9] but so far, the subependymoma has never been reported.

Herein, we report the first case of an 11-year-old Thai boy with *PTPN11* mutation-associated NS who developed subependymoma (WHO grade I) in Phramongkutklao hospital, Thailand.

2. Patients and Methods

2.1. Patients. A male patient was born at term with an uneventful pregnancy. His birth weight was 3,190 g (P50) and his birth length was 49 cm (P25). Physical examination at birth revealed dysmorphic facial features including left eye ptosis and triangular face, webbed neck, mild pectus deformity, and widely spaced nipples. The atrial septal defect was detected at the age of 9 months and surgical closure was performed at the 2 years of age. Short stature was detected at the age of 5 years. Owning to facial dysmorphism, a congenital heart defect,

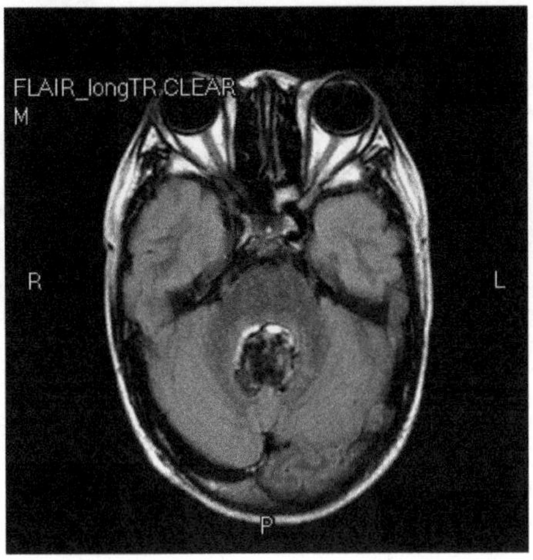

FIGURE 1: Magnetic resonance imaging (FLAIR, axial view) showing a lobulated, well-defined intraventricular mass (arrow) with no paraventricular extension attaching the fourth ventricular floor.

and short stature, he was diagnosed with Noonan syndrome. Growth hormone (GH) study revealed partial GH deficiency and GH treatment has been started since then.

At 11 years of age, he presented with one week of progressive headache and repeated vomiting, especially in the morning. Neither history of weakness nor seizures were noted. Neurological examination revealed only bilateral papilledema, the rest of the detailed neurological examination was normal. Magnetic resonance imaging (MRI) of the brain revealed a lobulated, well-defined intraventricular mass with no paraventricular extension attaching the fourth ventricular floor causing obstructive hydrocephalus (Figure 1). He underwent craniotomy and complete macroscopic removal of the tumor. Postoperative tumor histopathology revealed characteristic features of subependymoma with delicately fibrillar stroma with clusters of nuclei (Figure 2(a)) and microcystic change (Figure 2(b)). Tumor nuclei are round to oval and isometric with salt and pepper chromatin (Figure 2(c)). No mitosis was seen. Focal area of increased vasculature with sclerotic change as well as hemorrhage and calcification are also observed (Figure 2(d)). His headache resolved postoperatively and no radiological evidence of recurrence was seen at 7 years of follow-up.

2.2. Mutation Analysis of the PTPN11 Gene and Result. After informed consent was obtained from the patient and the parents, genomic DNA was extracted from peripheral blood lymphocytes. All 15 coding exons and exon-intron boundaries of *PTPN11* were amplified by PCR as described previously(14). All PCR products were directly sequenced in both directions.

A heterozygous missense; c.922A>G (p.Asn308Asp), mutation of *PTPN11* has been identified in the patient DNA. This mutation was not identified in both paternal and maternal DNA suggesting *de novo* mutation in the patient.

3. Discussion

Noonan syndrome (NS) is an autosomal dominant disorder which was characterized by characteristic facial features, short stature, and congenital cardiac defects. Missense mutations in *PTPN11* accounted for 31%–60% of NS cases [10]. These mutations were demonstrated to be gain-of-function resulting in excessive SHP-2 activity. Generally, overall children with NS have an estimated 8.1-fold increased risk of childhood cancers, whereas individuals with *PTPN11* mutation-associated NS have approximately 3.5-fold increased risk of all cancers including both hematologic and solid malignancies compared with the general population [11, 12]. Hematologic cancers widely accepted to be associated with NS include juvenile myelomonocytic leukemia (JMML), acute myelogenous leukemia (AML) and acute lymphoblastic leukemia (ALL) [2, 5]. Solid tumors including rhabdomyosarcoma, neuroblastoma, and CNS tumors were also reported [11, 12]. The majority of brain tumors associated with NS are low-grade glial and glioneural tumors, primarily dysembryoplastic neuroepithelial tumors (DNET) and low-grade gliomas [8, 9].

To date, a total of 27 cases of brain tumor associated with NS have been reported in the literature [8, 9]. The mean age at the time of brain tumor diagnosis for all patients was 16 years (ranging from 6–37 years). Majority of the patients were male. Approximately 80 percent of cases were caused by a heterozygous missense mutation in *PTPN11*, whereas, NS was diagnosed by clinical phenotypes only in the remaining (20%) of the patients. As in our patient who was a boy with NS, subependymoma (WHO grade I) was detected at the age of 11 years. Mutation analysis of *PTPN11* revealed a previously reported heterozygous missense p.Asn308Asp mutation [10]. This mutation has been previously identified in 3 NS associated CNS tumor patients. The first patient was a 6-year-old girl with dysembryoplastic neuroepithelial tumor (DNET), which is a rare CNS neoplasm [11]. The second patient was a 14-year-old female with anaplastic astrocytoma at the left brainstem and cerebellar peduncle [8]. The last patient was a 16-year-old male with DNET at left temporal and frontal lobe, and right thalamus [9]. Our study was the first report of subependymoma in the fourth ventricle in NS patients. Subependymoma is an extremely rare benign tumor accounting for less than 1% of all intracranial tumors and slow progression of symptoms in nature [13, 14]. Contrary to our patient, he developed symptoms related to hydrocephalus at the early age of presentation. This finding may explain from the moderate size of the tumor and location in the fourth ventricle which easily obstruct the cerebrospinal fluid (CSF) pathway. Common imaging characteristics of subependymoma include a lobulated, well-defined intraventricular mass with no paraventricular extension which was similar to our case [15]. The standard treatment is complete tumor resection which influenced the good prognosis. Our case confirmed this statement; he underwent total tumor resection without post-operative complication and achieved an excellent surgical outcome. Post-operative MRI brain was performed annually, no evidence of tumor recurrence was seen at 7 years of follow-up.

4. Conclusion

Our study demonstrates the first case of symptomatic subependymoma in *PTPN11* mutation-associated NS. Even though, there is no correlation between the specific mutation in

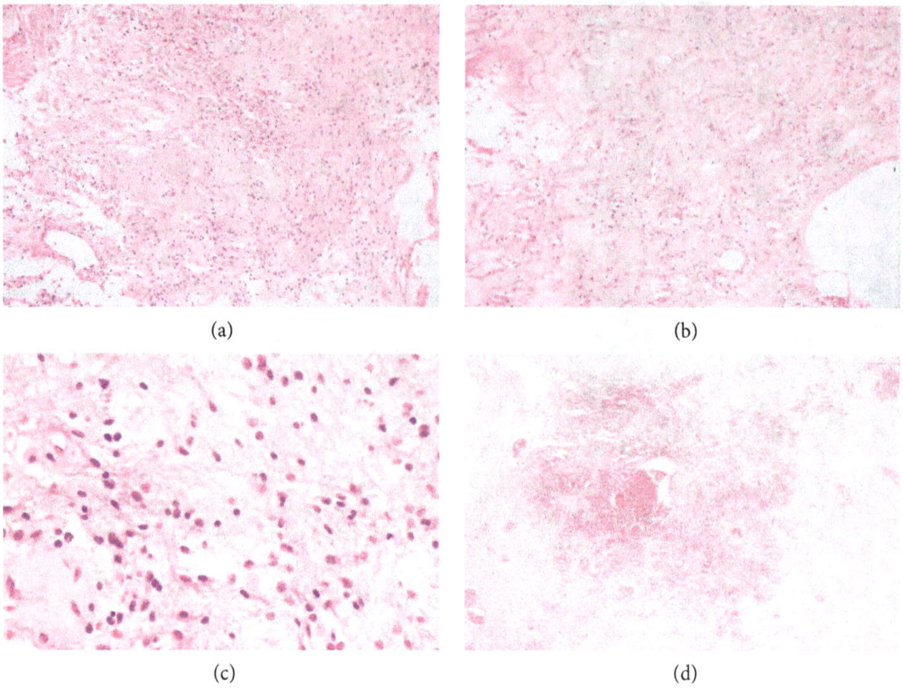

FIGURE 2: The mass showed delicately fibrillar stroma with clusters of nuclei (a, H&E 100x) and microcystic change (b, H&E 100x). Tumor nuclei are round to oval and isometric with salt and pepper chromatin (c, H&E 400x). Area of tumor hemorrhage (d, H&E 100x).

PTPN11 and the occurrence of cancer, approximately 15 percent of brain tumors in *PTPN11* mutation-associated NS were caused by heterozygous of p.Asn308Asp mutation in *PTPN11*. A high index of suspicion is required to explore CNS tumors in Noonan syndrome with *PTPN11* mutation patients who present with progressive headache as well as before starting GH therapy.

References

[1] J. A. Noonan, "Hypertelorism with turner phenotype. A new syndrome with associated congenital heart disease," *American Journal of Diseases of Children*, vol. 116, no. 4, pp. 373–380, 1968.

[2] A. E. Roberts, J. E. Allanson, M. Tartaglia, and B. D. Gelb, "Noonan syndrome," *The Lancet*, vol. 381, no. 9863, pp. 333–342, 2013.

[3] M. Tartaglia, E. L. Mehler, R. Goldberg et al., "Mutations in *PTPN11*, encoding the protein tyrosine phosphatase SHP-2, cause Noonan syndrome," *Nature Genetics*, vol. 29, no. 4, pp. 465–468, 2001.

[4] M. Tartaglia, K. Kalidas, A. Shaw et al., "*PTPN11* mutations in Noonan syndrome: molecular spectrum, genotype-phenotype correlation, and phenotypic heterogeneity," *The American Journal of Human Genetics*, vol. 70, no. 6, pp. 1555–1563, 2002.

[5] M. Tartaglia, C. M. Niemeyer, A. Fragale et al., "Somatic mutations in *PTPN11* in juvenile myelomonocytic leukemia, myelodysplastic syndromes and acute myeloid leukemia," *Nature Genetics*, vol. 34, no. 2, pp. 148–150, 2003.

[6] K. S. Grossmann, M. Rosário, C. Birchmeier, and W. Birchmeier, "The tyrosine phosphatase Shp2 in development and cancer," *Advances in Cancer Research*, vol. 106, pp. 53–89, 2010.

[7] P. Smpokou, D. J. Zand, K. N. Rosenbaum, and M. L. Summar, "Malignancy in Noonan syndrome and related disorders," *Clinical Genetics*, vol. 88, no. 6, pp. 516–22, 2015.

[8] M. El-Ayadi, M. Ansari, C. D. Kühnöl et al., "Occurrence of high-grade glioma in Noonan syndrome: report of two cases," *Pediatric Blood & Cancer*, vol. 66, no. 5, e27625 pages, 2019.

[9] A. Siegfried, C. Cances, M. Denuelle et al., "Noonan syndrome, *PTPN11* mutations, and brain tumors. A clinical report and review of the literature," *American Journal of Medical Genetics Part A*, vol. 173, no. 4, pp. 1061–1065, 2017.

[10] M. Zenker, G. Buheitel, R. Rauch et al., "Genotype-phenotype correlations in Noonan syndrome," *The Journal of Pediatrics*, vol. 144, no. 3, pp. 368–374, 2004.

[11] C. P. Kratz, L. Franke, H. Peters et al., "Cancer spectrum and frequency among children with Noonan, Costello, and cardio-facio-cutaneous syndromes," *British Journal of Cancer*, vol. 112, no. 8, pp. 1392–1397, 2015.

[12] M. C. Jongmans, I. van der Burgt, P. M. Hoogerbrugge et al., "Cancer risk in patients with Noonan syndrome carrying a *PTPN11* mutation," *European Journal of Human Genetics*, vol. 19, no. 8, pp. 870–874, 2011.

[13] M. Kurukumbi, A. Muley, G. Ramidi, Z. Wynn, and A. J. Trouth, "A rare case of subependymoma with an atypical presentation: a case report," *Case Reports in Neurology*, vol. 3, no. 3, pp. 227–232, 2011.

[14] R. Jooma, M. J. Torrens, J. Bradshaw, and B. Brownell, "Subependymomas of the fourth ventricle: surgical treatment in 12 cases," *Journal of Neurosurgery*, vol. 62, no. 4, pp. 508–512, 1985.

[15] R. Lobato, M. Sarabia, S. Castro et al., "Symptomatic subependymoma: report of four new cases studied with computed tomography and review of the literature," *Neurosurgery*, vol. 19, no. 4, pp. 594–598, 1986.

7

Intravascular Lymphoma with Progressive CNS Hemorrhage and Multiple Dissections

Ricky Chen[1] **Gurjeet Singh,**[2] **J. Scott McNally**[3] **Cheryl A. Palmer**[4] **and Adam de Havenon**[5]

[1]*Providence Brain & Spine Institute, Providence St. Vincent Medical Center, 9135 SW Barnes Road, Suite 461, Portland, OR 97225, USA*
[2]*Legacy Medical Group Neurology, Salmon Creek Medical Center, 2121 NE 139th St., Suite 205 Medical Office Building A, Vancouver, WA 98686, USA*
[3]*Department of Radiology and Imaging Sciences, University of Utah, 30 N 1900 E, Salt Lake City, UT 84132, USA*
[4]*Department of Pathology, University of Utah, Huntsman Cancer Institute, 2000 Circle of Hope Dr., Salt Lake City, UT 84112, USA*
[5]*Department of Neurology, University of Utah, 175 N Medical Dr., Salt Lake City, UT 84132, USA*

Correspondence should be addressed to Ricky Chen; ricky.chen2@providence.org

Academic Editor: Isabella Laura Simone

Introduction. Intravascular lymphoma (IVL) is an uncommon and often fatal disease characterized by intraluminal proliferation of lymphomatous cells within blood vessels. Because of a heterogeneous clinical presentation and lack of sensitive diagnostic protocols, diagnosis of IVL is most often made at autopsy. However, with early diagnosis and appropriate chemotherapy, the prognosis is greatly improved and complete remission is possible. In order to broaden the possible presentations of IVL, we present a patient with an atypical manifestation of biopsy-proven intravascular large B-cell lymphoma who suffered dissections of both intracranial and extracranial arteries in addition to progressive intracranial hemorrhages. *Case Report.* A 47-year-old woman presented with unilateral paresthesias. She developed progressive multifocal infarcts and hemorrhage with dissections of both intracranial and extracranial arteries, resulting in coma. Brain biopsy revealed IVL. She received aggressive chemotherapy and remains in complete remission with good neurologic recovery. *Conclusion.* IVL is known to exert its pathology on small arteries and capillaries, but is not known to cause dissections of large vessels. The diagnosis should be considered in cases with unexplained arterial dissections and progressive strokes. Early diagnosis with appropriate laboratory screening and tissue confirmation by biopsy can lead to greatly improved outcomes.

1. Introduction

Intravascular lymphoma (IVL) is recognized by the World Health Organization (WHO) as an extremely rare subtype of diffuse extranodal large B-cell non-Hodgkin's lymphoma with an estimated annual incidence of 0.5 cases per 1,000,000 [1]. IVL leads to intraluminal proliferation of neoplastic lymphoid cells in small and medium vessels [2]. These cells have lost the ability for transvascular migration due to defects in adhesion molecules [3]. IVL can involve any organ system, particularly the central nervous system (CNS), and its protean neurological manifestations often hinder diagnosis. Patients can present with subacute encephalopathy or dementia, paralysis, seizures, or multifocal cerebrovascular events, by order of frequency [1, 4, 5]. Systemic symptoms vary, but fever and skin lesions are the most common, whereas lymphadenopathy is usually absent [2].

Serologic abnormalities include anemia (63%), high lactate dehydrogenase (LDH) (82%) and beta 2-microglobulin levels (86%) [6]. Bone marrow involvement occurs in 32% of patients, and cerebrospinal fluid (CSF) rarely contains malignant cells [6]. Magnetic resonance imaging (MRI) is nonspecific and can be normal, though there are numerous reports of rapid progression of cerebral infarcts [5]. Organ biopsy is the gold standard for diagnosis of IVL but is frequently performed too late, and cases with CNS involvement are most

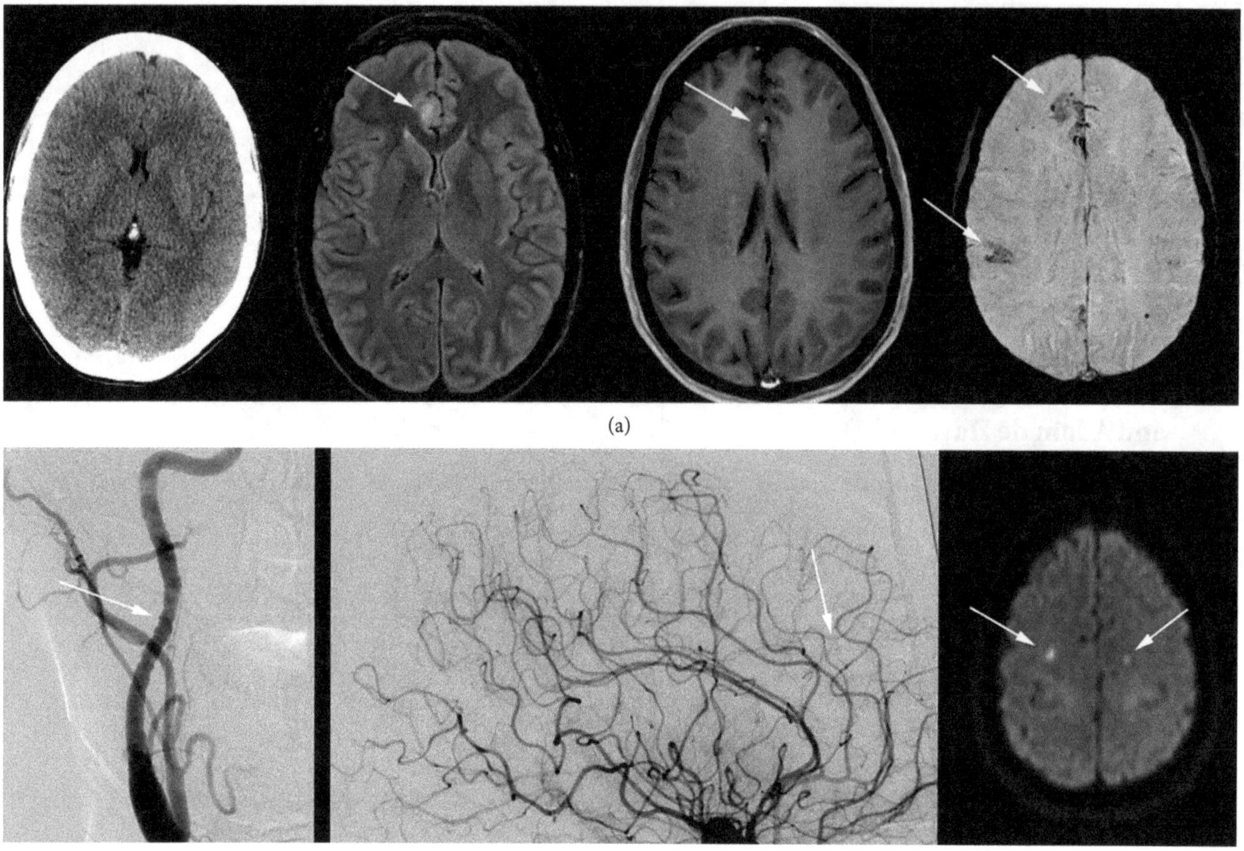

FIGURE 1: (a) Left to right: computed tomography (CT), fluid-attenuated inversion recovery (FLAIR), T1 post-contrast, and susceptibility-weighted imaging (SWI) 13 days after admission showed minimal findings on CT, but FLAIR hyperintensities and petechial hemorrhages on T1 and SWI images (arrows). These had progressed compared to initial imaging (not shown). (b) Left to right: Carotid and cerebral angiography showing irregular corrugated and beaded appearance of the cervical carotid arteries and subtle intracranial vessel narrowing (arrows), and two new foci of restricted diffusivity on diffusion weighted imaging (DWI) in the bilateral centrum semiovale consistent with interval infarcts (arrows). Note: there was another infarct in the left centrum semiovale on an adjacent slice not shown above.

often diagnosed post-mortem (60%) [7]. Random skin biopsies may help make the diagnosis earlier, with up to 83% sensitivity even without skin findings on exam [8, 9]. While IVL can have a grim prognosis with average untreated survival only a few months from diagnosis, chemotherapies containing rituxumab and doxorubicin have improved three-year survival rates to 60%, which may be further increased when methotrexate is added [1, 10]. When diagnosed and treated promptly, complete remission is seen in up to 42% of cases, although recent survival data with adequate treatment are lacking [11]. We describe an unusual presentation of IVL with multiple dissections of both intracranial and extracranial blood vessels and progressive intracranial hemorrhages (ICH).

2. Case Report

A 47-year-old woman with a history of delayed gastric emptying presented with migratory paresthesias traveling up her right side. These episodes occurred daily, lasted 20 minutes, and were associated with headache and confusion. During the month preceding her admission, she was admitted to an outside hospital with right-sided paresthesias, worsening migraines with visual aura, and somnolence. Initial contrast-enhanced MRI of the brain did not have acute findings, and showed minimal background nonspecific T2-weighted-fluid-attenuated inversion recovery (FLAIR) hyperintensities in the subcortical white matter.

After concern of a focal motor seizure, the patient was transferred to our hospital. She had no lymphadenopathy, skin lesions, or edema. Neurologically, she was initially somnolent but easily arousable, and once alert remained interactive and oriented sufficient to participate in the Montreal cognitive assessment (MOCA). Her MOCA score was 22/30 with notable deficits in attention, language and abstraction – a marked departure from her high-functioning baseline. The remainder of her neurologic exam was unremarkable. Laboratory evaluation including cerebrospinal fluid analysis was unrevealing (Table 1).

MRI of the brain was repeated 13 days after the initial scan (Figure 1(a)), showing two new foci of restricted diffusivity in the left centrum semiovale consistent with interval infarcts. There was also progression of FLAIR hyperintensities in the right anterior cingulate gyrus and inferior right and posterior left frontal lobes, with corresponding areas of petechial

Table 1: Additional laboratory findings.

	Value	Interpretation
Comprehensive metabolic panel		
Sodium	142 mmol/L	
Potassium	3.6 mmol/L	
Chloride	108 mmol/L	
CO_2	26 mmol/L	
BUN	10 mg/dL	
Creatinine	1.24 mg/dL	*High
Glucose	103 mg/dL	
Calcium	9.2 mg/dL	
Protein, total	6.1 g/dL	*Low
Albumin	4.1 g/dL	
Bilirubin	0.7 mg/dL	
Alkaline phosphatase	60 U/L	
AST	17 U/L	
ALT	11 U/L	
Anion gap	8 mmol/L	
Complete blood count		
WBC	3.73 k/μl	
RBC	4.47 M/μl	
HGB	13.3 g/dL	
HCT	38.9%	
MCV	86.9 fL	
MCH	29.7 pg	
MCHC	34.2 g/dL	
RDW	14.8%	*High
Platelet	152 k/μl	*Low
MPV	6.9 fL	
Granulocyte %, #	63.4, 2.4 k/μl	
Monocyte %, #	9.1, 0.3 k/μl	%*High
Eosinophil %, #	3.1, 0.1 k/μl	
Basophil %, #	0.4, 0.0 k/μl	
Lymphocyte %, #	24, 0.9 k/μl	
Paraneoplastic autoantibody evaluation (CSF)		
Neuronal nuclear Ab, Type 1	Negative	
Neuronal nuclear Ab, Type 2	Negative	
Neuronal nuclear Ab, Type 3	Negative	
Glial Nuclear Ab	Negative	
Purkinje cell cytoplasmic Ab, Type 1	Negative	
Purkinje cell cytoplasmic Ab, Type 2	Negative	
Purkinje cell cytoplasmic Ab, Type Tr	Negative	
Amphiphysin Ab	Negative	
CRMP-5 IgG	Negative	
Additional laboratory tests		
LDH[a]	427 U/L	*High
Ferritin[b]	1,107 ng/mL	*High
TSH	1.83 mU/L	
CRP	0.1 mg/dL	
Prothrombin time	13.7 sec	
INR	1.1	
Sed rate, Westergren	2 mm/hr	

[a]LDH was analyzed 45 days after initial test results. [b]Ferritin was analyzed 20 months after initial test results.

hemorrhage on T2*-weighted imaging. Continuous electroencephalograms (EEG) confirmed encephalopathic slowing without epileptiform discharges. Cerebral angiography showed irregular corrugated and beaded appearance of the cervical carotid arteries, thought to be consistent with chronic fibromuscular dysplasia (Figure 1(b)). High-resolution vessel wall MRI did not show arterial wall enhancement to suggest vasculitis. 18F-fluorodeoxyglucose positron emission tomography (FDG-PET) scan of the brain (Figure 2) and computed tomography (CT) of the chest, abdomen, and pelvis were unrevealing.

As an extensive workup was thus far negative (CSF OCB, flow, cytology, HSV/VZV, ANA, ANCA, Mayo paraneoplastic panel, VGKC, AQ4, NMDA, tox screen, EEG without obvious seizure), the patient received a presumptive diagnosis of idiopathic encephalitis and was treated empirically with a five-day trial of intravenous methylprednisolone followed by a prednisone taper. She improved clinically for one month after discharge and returned to work, but gradually developed worsening headache, vomiting, lethargy, and episodic left facial droop. Repeat MRI (Figure 3(a)) showed marked interval progression with new areas of cytotoxic edema/infarction, vasogenic edema, and a moderate-sized right temporoparietal hemorrhage causing cerebral edema and midline shift, with additional petechial hemorrhages on T2*-weighted imaging. There was extensive new sulcal FLAIR signal and enhancement compatible with blood-brain barrier breakdown.

CSF analysis demonstrated marked protein elevation (140 mg/dL) without pleocytosis. Repeat catheter angiography showed a new right cervical internal carotid artery dissection in the distal extracranial portion as well as progression of luminal irregularities indicative of progressive vasculopathy (Figure 3(b)). Magnetic resonance angiography (MRA) of the head and neck the same day revealed additional bilateral vertebral artery dissections involving the entire right vertebral artery and the left V3/4 segments, as well as new narrowing of the bilateral temporal arteries. There was no instrumentation above the level of the common carotid arteries or vertebral artery origins during the initial catheter angiogram to explain this finding. Our differential diagnosis expanded to include atypical vasculitides, inflammatory amyloid angiopathy, complicated Posterior reversible encephalopathy syndrome (PRES), and reversible cerebral vasoconstriction syndrome (RCVS), or IVL (Table 2). Because an elevated LDH level in an atypical case without infection can be suggestive of IVL, we measured LDH and found hers to be elevated to 450 U/L (Table 1).

The patient's clinical course progressed to coma due to cerebral edema and hematoma expansion. A right temporoparietal brain biopsy was obtained. Sections stained with hematoxylin-and-eosin showed small cortical vessels pathologically distended with neoplastic lymphocytes. These cells were pleomorphic, hyperchromatic, and displayed prominent nucleoli and occasional mitoses (Figure 4(a)). They did not spill out into the surrounding neuropil. Immunohistochemistry revealed these malignant cells to be diffusely positive for CD20, a B-cell marker (Figure 4(b)). The tumor cells also labeled widely for Mindbomb E3 Ubiquitin Protein Ligase 1 (MIB-1), a marker of proliferation. Based on these findings, the patient was diagnosed with IVL. The patient was urgently

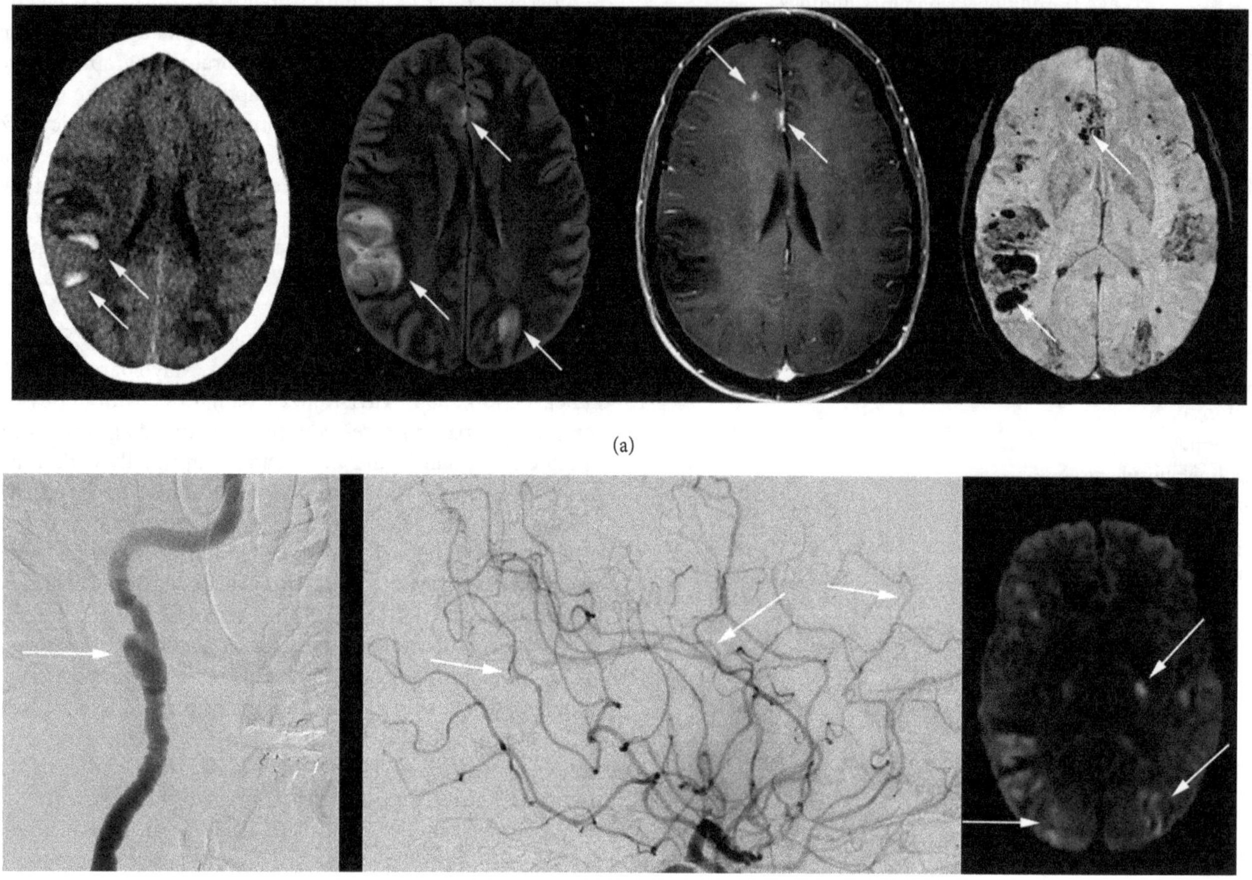

FIGURE 2: (a) Left to right: Repeat CT, FLAIR, T1post, and SWI showing marked interval progression of hemorrhages on CT and SWI with surrounding edema on FLAIR and subtle foci of enhancement on T1 post-contrast images (arrows). The vasogenic edema and moderate-sized right temporoparietal hemorrhage caused cerebral edema and midline shift, and there were multiple additional petechial hemorrhages. There was also new sulcal FLAIR signal with subtle enhancement consistent with blood-brain barrier breakdown. (b) Left to right: Repeat catheter angiography showed a new right cervical internal carotid artery dissection on carotid angiography (arrow), progression of luminal irregularities in the distal the middle cerebral artery and the anterior cerebral artery branches (arrows), and new areas of cytotoxic edema/infarction on DWI (arrows).

started on chemotherapy with rituximab, cyclophosphamide, doxorubicin, vincristine, and prednisone (R-CHOP) along with decompressive craniectomy, which led to reversal of coma and liberation from the ventilator several days later. She then received methotrexate, which halted progression of her disease and allowed her to return home with a modified Rankin Scale of 1. The patient remains in remission today, four years later.

3. Discussion

IVL involving the CNS is an aggressive condition with a poor prognosis because its protean clinical manifestations frequently preclude diagnosis. Laboratory and imaging tools provide clues to the etiology, but lack adequate sensitivity and specificity. Our patient exhibited an unusual presentation of multiple arterial dissections and progressive ICH. She underwent an extensive workup for progressive encephalopathy until her decline into coma necessitated a brain biopsy. The pathological proliferation of intraluminal lymphocytes in the small intracranial vessels explains our patient's symptoms and imaging findings. As arterioles, venules, and capillaries stagnate with malignant cells, intraparenchymal hemorrhage and infarction can occur. However, the formation of multiple large-artery dissections in her clinical course remains unexplained. Microvessels are a known source of intramural hematomas in the setting of arterial dissection and intraplaque hemorrhage, attributed to vasa vasorum leakage or rupture within the wall of carotid and vertebral arteries [12]. It is unclear whether IVL is capable of infiltrating these small vessels (vasa vasorum) within the arterial wall to cause rupture and dissection of the intima and adventitia of the artery.

Given the limitations of an individual reported case, we cannot rule out an alternative etiology for her dissections. It is possible that she had either underlying fibromuscular dysplasia (FMD) or another condition explaining her dissections, in addition to IVL explaining her brain findings. However, her angiographic studies showed interval development of new

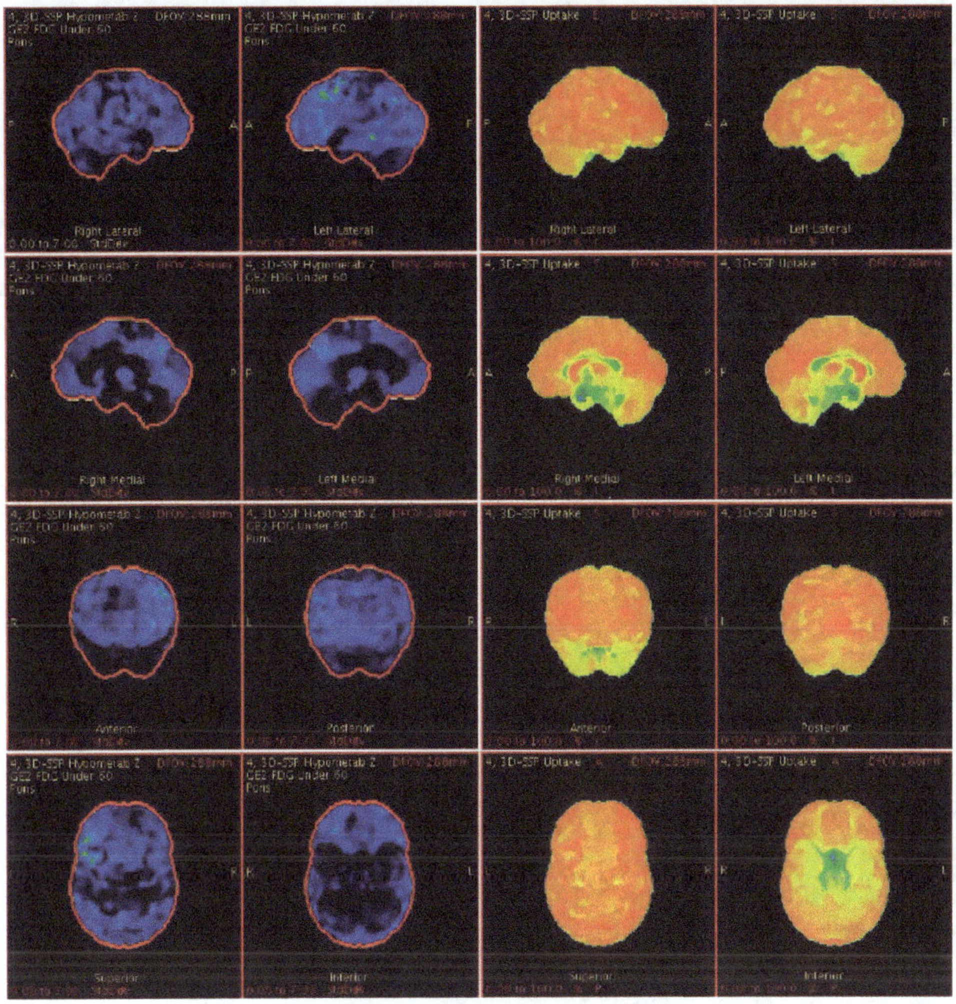

(a)

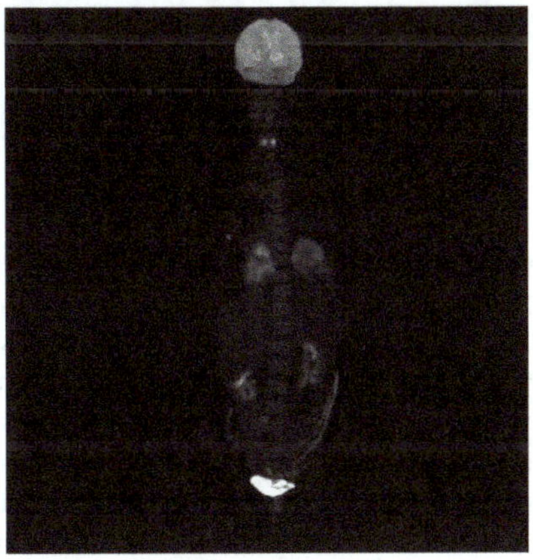

(b)

FIGURE 3: (a) FDG-PET scan of the brain demonstrated mildly diminished FDG uptake in the left more than right bilateral temporal, frontal, and parietal lobes as well as the in the posterior cingulate, precuneus and the primary visual and visual association cortices. The most prominent metabolic reduction was in the left frontal association cortex. There were no focal areas of hypermetabolism in the mesial temporal lobes or elsewhere. This diffuse pattern of mild metabolic changes was not specific for any inflammatory disease or other process, and most suggestive of a global encephalopathy with asymmetry due to more pronounced deficits in the left hemisphere. (b) PET scan of the body was notable for bilateral pleural effusions as well as pericardial effusion and scattered nonspecific ill-defined hypermetabolic pulmonary nodules with differential including infectious/inflammatory process or pulmonary lymphoma with max SUV (standard uptake value) of 6.8.

TABLE 2: Laboratory/imaging workup.

Differential diagnosis	Labs/imaging
Neurosarcoidosis	ACE
Cerebral sinus thrombosis	Catheter angiogram
Vasculitis	ANA, ANCA, SSA, SSB, ESR, CRP, Hepatitis panel
Reversible cerebral vasoconstriction syndrome	Catheter angiogram and high resolution vessel wall MRI
Autoimmune and paraneoplastic encephalitis	VGKC, NMDA, CASPR2, LGI1 paraneoplastic antibody panel, Cerebral FDG PET scan
CNS malignancy or metastasis	CSF cytology and flow cytometry, CT of the chest, abdomen, pelvis. PET of the brain
Infectious endocarditis with septic emboli	ESR, CRP, lactate
Encephalitis (Infectious etiologies)	TB, RPR, HIV, VZV, HSV, EBV, WNV, HTLV1/2, and others
Cerebral autosomal dominant arteriopathy with subcortical infarcts and leukoencephalopathy (CADASIL)	MRI
Drug-induced vasculopathy	Urine drug screen
Amyloid angiitis	Congo red and thioflavin on biopsy, MRI with Susceptibility-weighted imaging
Progressive multifocal leukoencephalopathy	HIV antibodies

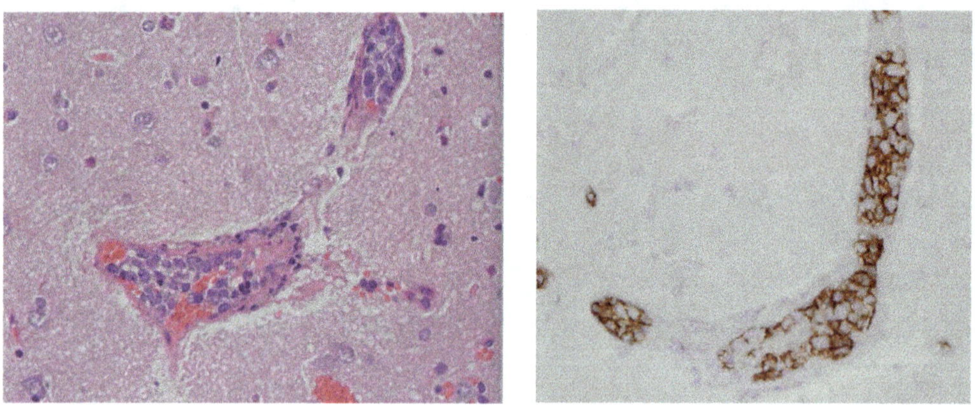

FIGURE 4: (a) Hematoxylin-and-eosin of the brain biopsy showed small cortical vessels pathologically distended with neoplastic lymphocytes (200X). (b) These cells were positive by immunohistochemistry for CD20, a B-cell marker (200X).

large-artery dissections associated with clinical and radiographic progression of her IVL. To date, there have been no reports in the literature to support IVL involving large arteries such as carotid and vertebral arteries, a disease known to involve mainly arterioles, venules, and capillaries.

This case highlights the need for a high index of suspicion for an underlying IVL in the setting of multiple intracranial and extracranial dissections and ICH, and progression of findings despite standard medical therapy. Our patient recovered from her coma and currently remains in remission four years later owing to accurate histopathological diagnosis and prompt treatment, which stands in stark contrast to the majority of patients who are diagnosed postmortem. In evaluating progressive encephalitis of unclear etiology, prompt brain biopsy proved essential in directing treatment. However, there may be reasons when brain biopsy may be delayed or inaccurate due to concerns regarding procedural risk or when there is little to no tumor mass formation, which could lead to nondiagnostic results that have the potential to critically delay the initiation of therapy. Imaging findings such as diffuse scattered foci of T2 hyperintensities and diffusion restriction, petechial and parenchymal hemorrhages, with or without arterial dissections should raise the suspicion for this elusive disease even in the absence of detectable mass lesions. Early clinical diagnostic strategies may enable treatment sooner. These strategies make the diagnosis by assimilating other important data including serum tumor markers, LDH (lactate dehydrogenase) and soluble IL2R (interleukin-2 receptor), as well as random skin and bone marrow biopsy with flow cytometry [6, 8, 9,13, 14]. In particular, CNS involvement of lymphoma at diagnosis portends a worse prognosis and these patients are thought to have a higher rate of relapse, especially in the CNS [15]. It has been proposed that positive findings on skin biopsy may be useful in cases without proven CNS disease as a risk factor for later relapse in the CNS, though further investigation is needed to prove this [15]. There remains a need for better pathophysiologic understanding of this elusive disease.

Acknowledgments

We humbly acknowledge the patient herself for exemplary generosity, courage, and patience throughout the course of diagnosis, treatment, and life after hospitalization. We would also like to thank Stefanie Linch for critical review of the manuscript and assistance with publication.

References

[1] E. Fonkem, S. Dayawansa, E. Stroberg et al., "Neurological presentations of intravascular lymphoma (IVL): meta-analysis of 654 patients," *BMC Neurology*, vol. 16, no. 1, p. 9, 2016.

[2] C. Cruto, R. Taipa, C. Monteiro, I. Moreira, M. Melo-Pires, and M. Correia, "Multiple cerebral infarcts and intravascular central nervous system lymphoma: a rare but potentially treatable association," *Journal of the Neurological Sciences*, vol. 325, no. 1-2, pp. 183–185, 2013.

[3] M. Ponzoni, G. Arrigoni, V. E. Gould et al., "Lack of CD 29 (β1 integrin) and CD 54 (ICAM-1) adhesion molecules in intravascular lymphomatosis," *Human Pathology*, vol. 31, no. 2, pp. 220–226, 2000.

[4] A. K. Panda and S. Malik, "CNS intravascular lymphoma: an underappreciated cause of rapidly progressive dementia," *BMJ Case Reports*, vol. 2014, Article ID bcr2014203772, 2014.

[5] L.-C. Hung, J.-H. Tsai, C.-S. Wu, Y.-C. Dai, C.-C. Chen, and S.-F. Sung, "Brain biopsy-proven intravascular lymphomatosis presenting as rapidly recurrent strokes-two case reports," *Acta Neurologica Taiwanica*, vol. 23, no. 1, pp. 11–18, 2014.

[6] A. J. M. Ferreri, E. Campo, J. F. Seymour et al., "Intravascular lymphoma: clinical presentation, natural history, management and prognostic factors in a series of 38 cases, with special emphasis on the "cutaneous variant"," *British Journal of Haematology*, vol. 127, no. 2, pp. 173–183, 2004.

[7] E. Fonkem, E. Lok, D. Robison, S. Gautam, and E. T. Wong, "The natural history of intravascular lymphomatosis," *Cancer Medicine*, vol. 3, no. 4, pp. 1010–1024, 2014.

[8] K. Matsue, N. Asada, J. Odawara et al., "Random skin biopsy and bone marrow biopsy for diagnosis of intravascular large B cell lymphoma," *Annals of Hematology*, vol. 90, no. 4, pp. 417–421, 2011.

[9] N. Asada, J. Odawara, S.-I. Kimura et al., "Use of random skin biopsy for diagnosis of intravascular large B-Cell lymphoma," *Mayo Clinic Proceedings*, vol. 82, no. 12, pp. 1525–1527, 2007.

[10] Y. Sekiguchi, A. Shimada, H. Imai et al., "Intravascular large B-cell lymphoma with pontine involvement successfully treated with R-CHOP therapy and intrathecal administration: a case report and review of literature," *International Journal of Clinical and Experimental Pathology*, vol. 7, no. 6, pp. 3363–3369, 2014.

[11] J. A. DiGiuseppe, W. G. Nelson, E. J. Seifter, J. K. Boitnott, and R. B. Mann, "Intravascular lymphomatosis: a clinicopathologic study of 10 cases and assessment of response to chemotherapy," *Journal of Clinical Oncology*, vol. 12, no. 12, pp. 2573–2579, 1994.

[12] R. R. Patel, R. Adam, C. Maldjian, C. M. Lincoln, A. Yuen, and A. Arneja, "Cervical carotid artery dissection: current review of diagnosis and treatment," *Cardiology in Review*, vol. 20, no. 3, pp. 145–152, 2012.

[13] M. Kitayama, M. Ueno, T. Itakura, and T. Yamashita, "Activated microglia inhibit axonal growth through RGMa," *PLoS One*, vol. 6, no. 9, Article ID e25234, 2011.

[14] Y. Masaki, L. Dong, A. Nakajima et al., "Intravascular large B cell lymphoma: proposed strategy for early diagnosis and treatment of patients with rapid deteriorating condition," *International Journal of Hematology*, vol. 89, no. 5, pp. 600–610, 2009.

[15] K. Shimada, T. Murase, K. Matsue et al., "IVL Study Group in Japan. Central nervous system involvement in intravascular large B-cell lymphoma: A retrospective analysis of 109 patients," *Cancer Science*, vol. 101, no. 6, pp. 1480–1486, 2010.

8

Ischemic Stroke and Ruptured Mycotic Aneurysm, Two Complications of Infective Endocarditis in One Patient

Alassane Mamadou Diop,[1,2] Ahmadou Bamba Mbodj,[3] Serigne Abdou Aziz Fall,[3] and Ibrahima Niang[4]

[1]*Cheikh Anta Diop University, Dakar, Senegal*
[2]*Neurology Department of the Pikine Hospital, Dakar, Senegal*
[3]*Neuroscience Department of the Fann Hospital, Dakar, Senegal*
[4]*Medical Imaging Department of the Fann Hospital, Dakar, Senegal*

Correspondence should be addressed to Alassane Mamadou Diop; alassanemamadou@hotmail.fr

Academic Editor: Isabella Laura Simone

The incidence of infective endocarditis is estimated to be around 30 cases per million inhabitants/year. It can be responsible for various neurological complications such as cerebral infarction, meningitis, cerebral abscesses, and cerebral hemorrhage due to ruptured mycotic aneurysms. Several germs have been incriminated in this condition including *Staphylococcus*, *Streptococcus*, and *Enterococcus*. We report the case of a 64-year-old patient who presented with an acute motor deficit of the left upper limb associated with dysarthria. MRI showed infarcts in both cerebral hemispheres, and the TOF sequence showed an amputation of M2. On transesophageal ultrasound, there was evidence of vegetations at the mitral valve. Blood culture isolated *Streptococcus oralis*. With antibiotic treatment, the evolution was marked by a stable apyrexia with regression of the dysarthria. Before her surgery, she suddenly developed aphasia with worsening of the motor deficit. CT scan showed a right fronto-parietal hematoma which was related to a ruptured cerebral aneurysm. She underwent endovascular embolisation and subsequent cardiac surgery.

1. Introduction

Infective endocarditis is responsible for neurological complications like ischemia, meningitis, brain abscess, and mycotic aneurysms, which are detected in 5% of patients in the acute and subacute phase of the infection and can be complicated by cerebral hemorrhage when ruptured [1]. Ischemic strokes due to vegetation embolism are considered the main neurological complication of endocarditis with two risk factors: the size and mobility of the vegetation [2]. Although recommendation of antibiotic therapy and surgical indications are now well defined in the recommendations, the ideal timing of surgery is still a matter of debate [3]. We report a case of streptococcal infective endocarditis complicated by ischemic stroke and cerebral hematoma due to a mycotic aneurysm rupture.

2. Observation

The patient was 64 years old and was admitted to hospital with sudden onset of motor deficit of the left upper limb associated with speech disorders. The examination on admission revealed a left brachial monoplegia, dysarthria, a fever of 41 degrees Celsius, and a mitral focus murmur. Brain MRI in FLAIR and diffusion sequences showed subacute ischemic lesions in both cerebral hemispheres with a more significant lesion in the right internal capsule (Figure 1). On the 3D TOF sequence, we found an amputation in the M2 segment of the left sylvian artery. A transthoracic cardiac echocardiography performed in emergency suspected vegetations of the mitral valve. Transesophageal echocardiography showed Oslerian graft of both mitral leaflets with a small prolapse over a probable cord rupture and vegetation

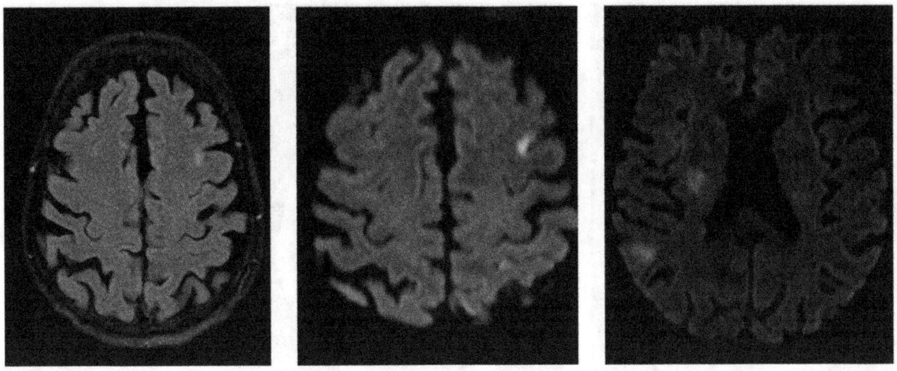

(a) (b) (c)

Figure 1: Bilateral ischemic lesions: at the left cortical frontal lobe in FLAIR and diffusion hypersignal (a, b) and in the right parietal and lenticular in diffusion hypersignal (c).

of 22 mm by 10 mm. The other valves and the myocardium were intact. The biology showed a CRP of 123 mg/l without hyperleukocytosis. Troponin and ProBNP were normal. Blood cultures were positive for *Streptococcus oralis*. The diagnosis of endocarditis complicated by stroke was retained and antibiotic therapy with penicillin at a dose of 4 million units every 6 hours was initiated at the beginning, followed by amoxicillin 2 g every 4 hours associated with preventive anticoagulation with 4000 IU of enoxaparin. The evolution was marked by apyrexia and disappearance of dysarthria. The patient was transferred to cardiology where a discussion for valve surgery was in progress with the surgeons when she presented with aphasia, headaches, and extension of the deficit to the lower limb giving a left hemiplegia. The brain scan showed a right fronto-parietal hematoma (Figure 2(a)) which was not present at admission (Figure 2(b)). Cerebral angiography revealed a probably mycotic aneurysm that ruptured, leading to this hematoma (Figure 2(c)). Endovascular embolisation of the aneurysm was performed. She was still aphasic and hemiplegic when she was transferred to cardiac surgery where a valve replacement was successfully performed.

3. Discussion

The incidence of infective endocarditis is estimated to be around 30 cases per million inhabitants per year in general population studies conducted in Western countries [4].

The diagnosis of endocarditis is based on a combination of clinical and microbiological criteria and additional examinations using the Duke criteria. Since the European recommendations in 2015, imaging is part of the diagnostic algorithm as a major criterion for endocarditis [3, 5]. *Staphylococcus* is now the most common organism causing infective endocarditis, followed by streptococci of oral origin and then enterococci [4]. Studies agree on the importance of finding the germ by repeated blood cultures to improve patient management [3]. Symptomatic ischemic stroke is reported in 10–35% of infective endocarditis and is the most common neurological complication: approximately 50% of neurological complications of infective endocarditis are strokes related to emboli from the vegetations [2, 6]. The pathogenesis of mycotic aneurysms results from the migration of septic emboli, which attach to the artery walls, leading to focal arteritis, necrosis, and pseudoaneurysm formation [7]. Our patient received preventive anticoagulation with enoxaparin at a dose of 4000 units per day. Elkaryoni et al. performed a large meta-analysis in the United States that included 41,545 patients with infective endocarditis, of whom 39,255 were not anticoagulated and 2290 were anticoagulated. After adjustment for potentially confounding variables, there was no significant difference in risk of death or embolic complications of IE with AC; however, risk of ICH was higher with use of AC but did not reach statistical significance. Our results do not support the use of AC in IE for reduction in risk of thromboembolic events [8].

Our patient could not benefit from thrombolysis due to the risk of hemorrhagic transformation and the ischemic lesions visible on the FLAIR sequence on cerebral MRI. In fact, during cerebral infarctions linked to infective endocarditis, thrombolysis multiplies the risk of intracranial hemorrhage by 4 and is therefore contraindicated. In contrast, thrombectomy has been shown to improve the functional prognosis of patients [3, 9].

Cerebral hemorrhage secondary to thrombolysis of cerebral ischemia has been described in patients with infective endocarditis. It is most often due to asymptomatic aneurysm rupture. Therefore, it is strongly recommended to perform CT angiography in addition to routine non-contrast head CT scan in patients with a history of infective endocarditis who present with acute neurologic symptoms, before they receive rtPA for acute ischemic stroke [10].

The main antibiotic treatment regimens according to the germs are defined in the ESC 2015 recommendations. For oral and bovis group streptococci, penicillin G 12–18 million·U/d intravenous (IV) in 4 or 6 injections or continuous administration, amoxicillin 100–200 mg/kg/d IV in 4 or 6 injections, or ceftriaxone 2 g/d IV in 1 injection can be used. The duration of treatment is 4 weeks for native valves and 6 weeks for prosthetic valves [3, 11].

The occurrence of cerebral hemorrhage due to aneurysm rupture in our patient delayed cardiac surgery. Patients with

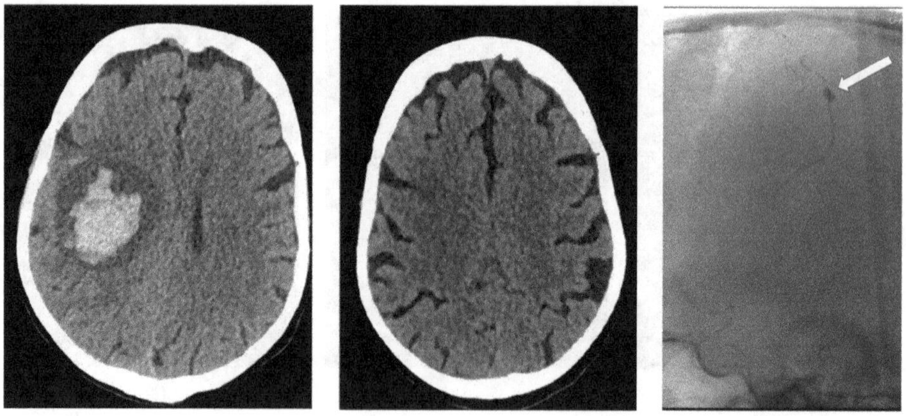

(a) (b) (c)

Figure 2: Hemorrhage from ruptured aneurysm right fronto-parietal hematoma (a); previously normal CT brain (b); angiography showing the aneurysm of a branch of the right middle cerebral artery (white arrow) (c).

radiographic evidence of ischemic stroke from septic emboli can safely undergo valvular surgery for IE without increased risk of symptomatic hemorrhage; as for thrombolysis, it is recommended to perform CT angiography to detect aneurysms [2, 12].

Heparin is the drug of choice for the mandatory anticoagulation during cardiopulmonary bypass (CPB), but the optimal heparin dose during CPB is not known. Compared with a lower dose of heparin during CPB, a high dose of heparin had little effect on the point-of-care measurements of hemostasis. Higher heparin dose does not seem to offer benefit during CPB [13].

4. Conclusion

Neurological complications are often life-threatening and may cause sequelae. Moreover, they are likely to radically modify the management of patients. Indeed, their occurrence must raise the question of possible specific diagnostic or therapeutic procedures and that of the indication and delay of a possible cardiac surgery.

References

[1] A. Consoli, O. Coskun, M. Perier et al., "[Therapeutic and endovascular management of cerebral mycotic aneurysms]," *Annales de Cardiologie et d'Angeiologie*, vol. 69, no. 6, pp. 411–414, 2020.

[2] R. Sonneville, I. Klein, L. Bouadma, B. Mourvillier, B. Regnier, and M. Wolff, "Complications neurologiques des endocardites infectieuses," *Reanimation*, vol. 18, no. 7, pp. 547–555, 2009.

[3] L. Duarte and A. Bouglé, "Endocardite aiguë," *Anesthésie & Réanimation*.vol. 7, no. 6, pp. 396–409, 2021.

[4] B. Iung, "[Infective endocarditis. Epidemiology, pathophysiology and histopathology]," *Presse Medicale*, vol. 48, no. 5, pp. 513–521, 2019.

[5] G. Habib, P. Lancellotti, M. J. Antunes et al., "2015 ESC Guidelines for the management of infective endocarditis," *Kardiologia Polska*, vol. 73, no. 11, pp. 963–1027, 2015.

[6] E. Ruttmann, J. Willeit, H. Ulmer et al., "Neurological outcome of septic cardioembolic stroke after infective endocarditis," *Stroke*, vol. 37, no. 8, pp. 2094–2099, 2006.

[7] P. Koch, H. A. Desal, E. Auffray-Calvier, and A. De Kersaint-Gilly, "Anévrysme mycotique cérébral: histoire naturelle et prise en charge thérapeutique," *Journal of Neuroradiology*, vol. 32, no. 4, pp. 258–265, 2005.

[8] A. Elkaryoni, S. S. Taduru, A. Barakat, H. F. Othman, and J. Enriquez, "Anticoagulation in infective endocarditis: insights from nationwide inpatient sample," *Journal of the American College of Cardiology*, vol. 73, 2019.

[9] K. L. Sloane, S. B. Raymond, J. D. Rabinov, and A. B. Singhal, "Mechanical thrombectomy in stroke from infective endocarditis: case report and review," *Journal of Stroke and Cerebrovascular Diseases*, vol. 29, no. 1, Article ID 104501, 2020.

[10] J. Glenn, M. Strecker-McGraw, I. McGraw, K. Jabbar, N. A. James, and C. K. Stone, "Rupture of an occult intracranial mycotic aneurysm after intravenous thrombolysis with recombinant tissue plasminogen activator for acute ischemic stroke," *Journal of Emergency Medicine*, vol. 53, no. 5, pp. 717–721, 2017.

[11] D. Luque-Paz, A. Le Bot, M. Sébillotte, S. Tchamgoué, D. Lebeaux, and P. Tattevin, "Antibiothérapie des endocardites infectieuses en 2021: actualités," *Archives des Maladies du Coeur et des Vaisseaux—Pratique*, vol. 2021, no. 298, pp. 2–6, 2021.

[12] C. N. Small, D. Laurent, B. Lucke-Wold et al., "Timing surgery and hemorrhagic complications in endocarditis with concomitant cerebral complications," *Clinical Neurology and Neurosurgery*, vol. 214, Article ID 107171, 2022.

[13] M. Lax, E. Pesonen, S. Hiippala, A. Schramko, R. Lassila, and P. Raivio, "Heparin dose and point-of-care measurements of hemostasis in cardiac surgery—results of a randomized controlled trial," *Journal of Cardiothoracic and Vascular Anesthesia*, vol. 34, no. 9, pp. 2362–2368, 1 sept 2020.

9

Immediate Response to Chemotherapy in an Adult Neuroblastoma Patient Presenting with Cord Compression

Nedal Bukhari,[1,2] Bachar Harfouch,[3] Majid Shallal Alotaibi,[4] Hulayel Al-Harbi,[1] and Omar Chamdine[5]

[1]*Department of Medical Oncology, King Fahad Specialist Hospital, Dammam, Saudi Arabia*
[2]*Department of Internal Medicine, King Fahd University Hospital, Imam Abdulrahamn Bin Faisal University, Dammam, Saudi Arabia*
[3]*Department of Neurosurgery, King Fahad Specialist Hospital, Dammam, Saudi Arabia*
[4]*Department of Neurology, King Fahad Specialist Hospital, Dammam, Saudi Arabia*
[5]*Department of Pediatric Hematology Oncology and Stem Cell Transplantation, King Fahad Specialist Hospital, Dammam, Saudi Arabia*

Correspondence should be addressed to Nedal Bukhari; nedal.bukhari36@gmail.com

Academic Editor: Norman S. Litofsky

We report a case of a 31-year-old female patient with high-risk neuroblastoma (NBL) who presented with a history of static back pain and bilateral lower limb weakness for almost a month. Her primary tumor was located in the right paraspinal region, causing spinal cord compression (SCC). Chemotherapy was administered with an immediate clinical improvement noted after 24 hours of starting treatment. We herein report the efficacy of chemotherapy in an adult neuroblastoma (aNBL) patient presenting with spinal cord compression.

1. Introduction

NBL is the most common extracranial solid tumor in childhood that originates from the neural crest. It is almost exclusively a disease of children. It affects them in early childhood (>90% of cases diagnosed before 5 years of age) and is rare among adolescents and adults [1].

Neuroblastomas can invade the spinal canal causing SCC. Our patient had symptoms and signs of epidural spinal cord compression (ESCC) and thus received chemotherapy [2, 3].

In this case, we describe the response to chemotherapy manifested by a marked improvement in the neurological symptoms within a very short period of time.

2. Case Report

A 31-year-old female, previously healthy, referred from a community hospital with a 4-week history of back pain, associated with bilateral lower limb weakness. No symptoms of paresthesia, urinary retention, or constipation reported. She was on dexamethasone 16 mg/day for 5 days prior to transfer to our hospital with no noticeable clinical improvement.

The patient was unable to stand on the first encounter. Positive findings on neurological examination revealed a muscle power of 2/5 on hip flexion, hip extension, knee flexion, foot dorsiflexion, and plantar flexion bilaterally. Hyperreflexia noted in lower extremities.

An ultrasound-guided biopsy was done at the referring hospital. Pathology was reviewed at our institute, and diagnosis of neuroblastoma was confirmed. MYCN amplification was present indicating unfavorable histology.

Upon arrival of the patient, magnetic resonance imaging (MRI) of the spine was done and indicated severe SCC at the 12th thoracic vertebra (T12) level (Figure 1).

A positron emission tomography (PET) scan was also done and revealed an $8 \times 13 \times 15$ cm, right FDG-avid suprarenal mass with an SUV uptake of 6.7.

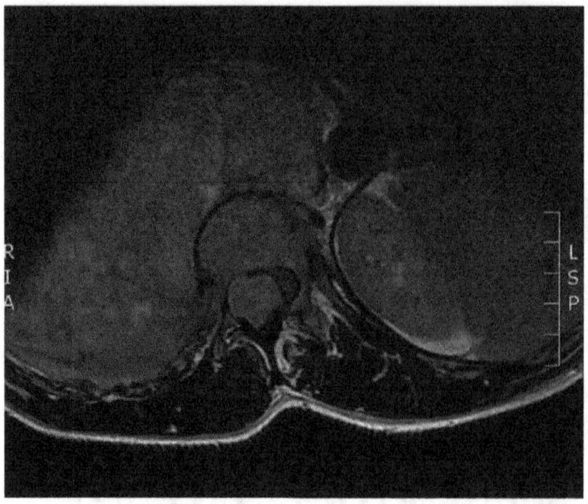

Figure 1: Severe compression of the cord with the absence of CSF around it.

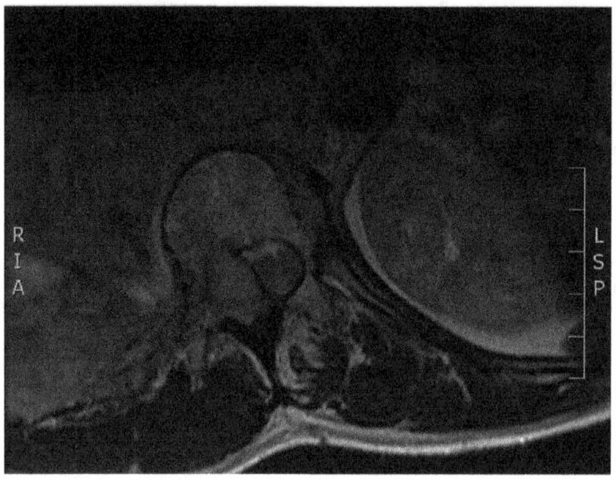

Figure 2: Image after the first cycle of chemotherapy indicating improvement in the compression with CSF present on the anterior aspect of the spinal cord.

Bone marrow biopsy was also performed and was remarkable for invasion by neuroblastoma cells.

The patient's case was discussed in a multidisciplinary fashion, and she started treatment as high-risk NBL with induction chemotherapy. The first cycle of induction chemotherapy consisted of vincristine, doxorubicin, and cyclophosphamide as per the Children's Oncology Group (COG) protocol A3973. The same dose of dexamethasone at 16 mg/day was continued.

She started noticing an improvement in her back pain 24 hours after administering chemotherapy. Neurological examination 72 hours after the first cycle of treatment showed a muscle power of 3/5 on hip flexion, hip extension, knee flexion, foot dorsiflexion, and plantar flexion bilaterally. We evaluated the patient one week after induction, and she was able to stand up and walk with assistance. The plan was to proceed as per the COG A3973 protocol which comprises vincristine, doxorubicin, and cyclophosphamide alternating with cisplatin and etoposide.

The patient continued chemotherapy treatments with further symptomatic improvement.

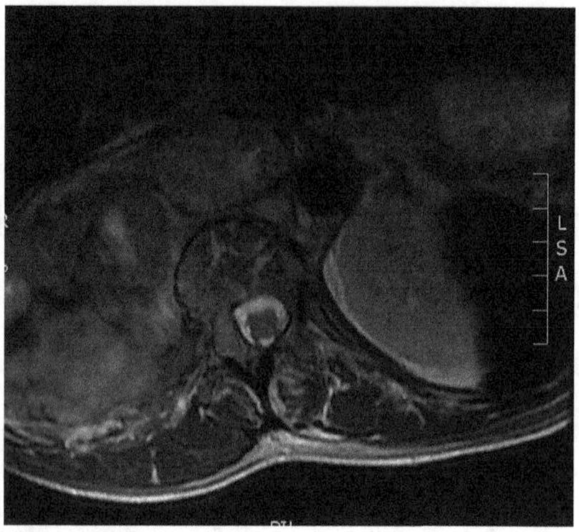

Figure 3: Complete decompression of the spinal cord with CSF surrounding it after 3 cycles of chemotherapy.

MRI thoracic spine was repeated after the first and third cycle of chemotherapy showed significant decompression of the spinal cord (Figures 2 and 3).

However, few days after cycle 6 of chemotherapy, she developed septic shock and unfortunately passed away shortly afterwards. Axial T2 cuts of thoracic spine MRI at T12 level taken 3 mm below the superior endplate of the vertebra.

3. Discussion

The term neuroblastoma (NBL) is used to refer to a spectrum of neuroblastic tumors that arise from the primitive sympathetic ganglion cells [1].

It is mainly a disease of the pediatric age group and is extremely uncommon in adults [3]. Due to the rarity of the adult NBL (aNBL), 1/10 million vs. 1/100,000 in children [4], the staging, risk assessment, and management in this age group are usually extrapolated from the pediatric literature [4]. In terms of biology, aNBL appears to be different from the pediatric counterpart. In one series of 44 adult patients, somatic mutations in *ATRX* and *ALK* were found in 58% and 42% of aNBL, respectively. Unlike our case, none of the patients harbored MYCN amplification. Treatment of high-risk neuroblastoma in the pediatric age group is intense and includes an induction chemotherapy, surgery, high-dose chemotherapy with autologous stem cell rescue, followed by radiation and biotherapy therapy with isotretinoin. More recently, targeted immune therapy with anti-GD2 monoclonal antibodies has become a standard of care in Europe and North America [5, 6]. The treatment of low and intermediate risk neuroblastomas is less intensive, and outcomes are typically better [6].

Spinal cord compression occurs approximately in 5–10% of newly diagnosed NBL patients, predominantly at the thoracic level [7]. Presenting symptoms can vary from loss of bowel and bladder control to complete paraplegia. This constitutes a neuro-oncological emergency and mandates urgent management to prevent irreversible long term deficits, especially if symptoms are of <4 weeks duration [8, 9]. The approach to such cases is debatable among physicians and varies from an institution to another. Available therapeutic options include surgery (decompressive laminectomy), chemotherapy, as well as radiation therapy. There is no clear evidence supporting the superiority of one modality over the other in terms of efficacy as evidenced by most studies [7, 9, 10]. We found two reported cases of adult patients with cord compression at presentation. Similar to our case, both patients underwent spinal cord decompression at diagnosis [11–14]. In general, it is advisable to limit surgery to patients who are progressing rapidly (within 24–72 hours), or if chemotherapy is not available, and in patients with low-grade tumors. Laminectomy and radiation therapy can be associated with a higher rate of spinal instability on the long term [10]. The use of glucocorticoids, after exclusion of lymphoma, may play a role in the improvement of early symptoms; however, it has not been shown to prevent late residual impairment [13]. In brief, treatment should be carefully tailored, taking into consideration the risk profile of the patient, as well as the factors mentioned above.

Additional Points

The case demonstrates the effectiveness of chemotherapy in treating adult neuroblastoma patients presenting with spinal cord compression.

References

[1] S. Davis, M. A. M. Rogers, and T. W. Pendergrass, "The incidence and epidemiologic characteristics of neuroblastoma in the United States," *American Journal of Epidemiology*, vol. 126, no. 6, pp. 1063–1074, 1987.

[2] R. P. Castleberry, "Biology and treatment of neuroblastoma," *Pediatric Clinics of North America*, vol. 44, no. 4, pp. 919–937, 1997.

[3] L. M. Francks, A. Bollen, R. C. Seeger, D. O. Tram, and K. K. Matthay, "Neuroblastoma in adults and adolescents: an indolent course with poor survival," *Cancer*, vol. 79, no. 10, pp. 2028–2035, 1997.

[4] H. J. Conter, V. Gopalakrishnan, V. Ravi, J. L. Ater, S. Patel, and D. M. Araujo, "Adult versus pediatric neuroblastoma: the M.D. Anderson cancer center experience," *Sarcoma*, vol. 2014, Article ID 375151, 6 pages, 2014.

[5] S. Sait and S. Modak, "Anti-GD2 immunotherapy for neuroblastoma," *Expert Review of Anticancer Therapy*, vol. 17, no. 10, pp. 889–904, 2017.

[6] N. R. Pinto, M. A. Applebaum, S. L. Volchenboum et al., "Advances in risk classification and treatment strategies for neuroblastoma," *Journal of Clinical Oncology*, vol. 33, no. 27, pp. 3008–3017, 2015.

[7] B. D. Bernardi, W. Balwierz, J. Bejent et al., "Epidural compression in neuroblastoma: diagnostic and therapeutic aspects," *Cancer Letters*, vol. 228, no. 1-2, pp. 283–299, 2005.

[8] A. Poretti and M. A. Grotzer, "Neuroblastoma with spinal cord compression: is there an emergency treatment of choice?" *Developmental Medicine & Child Neurology*, vol. 54, no. 4, pp. 297-298, 2012.

[9] M. Fawzy, M. El-Beltagy, M. E. Shafei et al., "Intraspinal neuroblastoma: treatment options and neurological outcome of spinal cord compression," *Oncology Letters*, vol. 9, no. 2, pp. 907–911, 2015.

[10] D. Plantaz, H. Rubie, J. Michon et al., "The treatment of neuroblastoma with intraspinal extension with chemotherapy followed by surgical removal of residual disease: a prospective study of 42 patients—results of the NBL 90 study of the French Society of Pediatric Oncology," *Cancer*, vol. 78, no. 2, pp. 311–319, 1996.

[11] J. I. Urios, L. R. Garceran, and T. V. Rosell, "Neuroblastoma in an adult causing spinal cord compression: report of a case and review of the literature," *Spinal Cord*, vol. 27, no. 5, pp. 394–401, 1989.

[12] G. Jost, S. Frank, N. Fischer, E. Taub, and L. Mariani, "An epidural neuroblastoma causing spinal cord compression in a 67-year-old woman," *Rare Tumors*, vol. 2, no. 2, pp. 74–77, 2010.

[13] T. Simon, B. Häberle, B. Hero, D. von Schweinitz, and F. Berthold, "Role of surgery in the treatment of patients with stage 4 neuroblastoma age 18 months or older at diagnosis," *Journal of Clinical Oncology*, vol. 31, no. 6, pp. 752–758, 2013.

[14] L. Patrick, D. B. Johnson, M. A. Thompson, V. L. Keedy, H. A. Frangoul, and K. M. Snyder, "Adult neuroblastoma complicated by increased intracranial pressure: a case report and review of the literature," *Case Reports in Oncological Medicine*, vol. 2014, Article ID 341980, 5 pages, 2014.

10

Early Aggressive Immunotherapy Improves Functional Outcome in Chronic Immune Sensory Polyradiculopathy

Jasmine Shimin Koh,[1] **James Wei Min Tung**,[2] **Genevieve Lynn Yu Tan-Yu**,[1] **and Thirugnanam Umapathi**[1]

[1]*Department of Neurology, National Neuroscience Institute, 11 Jalan Tan Tock Seng, Singapore, 308433*
[2]*Lee Kong Chian School of Medicine, Nanyang Technological University, 59 Nanyang Dr., Experimental Medicine Building, Singapore, 636921*

Correspondence should be addressed to Jasmine Shimin Koh; jasmine.koh.s.m@singhealth.com.sg

Academic Editor: Giuliana Galassi

Chronic immune sensory polyradiculopathy (CISP) is an uncommon and treatable inflammatory disorder of the proximal sensory nerve roots. Patients typically present with severe sensory ataxia, normal motor examination, unsteady gait, and normal nerve conduction studies (NCS). We describe an elderly man who presented with a two-week history of progressive numbness of both legs and recurrent falls. He had hyporeflexia, normal strength, severe proprioceptive, and vibration sense loss in both lower limbs and was unable to stand or walk because of severe sensory ataxia. The NCS and MR scan of the spine were normal. Tibial somatosensory evoked potentials revealed proximal conduction defect and localized the pathology to the lumbar sensory nerve roots proximal to the dorsal root ganglion. Cerebrospinal fluid showed cytoalbuminergic dissociation suggestive of inflammation. CISP was diagnosed; he was given aggressive immunotherapy consisting sequentially of corticosteroids with mycophenolate mofetil and three cycles of intravenous immunoglobulin after which he regained independent mobility. Unlike previous reports where patients presented months-years after symptom onset and improved after single-line immunotherapy, our patient presented fairly acutely and made dramatic improvement only after aggressive combination therapy. We urge physicians to recognize this uncommon neurologic cause of sensory ataxia where early aggressive treatment is crucial for better functional outcomes.

1. Introduction

First described by Sinnreich et al. in 2004 [1], chronic immune sensory polyradiculopathy (CISP) is an uncommon and probably underrecognized cause of peripheral sensory ataxia affecting the sensory nerve roots proximal to the dorsal root ganglion (DRG). Though some patients may have concomitant involvement of the proximal motor nerve roots and are termed chronic immune sensorimotor polyradiculopathy (CISMP) [2–5], others have disease strictly confined to the proximal sensory nerve roots. Publications related to CISP [6–8] remain rare and limited since the entity was first described. Here, we describe a case report of an elderly man who was diagnosed with CISP and improved remarkably only after several courses of combination immunotherapy, emphasizing the importance of prompt recognition and aggressive treatment.

2. Case Presentation

In this study, we describe an 80-year-old man presented with progressive feet numbness, unsteady gait, and recurrent falls for two weeks. He did not have limb weakness and bladder or bowel disturbance. He had severely impaired lower limb position and vibration sense as well as decreased deep tendon reflexes. Strength was normal, and Babinski's sign was absent. Cerebellar and cranial nerve examinations were normal. He was unable to stand or walk due to severe sensory ataxia. Initial differential diagnoses were sensory neuronopathy, CIDP, and dorsal spinal column pathology. Nerve conduction study (NCS), syphilis and HIV serologies, serum neuronal antibodies (anti-Hu, anti-Yo, anti-Ri, anti-CRMP5, antiamphiphysin, anti-Ma, anti-Ta, anti-SOX-1, and anti-GAD65), extractable nuclear antigen antibodies, vitamin B12, folate, and copper levels were normal. A nonenhanced MR scan of the spine showed normal spinal cord structure and signal and chronic lumbar degenerative changes with osteophyte and disc bulges. This did not explain the patient's relatively acute sensory ataxia. There was no nerve root thickening, enlargement, or enhancement seen possibly related to not administering contrast for the scan. CT brain showed normal brain parenchyma and cerebellum. Somatosensory evoked potentials (SSEP) and lumbar puncture were subsequently performed. Tibial SSEP (Table 1) revealed absent responses at lumbar, subcortical, and cortical points, suggesting proximal conduction defect and localizing the pathology to the lumbar sensory nerve roots proximal to the dorsal root ganglion. Median SSEP was normal at Erb's, cervicomedullary, and cortical points. Cerebrospinal fluid (CSF) showed cytoalbuminergic dissociation (nucleated cell 2 cells/μL (reference range 0–5 cells/μL) and protein 0.93 g/L (reference range 0.10–0.40 g/L)), indicative of inflammation. Ganglioside antibodies such as GD1b seen in acute and chronic sensory neuropathy with ataxia were not available. The constellation of clinical features, normal NCS, characteristic SSEP abnormalities, and raised CSF protein prompted a diagnosis of CISP.

Four days after admission, he was given 1 g of intravenous methylprednisolone daily for five days followed by oral prednisolone 1 mg/kg. He did not improve; hence, intravenous immunoglobulins (IVIg) were added at a dose of 0.4 g/kg daily for five days. Mycophenolate mofetil was also started as a steroid-sparing agent while the prednisolone dose was slowly tapered. He made minimal improvement over several weeks and remained functionally impaired. He was treated with another two courses of monthly IVIg before significant improvement in function was observed. Modified Rankin scale (mRS) improved from 4 to 1, while Berg balance score improved from 31/56 to 44/56 (Table 2). A repeat NCS remained normal (Table 3) while tibial SSEP suggested improvement with nonlocalized slowing (Table 1). Four months after the last IVIg course, he was able to walk independently. He is maintained on mycophenolate mofetil and has been in remission since.

3. Discussion

CISP is an immune-mediated inflammation of the proximal sensory nerve roots characterized by peripheral sensory ataxia, normal motor examination, normal motor and sensory NCS, characteristic SSEP abnormalities, raised CSF protein on spinal tap, and thickened nerve roots on MR imaging [1].

Initial symptoms may be asymmetric and start with paresthesia, numbness, or pain of the distal lower limbs.

Table 1: Initial and repeat tibial somatosensory evoked potentials.

	Initial		Repeat (four months after treatment)		
Waveform	Left (ms)	Right (ms)	Left (ms)	Right (ms)	Normal reference
Popliteal fossa	8.40	8.90	9.1	9.1	—
Lumbar point (N21)	Absent	Absent	Absent	Absent	<22.0
Subcortical (P31)	Absent	Absent	32.3	34.5	<31.6
Cortical (P37)	Absent	Absent	Absent	Absent	<40.2

These symptoms gradually worsen and spread proximally to the hips and upper limbs with more symmetric involvement. Duration from symptom onset to medical consult ranges from few months to 18 years [1,6–8]. Neurologic examination indicates large-fibre sensory loss and sensory gait ataxia. Muscle strength is often preserved except in CISMP where there is concomitant motor nerve root involvement [2–5].

Histologic findings of three cases from the largest series [1] diagnosed with CISP that underwent lumbar sensory rootlet biopsy showed presence of endoneurial macrophages, lack of degenerating profiles, and features of chronic demyelination and remyelination with numerous onion-bulb formations. These features support primary demyelination of proximal sensory nerve roots, similar to changes observed in the peripheral nerves of patients with CIDP suggesting that CISP may be an additional phenotype along the CIDP spectrum [8–10]. However, unlike CIDP, the distal nerve segments are spared in CISP, as evidenced by normal NCS. Characteristic SSEP abnormalities include absent or delayed proximal lumbar/cervical responses, while the contrast-enhanced MR scan of the spine could show thickened enhancing nerve roots. Spinal tap typically shows cytoalbuminergic dissociation [1, 6–8].

Through this case, we would like to raise awareness of this treatable immune-mediated condition among physicians and caution against wrongly attributing the sensory ataxia and unsteady gait to a functional gait disorder especially when routine NCS and spine imaging are normal. Prompt recognition in addition to specific evaluation with SSEP, spinal tap, and contrast-enhanced MR scan of the spinal nerve roots will help clinch the diagnosis.

In addition, we emphasize the importance of early and aggressive immunotherapy. The immunopathology in CISP is at the central processes of the spinal sensory nerve roots, proximal to the dorsal root ganglion. Nerve regeneration here is likely to be less robust because of the need to form connections with the central nervous system [11], possibly inhibited by factors such as Nogo-A [12]. Other pathologies at this site, e.g., traumatic nerve root avulsion, likewise have poor regenerative prognosis. Although there are currently no randomized trials to guide treatment in CISP owing to its rarity, we believe the importance of aggressive and early immunotherapy in CISP before Wallerian degeneration is advanced in the spinal

Table 2: Functional scores in relation to time course and treatment.

	On admission	1.5 weeks	5 weeks	2.5 months	4 months	7 months
Immunosuppressant		Corticosteroids and mycophenolate mofetil				
Intravenous immunoglobulins (IVIg)	—	1st IVIg	2nd IVIg	3rd IVIg	—	—
Modified Rankin scale (mRS)	4	4	4	4	1	0
Berg balance score	Not assessed	31/56	34/56	39/56	44/56	Not assessed

Table 3: Initial and repeat (performed 4 months apart) nerve conduction study parameters.

Sensory nerve conduction						
	Right median nerve (antidromic)			Right ulnar nerve (antidromic)		
	Initial	Repeat	Normal limit*	Initial	Repeat	Normal limit*
Peak latency (ms)	3.6	3.2	<3.9	3.0	3.0	<3.0
Amplitude (μV)	35	26	>14	20	23	>9.0
Velocity (m/s)	50	55	>50	50	51	>50
	Right sural (antidromic)					
	Initial	Repeat	Normal limit*			
Peak latency (ms)	3.8	3.7	<4.5			
Amplitude (μV)	7	8	>7.0			
Velocity (m/s)	48	49	>40			
Motor nerve conduction^						
	Right median nerve (antidromic)			Right ulnar nerve (antidromic)		
	Initial	Repeat	Normal limit*	Initial	Repeat	Normal limit*
Distal latency (ms)	3.7	—	<4.5	2.9	—	<3.0
Amplitudes (mV) (distal/proximal)	7.7/6.6#	—	>5.5	11.1/9.5#	—	>7.0
Velocity (m/s)	50	—	>50	56	—	>50
F-wave latency (ms)	26.2	—	22–32	27.4	—	21–29
	Right tibial nerve (antidromic)					
	Initial	Repeat	Normal limit*			
Distal latency (ms)	4.6	—	<4.6			
Amplitudes (mV) (distal/proximal)	8.7/7.9#	—	>5.0			
Velocity (m/s)	40	—	>42			
F-wave latency (ms)	47.8	—	38–52			

*Normative data derived from 245 age-height matched controls; #measurements following stimulation at the wrist/antecubital fossa for median nerve, at the wrist/above elbow for ulnar nerve, and at the ankle/popliteal fossa for tibial nerve; ^repeat motor nerve conduction study was not performed as the patient had no motor deficits.

sensory nerve roots. Our patient presented early compared with other cases in the literature [1,6,7]. This and the use of combination immunotherapy which has not been described before in CISP, we believe, led to his good and complete recovery after seven months of treatment.

Finally, we suggest incorporating follow-up SSEP in addition to clinical functional scores (mRS and Berg balance scale) to gauge treatment response. Our experience corroborates with a previous report that SSEP may serve as an additional aid for modulation of immunotherapy [7].

4. Conclusion

CISP is a rare and treatable cause of peripheral sensory ataxia. Prompt recognition and early institution of aggressive combination immunotherapy improve functional outcomes.

Consent

Written informed consent was obtained from the patient.

Authors' Contributions

All authors had access to data and a role in writing the manuscript.

References

[1] M. Sinnreich, C. J. Klein, J. R. Daube, J. Engelstad, R. J. Spinner, and P. J. B. Dyck, "Chronic immune sensory polyradiculopathy: a possibly treatable sensory ataxia," *Neurology*, vol. 63, no. 9, pp. 1662–1669, 2004.

[2] S. Khadilkar, B. Patel, K. A. Mansukhani, and S. Jaggi, "Two cases of chronic immune sensorimotor polyradiculopathy: expanding the spectrum of chronic immune polyradiculopathies," *Muscle & Nerve*, vol. 55, no. 1, pp. 135–137, 2017.

[3] T. Thammongkolchai, O. Suhaib, P. Termsarasab, Y. Li, and B. Katirji, "Chronic immune sensorimotor polyradiculopathy: report of a case series," *Muscle & Nerve*, vol. 59, no. 6, pp. 658–664, 2019.

[4] R. Rojas-Garcia, E. Gallardo, C. De La Torre, L. Sanvito, and I. Illa, "Chronic sensorimotor polyradiculopathy with antibodies to P2: an electrophysiological and immunoproteomic analysis," *Muscle and Nerve*, vol. 38, no. 1, pp. 933–938, 2008.

[5] C. M. Caporale, C. Staedler, C. Gobbi, C. L. Bassetti, and A. Uncini, "Chronic inflammatory lumbosacral polyradiculopathy: a regional variant of CIDP," *Muscle & Nerve*, vol. 44, no. 5, pp. 833–837, 2011.

[6] S. A. Trip, T. Saifee, W. Honan et al., "Chronic immune sensory polyradiculopathy with cranial and peripheral nerve involvement," *Journal of Neurology*, vol. 259, no. 6, pp. 1238–1240, 2012.

[7] A. M. Clerici, E. Nobile-Orazio, M. Mauri, F. S. Squellati, and G. G. Bono, "Utility of somatosensory evoked potentials in the assessment of response to IVIG in a long-lasting case of chronic immune sensory polyradiculopathy," *BMC Neurology*, vol. 17, no. 1, pp. 1–8, 2017.

[8] S. Khadilkar, P. Dhonde, and S. Deshmukh, "Chronic dysimmune neuropathies: beyond chronic demyelinating polyradiculoneuropathy," *Annals of Indian Academy of Neurology*, vol. 14, no. 2, pp. 81–92, 2011.

[9] E. K. O'Ferrall, D. Gendron, M. C. Guiot, J. Hall, and M. Sinnreich, "Lower motor neuron syndrome due to cauda equina hypertrophy with onion bulbs," *Muscle and Nerve*, vol. 48, no. 2, pp. 301–305, 2013.

[10] X. Ayrignac, K. Viala, R. M. Koutlidis et al., "Sensory chronic inflammatory demyelinating polyneuropathy: an under-recognized entity?" *Muscle & Nerve*, vol. 48, no. 5, pp. 727–732, 2013.

[11] P. K. Thomas, "Selective vulnerability of the centrifugal and centripetal axons of primary sensory neurons," *Muscle and Nerve*, vol. 5, no. 9S, pp. S117–S121, 1982.

[12] A. B. Huber and M. E. Schwab, "Nogo-A, a potent inhibitor of neurite outgrowth and regeneration," *Biological Chemistry*, vol. 381, no. 5-6, pp. 407–419, 2000.

11

A Case of Dysgraphia after Cerebellar Infarction Where Functional NIRS Guided the Task Aimed at Activating the Hypoperfused Region

Mutsumi Fujii[1] **Kazumi Tanigo**,[2] **Hirokazu Yamamoto**,[2] **Keijyu Kikugawa**,[2] **Masayuki Shirakawa**,[2] **Miki Ohgushi**,[1] **and Takaaki Chin**[3]

[1]*Department of Physical Medicine and Rehabilitation, Hyogo Rehabilitation Center, Kobe, Japan*
[2]*Department of Rehabilitation, Hyogo Rehabilitation Center, Kobe, Japan*
[3]*Hyogo Rehabilitation Center, Kobe, Japan*

Correspondence should be addressed to Mutsumi Fujii; mutsu-ygc@umin.ac.jp

Academic Editor: Dominic B. Fee

Background. Linguistic impairment following cerebellar lesions is characterized by a marked cerebellocerebral diaschisis with decreased perfusion in the left cerebral hemisphere. *Case.* We report on a 60-year-old right-handed French chef who presented with linguistic deficits following a right cerebellar infarction. Neurolinguistic examinations in the acute phase showed impaired graphomotor planning, especially for kanji (Japanese morphograms). Despite the absence of any structural damage to the supratentorial brain regions, a quantitative ^{123}I-IMP SPECT study revealed a relative hypoperfusion, mainly around the left posterior middle temporal gyrus, considered to be a crossed cerebellar-cerebral diaschisis. We performed functional near-infrared spectroscopy (fNIRS) and observed that a picture card task could increase blood perfusion in the affected area. This task was as follows: once he saw a picture card depicting a dish, the patient had to list the ingredients that make up the dish. For example, he had to name vegetables, meat, and spices upon seeing a "curry" picture card. We added this task to his daily speech-hearing therapy regimen. In the chronic phase, we confirmed symptom amelioration in linguistic performance-paralleled reduction in the level of hypoperfusion on SPECT study. *Discussion.* This case is the first report of an fNIRS approach used to evaluate evidence-based prospective speech-hearing tasks by observing blood flow to the hypoperfused area of the cerebral cortex surface.

1. Introduction

Schmahmann and Sherman introduced the concept of Cerebellar Cognitive Affective Syndrome, defining a group of deficits characterized by impairment of executive functions, difficulties with spatial cognition, personality change, and language deficits such as agrammatism and dysprosody following cerebellar damage [1]. Moreover, the recent results of neuroanatomical, clinical, and neuroimaging studies have demonstrated that the cerebellum appears to be involved in the modulation of a broad spectrum of linguistic functions such as verbal fluency, word retrieval, syntax, reading, and writing [2].

In recent years, data supporting participation of the cerebellum in language have come from a number of functional neuroimaging studies such as positron emission tomography (PET), functional magnetic resonance imaging (fMRI), and single photon emission computed tomography (SPECT). These techniques are important because they represent the only relatively noninvasive means of monitoring neuronal activity in humans by directly measuring associated changes in blood flow and oxygenation [2]. SPECT studies demonstrated a decrease in blood flow in the left cerebral hemisphere after hemorrhage or infarction mostly in the right cerebellum [3–7]. The effects of diaschisis are well known, that is, hypometabolism in otherwise unaffected brain regions functionally connected to brain areas involved by the stroke [8]. These changes in hypoperfusion provide evidence for cortical involvement in dysgraphia after cerebellum stroke. However, it is unclear whether this hypoperfused area can be activated by some other sort of stimulation instead of word generation task.

Functional near-infrared spectroscopy (fNIRS) is another useful system to observe neuronal activation especially in a clinical setting. The advantages of fNIRS are as follows: it is relatively robust with regard to subject motion, it requires relatively little time for attachment with less onerous constraints, and it can be used in a sitting position [9]. Here we report a patient who presented with writing disruption after a right cerebellar infarction considered to be a result of crossed cerebellar-cerebral diaschisis on SPECT. Then we performed fNIRS study with the patient to determine a task that can stimulate the left cerebrum hypoperfused area shown by the SPECT study, and the task was added to the daily speech and language therapy (ST). This is the first case report where ST was associated with the fNIRS approach.

2. Case

2.1. History. A 60-year-old native Japanese-speaking right-handed man, with 12 years of education, was admitted to an emergency hospital with vertigo and postural instability. He was a French chef. Apart from atrial fibrillation without medication, his medical history was unremarkable. Neurologic examination on admission showed a diplopia, dysarthria, and right cerebellar ataxia. Magnetic resonance images (MRI) on brain (GE Healthcare Japan; Sigma HDxt 1.5T) revealed a new infarction in the right cerebellar hemisphere involving cortex and the medullary core due to the obstructions of the right superior cerebellar artery and the right posterior inferior cerebellar artery (Figure 1(a)). He underwent subtentorial open decompressive craniectomy for brain edema. He was transferred to our rehabilitation hospital on day 35. Neurological assessment revealed gait ataxia and right-sided hemiataxia. The score in the simple test for evaluating hand function (STEF) that was designed to evaluate the speed of manipulating (catching, pinching, and carrying) objects (10 different shapes and sizes) using an upper limb [10] was 62 out of a maximum 100 points for the right hand. Speech was slightly dysarthric. On neurological examination, writing kanji (Japanese morphograms, originally adopted from Chinese characters) words and naming were defective, but the dysgraphia was too pronounced to be explained by hemiataxia. Although no evidence of supratentorial damage was found on MRI (General Electric Company; Sigma Excite 1.5T) (Figure 1(b)), SPECT using ^{123}I-N-isopropyl-p-iodoamphetamine (^{123}I-IMP SPECT) perfusion scans (Toshiba Medical Systems Corporation; Symbia E) on day 98 revealed lower levels of perfusion, mainly in the left posterior middle temporal gyrus, left superior and middle temporal gyrus, and right cerebellar hemisphere (the current infarct area), than those observed in normal individuals (normal database findings) (Figure 2(a)). We proposed that hypoperfusion due to crossed cerebellar-cerebral diaschisis is a cause of his poor kanji writing.

2.2. Neurolinguistic and Neurocognitive Assessments. ST was started on a daily basis, and the first in-depth neuropsychological investigations were performed 1.5 months after stroke. The language assessments of the Standard Language Test of Aphasia (SLTA), which is a formal neurolinguistic approach administered in Japanese [11], showed impaired writing, especially for kanji and verbal word fluency tests (Table 1). Articulation, repetition, oral reading, writing kana (the other type of syllabographic Japanese characters), and reading comprehension were almost normal. During a conversation, a listener was required to speculate and accordingly make a deduction in order to adequately comprehend the patient's response owing to the lack of subjects in his sentences or a frequent and abrupt change of topics. As verbal fluency tasks, we conducted category fluency tasks (semantic generation) and letter fluency tasks (phonological generation) in one minute. We regarded 15 or more word generation as normal. Results of verbal fluency tasks were moderately impaired: the number of words expressed aloud in semantic generation ("transportation" and "cooking tools") were 7 and 2, and in phonological generation (started with "Sa" and "Ra") were 4 and 6 at 4 months after the onset. Written kanji skills were also examined in more detail. In Japan, children between the ages of 6 (the 1st grade) and 12 (the 6th grade) are taught a total of 1006 kanji characters in elementary school, and the upper grade students gradually tend to learn more difficult kanji characters. The patient obtained a deficient score of 12/20 on a kanji screening writing test (that consisted of 1 or 2 kanji characters that were taught before the 5th grade) at 4 months after the onset. His dysgraphia in the poor kanji writing constituted difficulty to recall correct letters with morphological, orthographical, or semantical errors, most of which resulted in nonwords (Figure 3). He was able to copy kanji characters in both spontaneous writing and dictation and the types of writing error were the same with both right and left hands. When it comes to the kanji character that he could not write correctly, it was difficult for him to recall it even after we offered hint of some radicals (the building components of kanji) or a part of the character. He also could not explain the shape of kanji characters or the stroke order, which means his letter recognition was impaired. Neurocognitive functions were evaluated by the trail making test and Kohs block design test at 1.5, 6, and 12 months after the onset and the Wechsler adult intelligence scale-III (WAIS-III) at 6 and 12 months after the onset (Table 2). Except for an attention disorder, the patient did not reveal prefrontal cortex dysfunction such as lack of spontaneity, loss of initiative, or flattened affect.

2.3. Rehabilitation Task Evaluation Using fNIRS. Since writing kanji words and naming did not improve 4 months after the onset, we performed fNIRS study to identify a task that would be able to recruit blood flow to the hypoperfused area in the left cerebral location. fNIRS is a noninvasive functional brain mapping method that uses near-infrared light. It can measure changes in regional cerebral blood flow induced by neural activity in the cerebral cortex based on absorbance at three wavelengths (780 nm, 805 nm, and 830 nm) according to the Beer-Lambert law. To detect task-related hemoglobin signal changes, a continuous-wave NIRS

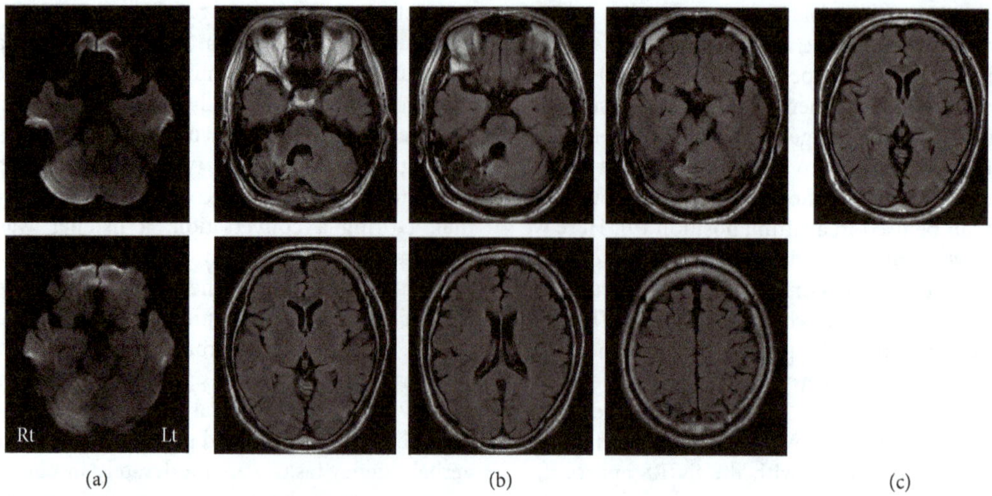

Figure 1: (a) Magnetic resonance (MR) images on day 0. Axial diffusion weighted images demonstrating a very new infarction in the right cerebellar hemisphere. Rt: right, Lt: left. (b) MR images on day 148. Axial FLAIR (fluid attenuated inversion recovery) MR images demonstrating no evidence of supratentorial damage without current infarction in the right cerebellar hemisphere. (c) A MR image 3 years after stroke onset. An axial FLAIR MR image demonstrating still no structural damage on the left posterior middle temporal gyrus.

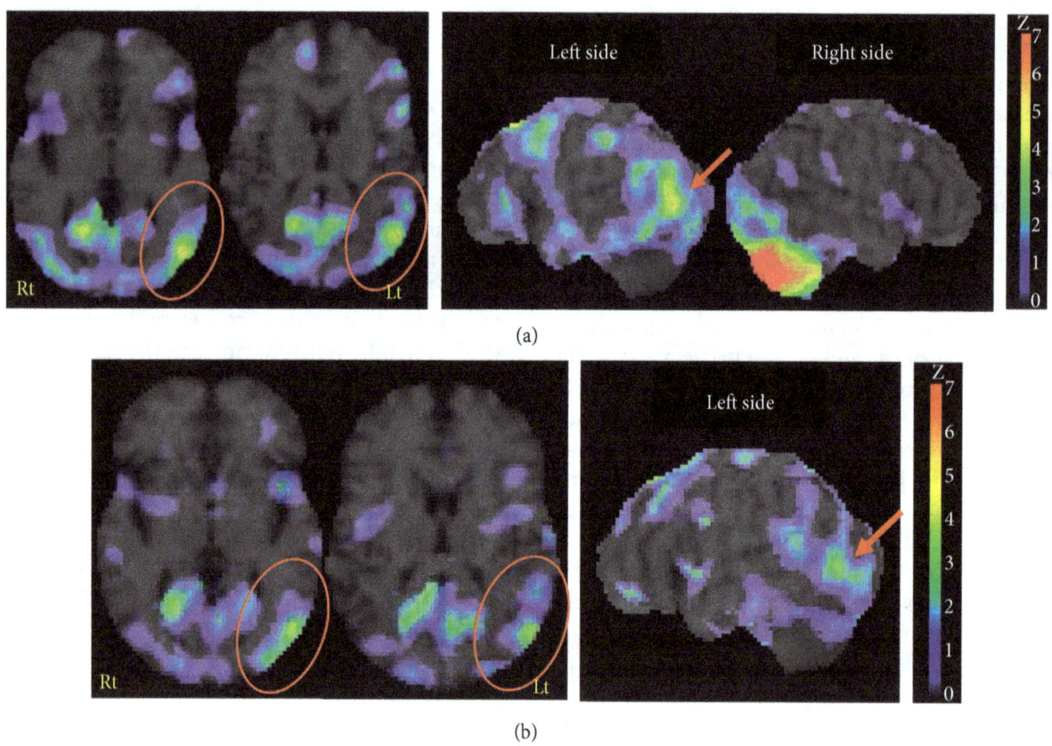

Figure 2: (a) A single photon emission computed tomography using ^{123}I-N-isopropyl-p-iodoamphetamine (^{123}I-IMP SPECT) perfusion scans on day 98. Compared with a standard normal database in perfusion findings, the *Z*-scores (SD) were calculated for each region and a regional *Z*-score of >2.0 was considered significant and indicated in green to red (compatible with the side color bar). The decreased perfusion was mainly observed in the left posterior middle frontal gyrus (pointed by red circles and arrows). (b) A following SPECT 3 years after stroke onset. The previous hypoperfusion showed an attenuation in both the area and degree on the left side view of this study.

system (SMARTNIRS, Shimadzu Corp., Kyoto, Japan) with 17 light emitter fibers and 16 light detectors was employed, and data were analyzed by LABNIRS (Shimadzu Corp., Kyoto, Japan). We determined the locations of the emitter/detector probes and measurement channels. Every channel was expected to measure the changes at the midpoint between two probes and at a depth of 20–30 mm under the scalp. We concluded that No. 10 and No. 13 channels were recording signals from the regions of interest that corresponded to the hypoperfused area in the left posterior middle temporal gyrus; this conclusion was based on a fusion map generated using an image of the patient's head

Table 1: The scores of the Japanese standard language test of aphasia (SLTA) at 1.5 months and 12 months after the onset.

Language modality	Test	Scores in 1.5 mo	Six-stage assessment on 1.5 mo						Scores in 1 yr	Six-stage assessment on 1 yr					
			6	5	4	3	2	1		6	5	4	3	2	1
Auditory comprehension	1, auditory word recognition	100	10	0	NA	0	NA	0	100	10	0	NA	0	NA	0
	2, sentence comprehension	100	10	0	NA	0	NA	0	100	8	2	NA	0	NA	0
	3, following verbal commands	90	9	0	1	0	0	0	90	9	0	1	0	0	0
	4, kana letter discrimination	100	10	0	NA	0	NA	0	100	10	0	NA	0	NA	0
Oral expression	5, object naming	90	17	1	0	0	0	2	90	18	0	0	1	0	1
	6, word repetition	100	10	0	0	0	0	0	100	10	0	0	0	0	0
	7, capability of explaining behaviors	100	8	2	0	0	0	0	100	8	2	0	0	0	0
	8, capability of explaining the content of comics	100			Stage 6				100			Stage 6			
	9, sentence repetition	80	4	0	1	0	0	0	100	5	0	0	0	0	0
	10, word fluency (listing)	73			11				87			13			
	11, reading aloud kanji words	100	5	0	0	0	0	0	100	5	0	0	0	0	0
	12, reading aloud kana letters	100	10	0	NA	NA	0	0	100	10	0	NA	NA	0	0
	13, reading aloud kana words	100	5	0	0	0	0	0	100	5	0	0	0	0	0
	14, reading aloud short sentences	100	5	0	0	0	0	0	100	4	1	0	0	0	0
Reading comprehension	15, matching written kanji word and picture	100	10	0	0	0	0	0	100	10	0	0	0	0	0
	16, matching written kana word and picture	100	9	1	0	0	0	0	100	10	0	0	0	0	0
	17, matching sentence and picture	100	7	3	NA	0	NA	0	90	9	0	NA	1	NA	0
	18, following written commands	80	6	2	1	0	0	1	90	9	0	0	1	0	0
Writing competence	19, writing kanji words	40	2	0	0	1	1	1	100	4	1	0	0	0	0
	20, writing kana words	80	1	3	0	1	0	0	100	3	2	0	0	0	0
	21, writing the story of a cartoon	60			Stage 4				80			Stage 5			
	22, dictating kana letters	100	10	0	0	0	0	0	100	10	0	0	0	0	0
	23, dictating kanji words	40	1	1	2	0	1	0	100	5	0	0	0	0	0
	24, dictating kana words	80	4	0	0	0	1	0	100	5	0	0	0	0	0
	25, dictating short sentences	100	1	4	0	0	0	0	100	5	0	0	0	0	0
Calculation	26, simple mathematical calculation	75			15				85			17			

The maximal score is 100 in every test. The score is considered 100% when the number of words reaches 15 words in "10, word fluency (listing)." Both stages 6 (perfect) and 5 (sluggish but good) in the six-stage assessment are considered "correct" in the score part, and stage 4 (a certain amount of error) to 1 (wrong answer) in the six-stage assessment are "incorrect" in the score part. The patient did not show any discontinuation over the tests. NA: not applicable.

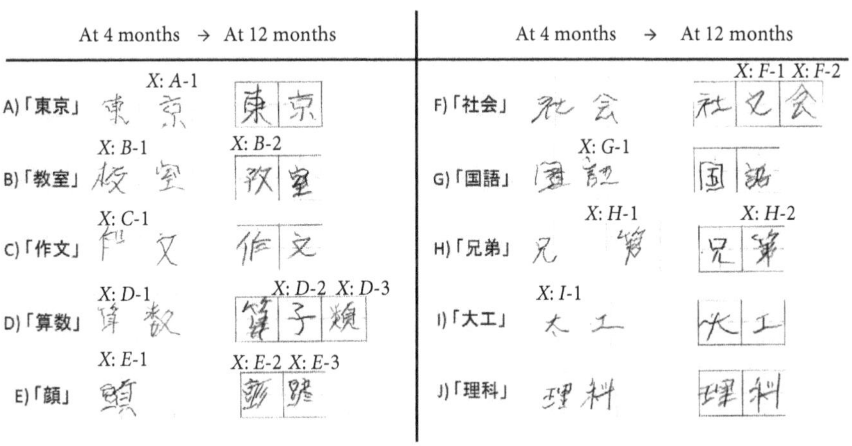

Figure 3: Samples of the patient's handwriting in the dictation ability between 4th and 12th month after onset. Kanji characters were chosen from the screening writing under the 4th grade test, (A)「東京」([Tokyo], Tokyo), (B)「教室」([kyoshitsu], classroom), (C)「作文」([sakubun], essay), (D)「算数」([sansu], mathematics), (E)「顔」([kao], face), (F)「社会」([shakai], society), (G)「国語」([kokugo], national language), (H)「兄弟」([kyodai], brother), (I)「大工」([daiku], carpenter), and (J)「理科」([rika], science). Underlined letters are kanji. Japanese pronunciation and meaning in English are noted. *X* is incorrect kanji letters. Red strokes are additional handwriting by a speech therapist. Phonologically related errors: *D*-2, *G*-1, *H*-1, and *H*-2; orthographically related errors: *A*-1, *B*-2, *C*-1, *D*-1, *D*-3, *E*-2, *E*-3, *F*-2, *F*-3, *G*-1, *H*-1, and *I*-1; semantically related errors: *B*-1 and *E*-1 (some were classified in combinations of these two types). Nonreal letters were as follows: *A*-1, *B*-2, *C*-1, *D*-1, *D*-3, *E*-2, *E*-3, *F*-3, *G*-1, and *H*-1.

Table 2: Neurocognitive functions were evaluated by the trail making test, Kohs block design test at 1.5, 6, and 12 months after the onset, and the Wechsler adult intelligence scale-III (WAIS-III) at 6 and 12 months after the onset.

Period from onset	1.5 months	6 months	12 months	Normal range
Trail making test				
Part A (sec)	125	88	91	157.6 ± 65.8
Part B (sec)	234	145	100	216.2 ± 84.7
Kohs block design test	108 (IQ115)	121 (IQ112)	128 (IQ119)	
Wechsler adult intelligence scale-III				
Total IQ (TIQ)		77	85	
Verbal IQ (VIQ)		78	82	
Performance IQ (PIQ)		80	91	
Verbal comprehension (VC)		88	92	
Perceptual organization (PO)		97	101	
Working memory (WM)		74	79	
Processing speed (PS)		66	66	

inside the fiber cap-type holder and a left-side SPECT view (Figure 4(a)). During the experiment, this holder was specifically placed for this patient so that it would position the probes at the same location every time. Channels corresponding to the left temporooccipital cortex are shown in Figure 4(b). The patient sat on a chair during the experiment. We considered the cortical oxygenated hemoglobin (oxy-Hb) signal increase as a real-time stimulatory response to a task [9]. After a long rest and the stabilization of the oxy-Hb level, we began a test. The operator ordered the patient to start the first task after 20 sec of resting. Before and after the 20 sec tasks, the patient was instructed to clear his mind and not move for 20 sec, and each 20 sec rest-task-rest cycle was repeated 5 times for averaging (Figure 4(c)).

After trying several tests such as word imaging tasks or difficult kanji recalling tasks over a few days, we finally identified a workable picture card task that could increase blood perfusion in the hypoperfused area of the left posterior middle temporal gyrus, where we presumed to be the anatomical location of pure agraphia of kanji (Figure 5) [12]. The task was as follows: upon being shown a card that pictured a dish prepared with various ingredients, the patient had to think and name the ingredients of the dish, while remaining motionless. For example, he had to name most vegetables, meat, and spices that he expected to be contained in the dish after seeing a "curry" picture card. We conducted a comparison kanji writing test between one week before and just after the first picture card naming task. These two tests were totally different but the difficulty was intentionally the same. They consisted of 1 or 2 kanji characters which were taught in 3rd and 4th grade, and each pair of the kanji characters had the same number of strokes and the same importance level based on the Japanese pedagogical wordlists. The kanji writing score improved from 5 (one week before) to 8 out of 20 points after the first card naming task. Since the task took about only 5 minutes to perform but seemed to be effective, it was incorporated into the daily ST a few times a week.

2.4. Outcome. The patient was discharged from our hospital on day 204, walking independently with a slight stagger. One year after the stroke, an overall improvement in linguistic and cognitive function was observed (Tables 1 and 2). Results on verbal fluency tasks were improved: the number of words expressed aloud in semantic generation ("transportation" and "cooking tools") were 10 and 8, and in phonological generation (started with "Sa" and "Ra") were 4 and 9. Spontaneous and dictational writing of kanji letters also resulted in a perfect recovery in the SLTA. And when we reassessed his writing kanji ability using the same kanji screening test that was previously used 4 months after the onset, the correct numbers of kanji characters improved to 14/20 (Figure 3). Since similar types of writing errors persisted, we concluded that his deficiencies in kanji writing slightly remained although he had no difficulty in dysphasia in his regular life. Follow-up MRI did not show any additional damage (Figure 1(c)) and previous hypoperfused areas were attenuated on SPECT study after 3 years (Figure 2(b)). Written informed consent was obtained from this individual participant included in the study.

3. Discussion

Here we report a case where fNIRS test was used to confirm brain blood flow changes in the hypoperfused area as a reflection of task stimulation. This area was defined by the ^{123}I-IMP SPECT study and resulted from crossed cerebellar-cerebral diaschisis. In the clinical practice, the assessment for impairment analysis of aphasia and the selection of corresponding tasks are performed by a trained speech and language therapist. This is the first report that an evidence-based task was selected by observing blood flow using fNIRS and was incorporated into the daily ST regiment of the patient.

Nine cases of dysgraphia after cerebellar hemorrhage or infarction have been reported to date (Table 3) [3–7, 13, 14]. Given the perfusion deficits in the structurally unaffected left cerebral hemisphere in most cases (including ours), crossed cerebellocerebral diaschisis has been identified as a possible pathophysiological mechanism to explain cerebellar involvement in dysgraphia. The follow-up period in most cases was 1 year or less, and it appears to be difficult to obtain a complete recovery in dysgraphia. We previously reported a patient with right cerebellar hemorrhage in kanji writing errors after as long as 7 years [14]. Her kanji dysgraphia was

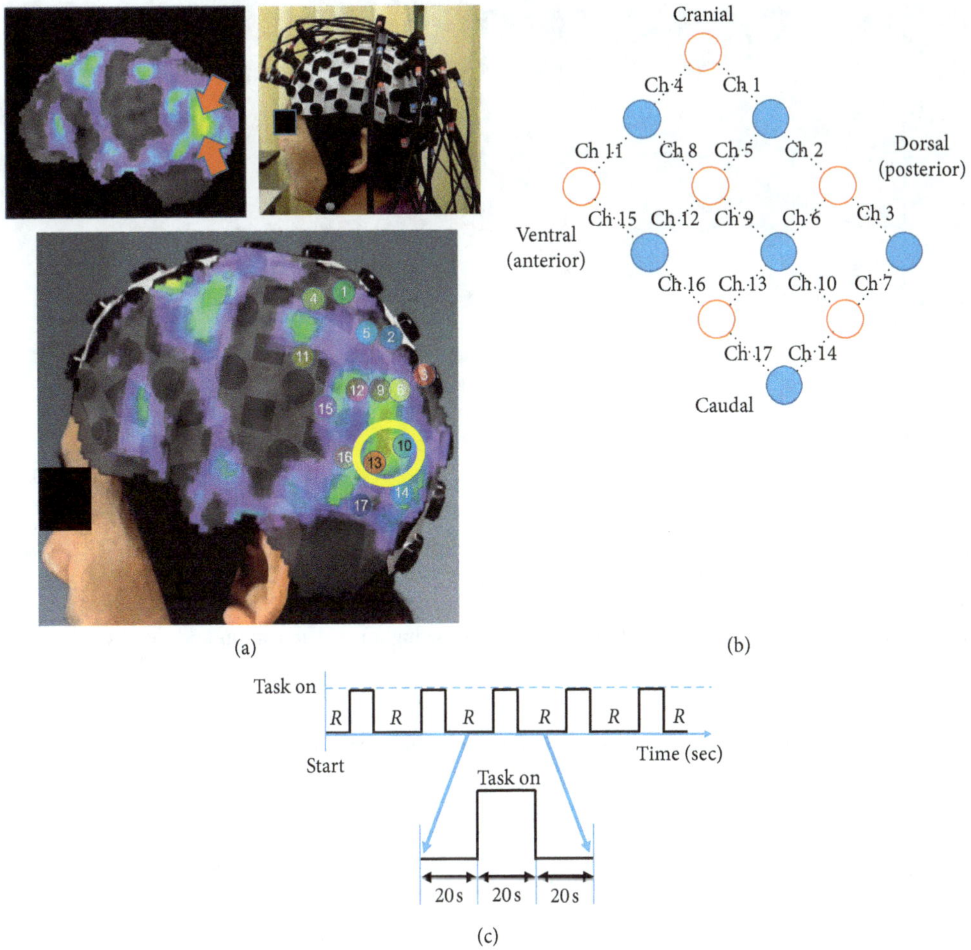

FIGURE 4: (a) Fusion map (lower photo) was comprised of left lateral side view of SPECT (upper left) and the patient's head photo in the fiber cap-type holder (upper right). The measurements were obtained from areas on both sides of the prefrontal and temporooccipital cortex (upper right). No. 10 and No. 13 channels (in a yellow circle) were considered to be receiving signals from the region of interest that corresponded to the hypoperfused area in the left posterior middle temporal gyrus. (b) Schematic figure of numbered channel arrangements that was indicated between the light detector (blue circle) and light source (red circle) on the left temporooccipital gyrus on fNIRS. (c) The procedure of tasks. The patient was instructed to empty his mind without movement for 20 sec, and then the operator prompted the patient to start a task. After a 20 sec task period, the patient was ordered to relax for another 20 sec: 5 cycles of 20 sec of rest, 20 sec of task, and 20 sec of rest were performed for averaging. For example, for the 5 times' task, we showed the patient the picture of curry, miso soup, ramen, a combination meal of rice and hamburger steak, and sukiyaki, respectively. R: rest period.

markedly improved but did not fully recover, suggesting even if no structural damage in the cerebrum can be seen after cerebellum stroke, appropriate rehabilitation therapy (including speech therapy) is essential to address the relevant symptoms.

Japanese writing system is biscriptal: it involves syllabographic kana and morphographic kanji. Every kana character has a consistent character-sound correspondence, whereas kanji characters have various degrees of character-sound correspondence. While most individual kana characters have no meaning, every kanji character conveys some meaning, even if it is not a word on its own [15]. This provides a basis for dissociation between residual ability for kana and kanji writing after stroke in Japanese patients. According to the anatomically based dual-route hypothesis for writing in response to dictation, agraphia of kanji can happen by a disruption of phonological pathways, orthographic pathways, interaction between phonology and orthography, and interaction between parietal graphemic area and frontal hand area [16]. These pathways include the primary auditory cortex (Heschl's gyri), the posterior superior temporal gyrus (Wernicke's area), the supramarginal gyrus, the angular gyrus and the adjoining lateral occipital gyri, the posterior inferior temporal cortex (Brodmann Area 37), and the posterior middle and inferior frontal gyri (Areas 44/45 and 6). Although the patient showed slight kana writing mistakes of kana writing competence at 1.5 months in SLTA (Table 1), the symptom nearly disappeared in the next few weeks and then there remained certain pure kanji dysgraphia. Sakurai et al. reported that agraphia (without alexia) for kanji arose from an isolated lesion in the left posterior middle temporal gyrus, where the visual images of words or output from the image were considered to be processed [17]. We concluded that the culprit lesion for

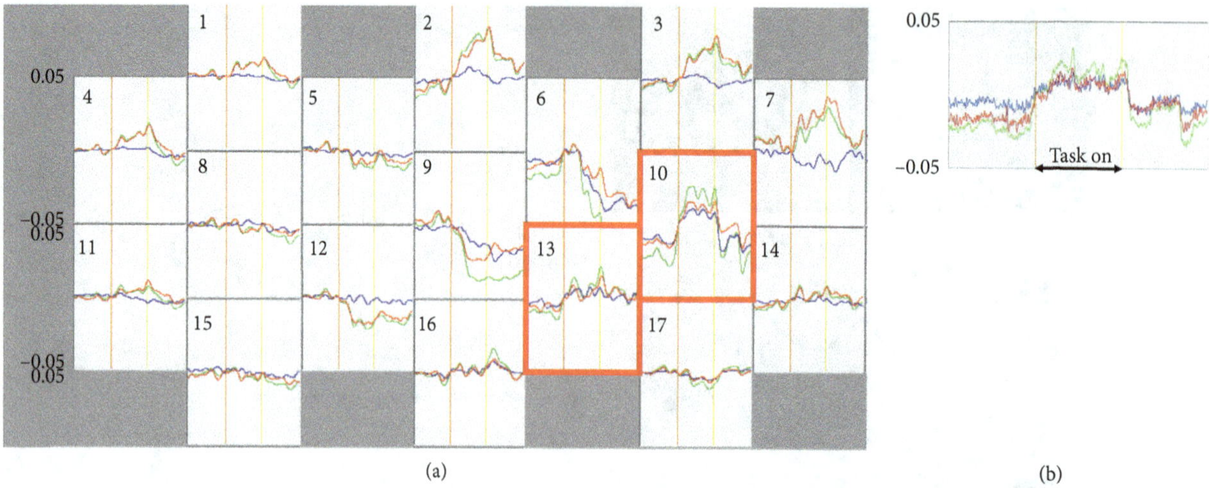

Figure 5: (a) Raw data after merging 5 continuous trials of the picture card task on fNIRS. Relative change in hemoglobin (Hb) (a.u.) is shown on the vertical axis, and a task was ongoing during the time period between the orange and yellow lines in the horizontal axis. The red, green, and blue lines indicate changes in oxy-Hb, total-Hb, and deoxy-Hb, respectively. No. 10 and No. 13 channels (surrounded by a red frame) were allocated to the region of interest according to the fusion map in Figure 4(a). (b) Group-averaged fNIRS recordings at No. 10 and No. 13 channels in response to the picture card task stimulation showing a rapid activation and deactivation corresponding to the picture task.

Table 3: Case reports of dysgraphia in patients with cerebellar stroke.

Author (year)	Age	Sex	Handedness	Lesion side	Disease	Putative mechanism	Follow-up	Outcome
Marien et al. [3]	73	Male	Right	Right	Infarction	Crossed cerebellocerebral diaschisis	1 year	Slightly amelioration of aphasic syndrome
Gasparini et al. [13]	51	Male	Right	Right	Infarction	The cerebellum's direct involvement (not showing any supratentorial abnormalities of perfusion distribution)	NA	NA
Marien et al. [4]	72	Male	Right	Right	Hemorrhage	Crossed cerebellocerebral diaschisis	6 months	Apraxic symptoms persisted in writing
Marien et al. [5]	58	Male	Right	Right	Infarction	Crossed cerebellocerebral diaschisis	4 weeks	Similar in writing to dictation
Fukunaga and Tokuda [6]	74	Male	Right	Right	Hemorrhage	Crossed cerebellocerebral diaschisis	3 months	Markedly improved
De Smet et al. [7]	74	Male	Right	Right	Hemorrhage	Crossed cerebellocerebral diaschisis	4 months	Amelioration
De Smet et al. [7]	86	Female	Right	Bilateral	Infarction	Same side hypoperfusion	6 months	Markedly improved
De Smet et al. [7]	76	Male	Right	Right	Infarction	Crossed cerebellocerebral diaschisis	NA (deceased)	NA
Fujii et al. [14]	48	Female	Right	Right	Hemorrhage	Crossed cerebellocerebral diaschisis	7 years	Markedly improved
Our case (2021)	60	Male	Right	Right	Infarction	Crossed cerebellocerebral diaschisis	1 year	Amelioration

NA: not applicable.

dysgraphia in our case should be coming from the dysfunction in the left posterior middle temporal gyrus. The region was also shown as a main hypoperfused area in the SPECT study.

Although fNIRS contains some strengths and limitations compared to other neuroimaging methods like functional magnetic resonance imaging in terms of temporal and spatial resolution, it is the most convenient and useful approach to supply blood perfusion information when the region of interest is limited to the cortical surface of the cerebrum [18]. Since the signals on the hypoperfused area in the posterior middle temporal gyrus was considered to correspond to channels No. 10 and No. 13 of fNIRS, we concentrated on their oxy-Hb signal trends during the task. First, we observed that more complicated kanji recall could increase oxy-Hb level in this region of interest (unpublished data). However, this task was too hard to administer because it loaded a substantial mental pressure for the dysgraphia patient to keep imaging increasingly difficult kanji letters. In fact, the patient did not want to deal with this task. In order to ensure that tasks can be administered on a daily basis, training tasks should avert excess effort for the patient. We had to set up alternative training task. We identified a good picture task wherein the patient looked at a card on which a type of dish consisting of various ingredients was depicted. Upon seeing the picture, the patient was requested to name food materials inside the dish. We considered the reasons behind this task being able to stimulate the left posterior middle temporal hypoperfused area. This region is thought to play a key role in both controlled aspects of semantic retrieval and the comprehension of events, relations, and actions [19]. It also supports controlled retrieval of weak conceptual combinations and associations [20]. The central role of the task is thought to be the work that we had the patient to perform when retrieving category-related objects from the picture (that is a categorically superordinate theme), after identifying the object illustrated on it. We also considered that the card task was not so hard for the patient, but sufficient to stimulate the left posterior middle temporal gyrus, in terms of the retrieval of relevant thematic associations. The patient accepted this food picture card task eagerly because he was a chef. And it is conceivable that this task could contribute to an amelioration in kanji dysgraphia as well as verbal fluency.

His writing and word fluency impairment were found to be attenuated one year after the onset. And we confirmed this improvement in linguistic performance paralleled reduction in the level of hypoperfusion. Since this attenuation had been improving even after 4 months of onset, we consider that the picture card task may make a favorable contribution to attenuate his impairment. To clarify this topic, we will have to accumulate kanji dysgraphia cases caused by the crossed cerebellar-cerebral diaschisis and evaluate rehabilitation effects in the future.

4. Conclusion

Here we report a case of linguistic deficits following a right cerebellar hemisphere infarction considered to be a result of crossed cerebellar-cerebral diaschisis. A quantified ^{123}I-IMP SPECT study revealed hypoperfusion mainly around the left posterior middle temporal gyrus, which we considered was a plausible cause of his kanji dysgraphia. fNIRS allowed us to identify a picture card task that could increase blood perfusion in the hypoperfused area, so that the task could be incorporated in the daily ST regimen of the patient. This is the first report of a plausible evidence-based task for such a diaschisis condition, which was selected by observing blood flow using fNIRS, and which might contribute to attenuate dysgraphia.

References

[1] J. D. Schmahmann and J. C. Sherman, "The cerebellar cognitive affective syndrome," *Brain*, vol. 121, no. 4, pp. 561–579, 1998.

[2] B. E. Murdoch, "The cerebellum and language: historical perspective and review," *Cortex*, vol. 46, no. 7, pp. 858–868, 2010.

[3] P. Mariën, J. Saerens, R. Nanhoe et al., "Cerebellar induced aphasia: case report of cerebellar induced prefrontal aphasic language phenomena supported by SPECT findings," *Journal of the Neurological Sciences*, vol. 144, no. 1-2, pp. 34–43, 1996.

[4] P. Mariën, J. Verhoeven, R. Brouns, L. De Witte, A. Dobbeleir, and P. P. De Deyn, "Apraxic agraphia following a right cerebellar hemorrhage," *Neurology*, vol. 69, no. 9, pp. 926–929, 2007.

[5] P. Mariën, H. Baillieux, H. J. De Smet et al., "Cognitive, linguistic and affective disturbances following a right superior cerebellar artery infarction: a case study," *Cortex*, vol. 45, no. 4, pp. 527–536, 2009.

[6] N. Fukunaga and Y. Tokuda, "A case of cerebellar cognitive affective syndrome exhibiting paragraphia," *The Japanese Journal of Rehabilitation Medicine*, vol. 48, no. 9, pp. 628–634, 2011.

[7] H. J. De Smet, S. Engelborghs, P. F. Paquier, P. P. De Deyn, and P. Mariën, "Cerebellar-induced apraxic agraphia: a review and three new cases," *Brain and Cognition*, vol. 76, no. 3, pp. 424–434, 2011.

[8] W.-J. Shih, W.-S. Huang, and P. P. Milan, "F-18 FDG PET demonstrates crossed cerebellar diaschisis 20 years after stroke," *Clinical Nuclear Medicine*, vol. 31, no. 5, pp. 259–261, 2006.

[9] M. Mihara, I. Miyai, N. Hattori et al., "Neurofeedback using real-time near-infrared spectroscopy enhances motor imagery related cortical activation," *PLoS One*, vol. 7, no. 3, Article ID e32234, 2012.

[10] K. Shindo, H. Oba, J. Hara, M. Ito, F. Hotta, and M. Liu, "Psychometric properties of the simple test for evaluating hand function in patients with stroke," *Brain Injury*, vol. 29, no. 6, pp. 772–776, 2015.

[11] Brain Function Test Committee of the Japanese Society for Higher Brain Dysfunction, *Standard Language Test for Aphasia (SLTA)*, Japanese Society for Higher Brain Dysfunction, Tokyo, Japan, 2nd edition, 2003, in Japanese.

[12] Y. Soma, M. Sugishita, K. Kitamura, S. Maruyama, and H. Imanaga, "Lexical agraphia in the Japanese language," *Brain*, vol. 112, no. 6, pp. 1549–1561, 1989.

[13] M. Gasparini, V. D. Piero, O. Ciccarelli, M. M. Cacioppo, P. Pantano, and G. L. Lenzi, "Linguistic impairment after right cerebellar stroke: a case report," *European Journal of Neurology*, vol. 6, no. 3, pp. 353–356, 1999.

[14] M. Fujii, K. Tanigo, M. Hayakawa et al., "A Case of Dysgraphia with Right Cerebellum Infarction Seven Years after Onset," Bulletin of Hyogo Social Welfare Corporation, Kobe, Japan, 2018.

[15] H. Sato, "Do different orthographies share the same mechanisms of reading? a review of research on and models for Japanese acquired dyslexia," *Aphasiology*, vol. 29, no. 10, pp. 1189–1218, 2015.

[16] Y. Sakurai, Y. Onuma, G. Nakazawa et al., "Parietal dysgraphia: characterization of abnormal writing stroke sequences,

character formation and character recall," *Behavioural Neurology*, vol. 18, no. 2, pp. 99–114, 2007.

[17] Y. Sakurai, I. Mimura, and T. Mannen, "Agraphia for kanji resulting from a left posterior middle temporal gyrus lesion," *Behavioural Neurology*, vol. 19, no. 3, pp. 93–106, 2008.

[18] V. Scarapicchia, C. Brown, C. Mayo, and J. R. Gawryluk, "Functional magnetic resonance imaging and functional near-infrared spectroscopy: insights from combined recording studies," *Frontiers in Human Neuroscience*, vol. 11, p. 419, 2017.

[19] J. Davey, H. E. Thompson, G. Hallam et al., "Exploring the role of the posterior middle temporal gyrus in semantic cognition: integration of anterior temporal lobe with executive processes," *Neuroimage*, vol. 137, pp. 165–177, 2016.

[20] H. Thompson, J. Davey, P. Hoffman et al., "Semantic control deficits impair understanding of thematic relationships more than object identity," *Neuropsychologia*, vol. 104, pp. 113–125, 2017.

12

Cerebral Sinus Thrombosis Secondary to SARS-CoV-2 Infection

Mojtaba Khazaei,[1] **Kiana Karimi**,[2,3] **Parinaz Sedighi**,[2,3] **and Salman Khazaei**[4]

[1]*Department of Neurology, Hamadan University of Medical Sciences, Hamadan, Iran*
[2]*Student Research Committee, Hamadan University of Medical Sciences, Hamadan, Iran*
[3]*Universal Scientific Education and Research Network (USERN), Tehran, Iran*
[4]*Research Center for Health Sciences, Hamadan University of Medical Sciences, Hamadan, Iran*

Correspondence should be addressed to Parinaz Sedighi; psedighi95@gmail.com

Academic Editor: Shahid Nimjee

Coronavirus disease-19 (COVID-19) is a novel infectious disease and every day we are learning more about its various clinical features and complications. Different studies during the pandemic have shown various neurological manifestations secondary to the infection such as stroke due to cerebral vessel thrombosis. Herein, we presented a 57-year-old man admitted to our hospital with gradual headache, seizure, and decreasing level of consciousness. Three weeks earlier, he was diagnosed with COVID-19 and mild to moderate respiratory problems. Decreased level of consciousness made physicians intubate the patient and initiate mechanical ventilation in the intensive care unit (ICU). Treatment was initiated with phenytoin. Brain CT scan showed right transverse sinus and cortical vein thrombosis with subarachnoid hemorrhage. He received successful anticoagulant therapy, with further improvement in oxygenation, and discharged with a good general condition. This case is important because several neurological complications of COVID-19 should be noticed and managed by appropriate treatment according to the patient's condition.

1. Introduction

Stroke is the second leading cause of death and one of the most debilitating neurological diseases [1]. Cerebral venous thrombosis is considered an important cause of ischemic stroke. The prevalence of this thrombosis in Iran is about 12 per million people, which is much higher than in European and American countries [2]. This condition used to be considered rare, but now it is one of the most common brain diseases, especially in the Middle East [3]. Symptoms vary from mild to severe headaches to focal brain symptoms and loss of consciousness. The first step in the management of this condition is to use intravenous heparin and replace it with oral warfarin after a few days, based on stroke guidelines [4]. There are several known causes for cerebral sinus thrombosis, including pregnancy, dehydration, hereditary thrombophilia, history of trauma or surgery, using oral contraceptives, vasculitis, and ulcerative colitis. Since the end of 2019, with the spread of the severe acute respiratory syndrome coronavirus-2 (SARS-CoV-2) disease, concerns about arterial and venous thrombosis and also neurological complications have increased in this viral disease [5]. Neurological complications due to COVID-19 have increased which can be related to the hyperinflammatory and hypercoagulable states of viral infection. Central nervous system (CNS) disorders include encephalopathy, encephalitis, meningitis, ischemic and hemorrhagic stroke, and venous sinus thrombosis [6]. Different mechanisms have been suggested to explain thrombosis secondary to COVID-19. One of the explanations is the hypercoagulation state, due to rises in interleukin-6 (IL-6) and C reactive protein (CRP) levels [7]. Evidence of coagulation abnormalities has been observed in some patients with COVID-19, including thrombocytosis, hyperfibrinogenemia, elevated prothrombin time (PT) and partial thromboplastin time (PTT), elevated fibrin D-dimer, and elevated von Willebrand factor levels [8]. Cardiac and peripheral arteries, as well as cerebral arteries, are at risk for thrombosis. A way to prevent thrombosis and its complications is the use of anticoagulants as prophylaxis. It is estimated that about 6% of COVID-19 patients develop cerebrovascular complications. Also, in these patients, CT scan and brain image studies strongly confirm the association of COVID-19 with stroke [9, 10]. Here, we present a 57-year-old man presenting with headache and lowering level of consciousness with a history of COVID-19 three weeks before admission, who was diagnosed with cerebral venous thrombosis and underwent successful anticoagulation therapy.

2. Case Presentation

A 57-year-old man was admitted to the emergency department of our hospital. Two days before admission, he had headache, followed by left hemiplegia. On the next day, he experienced two episodes of seizure (generalized tonic-clonic) and each one continued for five minutes and he was not conscious between the two episodes. After the seizures, the patient's consciousness remained low. On admission, the patient was unconscious and agitated. His past medical history was unremarkable for any chronic diseases including diabetes mellitus, hypertension, and ischemic heart disease. The only considerable point was the SARS-CoV-2 infection three weeks ago and his symptoms were completely recovered. He did not have a history of head trauma. He did not smoke and did not use any kind of drugs before admission. On the first visit, the Glasgow Coma Scale (GCS) was two, vital signs including blood pressure, respiratory rate, heart rate, and temperature were within normal ranges, and O_2 saturation was 87.5%. The pupils were mid-dilated and were not responsive to light. The doll's eye reflex was positive. Respiratory, abdominal, heart, and other physical examinations were unremarkable. The patient was admitted to the intensive care unit (ICU) and was intubated due to unconsciousness and agitation. Also, the first dosage of diazepam and sodium valproate was administered. Initial laboratory evaluations were performed, and the results are provided in Table 1. Midazolam, dexamethasone, phenytoin, sodium valproate, vancomycin, and meropenem were administered. On the second day of admission, the patient was auto-extubated due to agitation. O_2 saturation was 96%, so after extubation, the patient was only supported by an O_2 face mask. A brain CT scan was requested, and it revealed thrombosis in cortical veins and right transverse sinus in addition to subarachnoid hemorrhage (SAH) (Figure 1). D-Dimer test was done, and the result was 4654 ng/ml. After the diagnosis of thrombosis in brain veins, 7000 units of heparin were prescribed as a single dose, followed by infusion at 1000 units/kg, and heparin was monitored by the PTT. After achieving the therapeutic goal of heparin therapy, it was changed to warfarin after three days. The challenging point in the management of the patient was the variations in the INR (international normalized ratio) level that raised over four even with the administration of 1.25 mg of warfarin. Fortunately, there was no life-threatening bleeding. On the third day of admission, the patient's consciousness improved and the GCS was 13. The patient continued to be monitored in the ICU for five days. On the fifth day, he was transferred to the neurology ward and the second brain CT scan was requested for follow-up and it revealed parenchymal hemorrhage in the middle and posterior right temporal lobe inconsistent with the previous finding on the first scan (Figure 2). Also, magnetic resonance imaging (MRI) and

Table 1: Initial laboratory evaluations.

	Result	Unit
Hematology tests		
White blood cells (WBC)	15700	$10^3/\mu l$
Red blood cells (RBC)	5.62	$10^6/\mu l$
Hemoglobin (HB)	17.2	g/dl
Platelets (PLT)	200	$10^3/\mu l$
Erythrocyte sedimentation rate (ESR)	22	m/h
Biochemistry tests		
Blood sugar	229	mg/dl
Urea	35	mg/dl
Aspartate aminotransferase (AST)	53	mg/dl
Alanine aminotransferase (ALT)	95	mg/dl
Sodium	135	mEq/L
Potassium	4.9	mEq/L
Calcium	8.5	mg/dl
Phosphorus	2.8	mg/dl
Creatine phosphokinase (CPK)	381	U/L
Lactate dehydrogenase (LDH)	658	U/L
Creatine kinase-MB (CK-MB)	32	IU/L
Troponin	Negative	Qualitative
Immunoserology test	Result	Unit
C-reactive protein (CRP)	+++	Qualitative
Coagulation tests	Results	Unit
Prothrombin time (PT)	10	Seconds
International normalized ratio (INR)	1	—
Partial thromboplastin time (PTT)	24	Seconds
Blood gas		
pH	7.4	—
pCO_2	42.1	mmHg
pO_2	54	mmHg
HCO_3^-	26.1	mmol/L
Urine analysis and culture		
Color	Yellow	—
Appearance	Semiturbid	—
Specific gravity	1.015	—
pH	8	—
Proteins	Negative	—
Glucose	Positive	—
Ketones	Negative	—
Blood	Positive	—
Bilirubin	Negative	—
Urobilinogen	Negative	—
Bacteria	Few	—
Urine culture	No bacterial growth after 24 hours	—

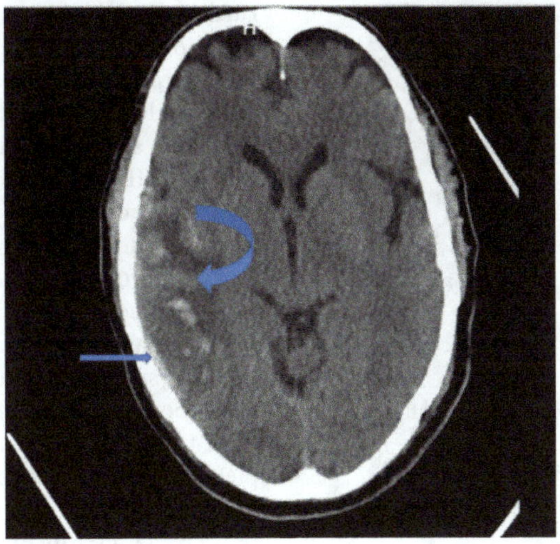

FIGURE 1: First brain CT scan showing cortical vein thrombosis (inferior anastomosis vein) (rectus arrow) with right temporal infarction in which transformation to hemorrhage occurs (curved arrow).

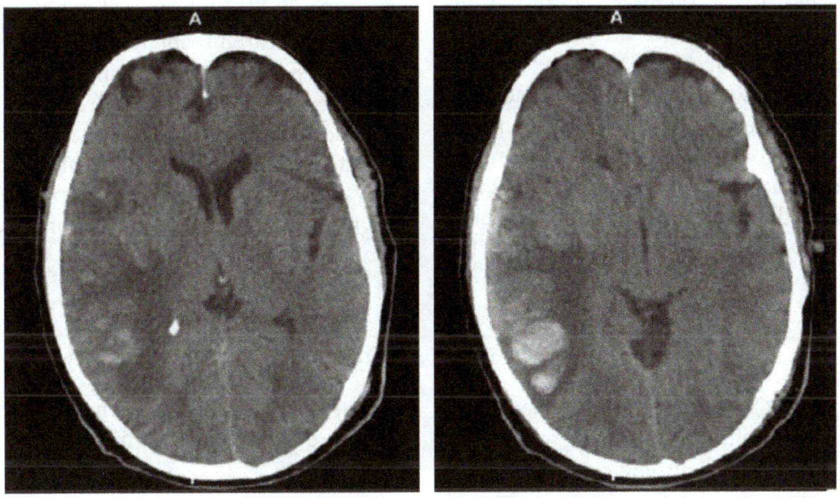

FIGURE 2: Second brain CT scan.

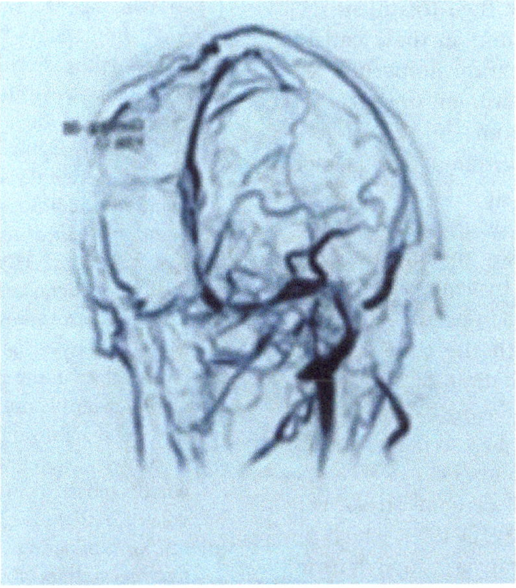

FIGURE 3: Brain MRV showing absence of right transverse sinus.

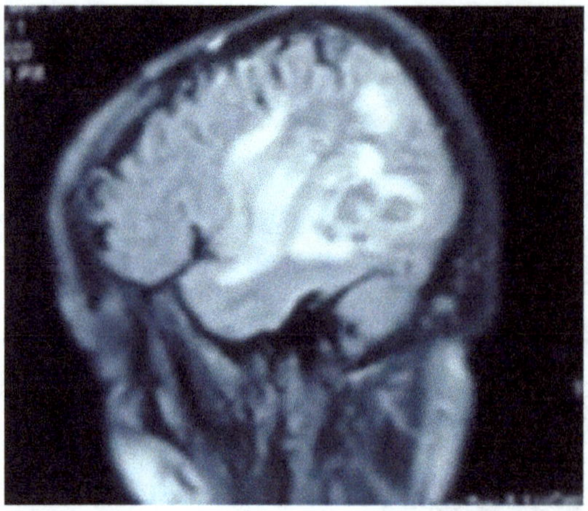

Figure 4: Brain MRI (FLAIR) in the sagittal plane showing hyperintensity in the right temporal lobe.

magnetic resonance venography (MRV) were done and confirmed the findings of CT scan (Figures 3 and 4). Additional examinations for vasculitis and thrombophilia including antiphospholipid syndrome (APS) profile, C and S protein, and factor V Leiden were all negative. Finally, the patient was discharged with a good general condition, and mild dysarthria which was completely recovered on the follow-up visit. Warfarin was changed to apixaban after two weeks due to variation in the therapeutic range of warfarin, and the patient did not present any signs of thrombosis on the follow-up visits.

3. Discussion

The outbreak of the SARS-CoV-2 infection has become a serious challenge to all healthcare settings worldwide. Various central and peripheral neurologic complications have been reported among patients with different degrees of infection severity. It is estimated that about 30% of patients who were hospitalized due to COVID-19 develop neurological complications at some point in their treatment [11]. The spectrum of neurological symptoms in these patients includes stroke, sinus thrombosis, encephalomyelitis, encephalopathy, meningitis, ageusia and anosmia, muscle injury, and the Guillain–Barre syndrome [6]. COVID-19-related ischemic strokes are more common than hemorrhagic strokes [12]. Therefore, in any patient with symptoms of stroke, it is necessary to conduct workup for COVID-19 while we are in the pandemic. Strokes are mostly due to arterial involvement and less frequent by venous thrombosis [13]. Venous strokes can be caused by sinus or cortical vein thrombosis, and in this patient, both the sinus and the cortical veins were blocked. Presentation of venous involvement can vary from a simple headache to a deep loss of consciousness, in which seizures and loss of consciousness were the main symptoms in our patient [14].

Zayet et al. reported two cases of cerebral stroke with multiple infarctions secondary to COVID-19 in which patients were under anticoagulation therapy as prophylaxis for atrial fibrillation due to the previous history of cardiovascular disease. Both cases developed alterations in consciousness and one of them presented with hemiplegia, the same manifestations as our patient, but none of them had seizures. Finally, one of the patients died, despite supportive care and anticoagulation therapy. The cases demonstrate that COVID-19-induced hypercoagulation state can be severe as it can cause thrombosis in patients even under anticoagulation therapy [15]. Also, Fara et al. reported three cases of thrombosis and stroke in patients with mild SARS-CoV-2 infection in which all of them first presented with hemiplegia. One of the patients was under anticoagulation therapy (subtherapeutic dosage) due to a history of deep vein thrombosis (DVT) two months before. Finally, all of them were treated by proper anticoagulation therapy with complete resolution of thrombosis. The three patients had mild respiratory symptoms and positive polymerase chain reaction (PCR) tests inconsistent with CNS manifestations, but in our patient, cerebral hemorrhage developed three weeks later. Hence, we can conclude that COVID-19 can have both acute and delayed-type CNS complications [16].

A considerable point about this patient is clinicians should be careful about various types of CNS (central nervous system) involvement in patients with COVID-19 and they should treat the CNS complications besides the infection. And also, the treatment plan may differ from the treatment of the same problem in individuals without SARS-CoV-2 infection. The treatment plans for CNS involvement might be modified as we get more experienced during the pandemic.

Consent

No written consent has been obtained from the patient as there are no patient identifiable data included in this case report.

References

[1] M. Khazaei, F. Ghasemian, M. Mazdeh, M. Taheri, and S. Ghafouri-Fard, "Comparison of administration of clopidogrel with aspirin versus aspirin alone in prevention of secondary stroke after transient ischemic attack," *Clinical and Translational Medicine*, vol. 8, no. 1, p. 6, 2019.

[2] A. Borhani Haghighi, N. Ashjazadeh, A. Safari, and S. Cruz-Flores, "Cerebral venous sinus thrombosis in Iran: cumulative data, shortcomings and future directions," *Iranian Red Crescent Medical Journal*, vol. 14, no. 12, pp. 805–810, 2012.

[3] K. Ghandehari, H. Akhbari, M. Shams et al., "Oral contraceptive pills consumption and cerebral venous thrombosis," *ARYA Atherosclerosis*, vol. 5, pp. 108–110, 2009.

[4] M. A. F. Fayyaz and T. Kashif, "The role of warfarin and rivaroxaban in the treatment of cerebral venous thrombosis," *Cureus*, vol. 11, no. 5, 2019.

[5] B. Shakibajahromi, A. Borhani-Haghighi, S. Haseli, and A. Mowla, "Cerebral venous sinus thrombosis might be under-diagnosed in the COVID-19 era," *eNeurologicalSci*, vol. 20, Article ID 100256, 2020.

[6] I. J. Koralnik and K. L. Tyler, "Covid -19: a global threat to the nervous system," *Annals of Neurology*, vol. 88, no. 1, pp. 1–11, 2020.

[7] A. Zakeri, A. P. Jadhav, B. A. Sullenger, and S. M. Nimjee, "Ischemic stroke in COVID-19-positive patients: an overview of SARS-CoV-2 and thrombotic mechanisms for the neurointerventionalist," *Journal of NeuroInterventional Surgery*, vol. 2020, Article ID 016794, 2020.

[8] T. E. Warkentin and S. Kaatz, "COVID-19 versus HIT hypercoagulability," *Thrombosis Research*, vol. 196, pp. 38–51, 2020.

[9] L. Mao, H. Jin, M. Wang et al., "Neurologic manifestations of hospitalized patients with coronavirus disease 2019 in Wuhan, China," *JAMA Neurology*, vol. 77, no. 6, pp. 683–690, 2020.

[10] P. Belani, J. Schefflein, S. Kihira et al., "COVID-19 is an independent risk factor for acute ischemic stroke," *American Journal of Neuroradiology*, vol. 41, no. 8, pp. 1361–1364, 2020.

[11] C. Iadecola, J. Anrather, and H. Kamel, "Effects of COVID-19 on the nervous system," *Cell*, vol. 183, no. 1, pp. 16–27, 2020.

[12] J. D. Spence, G. R. de Freitas, L. C. Pettigrew et al., "Mechanisms of stroke in COVID-19," *Cerebrovascular Diseases*, vol. 49, no. 4, pp. 451–458, 2020.

[13] C. Hui, T. Prasanna, and P. Laryssa, *Ischemic Stroke*, StatPearls Publishing, 2020.

[14] A. A. Divani, S. Andalib, M. Di Napoli et al., "Coronavirus disease 2019 and stroke: clinical manifestations and pathophysiological insights," *Journal of Stroke and Cerebrovascular Diseases*, vol. 29, no. 8, Article ID 104941, 2020.

[15] S. Zayet, T. Klopfenstein, R. Kovács, S. Stancescu, and B. Hagenkötter, "Acute cerebral stroke with multiple infarctions and COVID-19, France, 2020," *Emerging Infectious Diseases*, vol. 26, no. 9, p. 2258, 2020.

[16] M. G. Fara, L. K. Stein, M. Skliut, S. Morgello, J. T. Fifi, and M. S. Dhamoon, "Macrothrombosis and stroke in patients with mild Covid-19 infection," *Journal of Thrombosis and Haemostasis*, vol. 18, no. 8, pp. 2031–2033, 2020.

13

Presentation of Bilateral Facial Paralysis in Melkersson–Rosenthal Syndrome

Gustavo Gaitan-Quintero,[1] **Loida Camargo-Camargo**,[1] **Norman López-Velásquez**,[2] **and Miguel González**[3]

[1]*Neurology Residency Program of Sinú University, Cartagena, Colombia*
[2]*Universidad de La Costa, Barranquilla, Colombia*
[3]*Duke University, Durham, NC, USA*

Correspondence should be addressed to Gustavo Gaitan-Quintero; gustavoagaitanq@hotmail.com

Academic Editor: Peter Berlit

Introduction. Melkersson–Rosenthal syndrome (MRS) is a neuromucocutaneous disorder characterized by the following classic symptom triad: peripheral facial paralysis, orofacial edema, and scrotal or fissured tongue. It is rare, and since most of the patients are oligo- or monosymptomatic, it makes it difficult to diagnose. *Clinical Case*. We present a 26-year-old male patient with a history of sickle cell trait, untreated snoring, and left peripheral facial paralysis when he was 11 years old. This was an overall 20-day clinical profile that started with left peripheral facial paralysis, which was accompanied by moderate-intensity occipital pulsatile headaches. Additionally, the patient experienced paresthesias in the tongue and feelings of labial edema. After one week, he manifested peripheral facial paralysis on the right side. Physical examination revealed bilateral peripheral facial paralysis, mild labial edema, and a scrotal or fissured tongue. The patient received corticosteroids, which resulted in improvement of the edema and facial paralysis. *Discussion*. MRS is a rare disorder that predominantly affects women, typically starting in their 20s or 30s. The etiology is unknown. However, a multifactorial origin that involves environmental factors and a genetic predisposition has been proposed, which causes a dysfunction of the local immune system and autonomic nervous system (ANS) and an appearance of granulomatous inflammation in the lips and tongue. Facial paralysis usually appears later on; however, it can occur from its clinical debut. There are no curative treatments. Therapy is focused on modulating the patient's immune response, and relapses are frequent.

1. Introduction

Melkersson–Rosenthal syndrome (MRS) is a neuromucocutaneous disorder without a known etiology. MRS is characterized by a late onset of peripheral facial paralysis with recurring incidences, orofacial edema, and a scrotal or fissured tongue [1]. Even though MRS is rare and has a low clinical presentation of 0.08% in the general population [2], it is estimated that only 8–25% of the patients present the classic symptom triad [3], making diagnosis difficult. Most MRS patients have a monosymptomatic presentation of reoccurring labial edema, which is also predominately found in Miescher syndrome and Miescher's cheilitis granulomatosa [4]. We present a case of MRS in a male patient who came with bilateral facial paralysis and who was also diagnosed with sickle cell trait.

2. Clinical Case

The patient is a 26-year-old Afro-Colombian male with a history of sickle cell trait and left peripheral facial paralysis from when he was 11 years old. He came for a 20-day clinical profile development that started with feelings of weakness in the right half of the face, causing difficulties in palpebral closure. As a result, the patient experienced moderate-intensity occipital pulsatile headaches that radiated to the mastoid process, feelings of paresthesias in the tongue, and labial edema. The following week, he started to manifest contralateral weakness on one side of his face and the inability for palpebral closure. The physical exam showed evidence of peripheral bilateral facial paralysis, House Brackmann 2 on the left side and 3 on the right side, slight labial edema, and a scrotal or fissured tongue (Figure 1). The blood analysis was normal, expect for sickle cell trait. The cerebral MRI did not present any alternations. The patient was treated with oral prednisolone for 7 days and resulted in complete symptom improvement of his facial paralysis and labial edema.

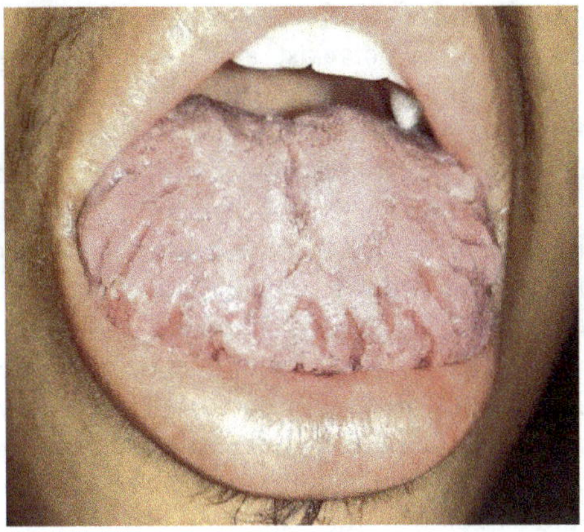

Figure 1: Slight labial edema and a scrotal or fissured tongue.

3. Discussion

Melkersson–Rosenthal syndrome (MRS) is a rare disorder described for the first time in 1929 by Ernst Gustaf Melkersson as peripheral facial paralysis and edema in the lips. In 1931, Curt Rosenthal completed the classic symptom triad by adding the presence of a scrotal or fissured tongue [1]. This syndrome predominately affects women in a 2 : 1 ratio, usually starting in their 20s or 30s, and has a range of 1–69 years of age [3, 5]. This clinical case presents a young adult Afro-Colombian male patient. Ethnic distribution for MRS has not been proven. Furthermore, more cases have been reported in the United States and Europe, which could be a misleading statistic according to some authors [6, 7].

The etiology of MRS is unknown. However, a multifactorial origin that involves environmental factors and a genetic predisposition has been proposed, which causes a dysfunction of the local immune and autonomic nervous system (ANS) [1, 8]. Multiple factors have been implicated in its pathogenesis: infectious agents and allergic reactions to a wide array of foods and dietary additives. This includes cobalt, monosodium glutamate, periodontal infections, tonsillitis, adenoidal hypertrophy, orofacial infections due to herpes type 1, and infections from influenza and mycobacteria [1, 5, 7]. There have been reports of familial occurrences that support a genetic etiology and autosomal dominant mutations in genes such as FATP1 (fatty acid transport protein) [9, 10]. The tissue damage from MRS is based on a noncaseating granulomatous inflammation in epithelial cells, Langhans multinucleated giant cells, perivascular lymphocytic infiltrate, and fibrosis [11]. The paralysis has been related to pressure due to edema that passes from the facial canal inside the temporal bone or the granulomatous infiltration from the nerve [1].

The clinical manifestations of MRS vary and are predominately monosymptomatic or oligosymptomatic (two symptoms). According to different case series, only 25–75% of patients with MRS present the classic symptom triad [3, 5]. Facial paralysis is observed in 30–90% of cases and is associated with orofacial edema that occurs in 13–50% of patients [5]. Additionally, facial paralysis is usually the last symptom to manifest, which can occur months or years after the orofacial edema [7]. However, it can develop from its clinical debut, which, almost always, is accompanied with orofacial edema or a fissured tongue [3, 7]. Characteristically, facial paralysis develops within hours or days and is always either partly or completely peripheral. Additionally, the clinical course can be monophasic or recurring, with possibilities of unilateral, bilateral, or alternating facial paralysis. As the clinical profile advances, facial paralysis can become permanent [1]. In this clinical case, the patient presented a bilateral facial paralysis. In a series of cases in China, up to 58% of patients with MRS had bilateral facial paralysis [12]. Peripheral bilateral facial paralysis is most commonly caused by trauma, Guillain–Barré syndrome, Bell's palsy, sarcoidosis, and types of neoplasticism or infectious meningitis [13].

Either in the form of facial edema, labial edema, or both, orofacial edema is present in 70–80% of patients [3, 12], making it the most common monosymptomatic presentation.

When labial edema is recurring, it is most often Miescher syndrome or Miescher's cheilitis granulomatosa [4]. The tongue alteration is present in 30–80% of cases [5] and has been described as scrotal, geographic, fissured, or plicated. It should be taken into account that the tongue alteration is present in 5% of the population, which could make it congenital in 30–80% of patients and of diagnostic value only when accompanied by the other two symptoms [7]. Other clinical neurological manifestations of MRS depend on the degree of inflammation and where structures are compromised near the facial and other cranial nerves. Different symptoms have been described, such as orolingual paresthesias, facial paresthesias, trigeminal neuralgia, weakness and atrophy in the masticatory musculature, dysgeusia, dry eye, hearing loss, vertigo, auricular pain, migraines predominately in the occipital region, lingual weakness and atrophy, anosmia, dysphagia, and diplopia [3, 7, 14–16].

MRS has been associated with other manifestations that are not neurological: lymphadenopathy, conjunctivitis, uveitis, keratitis, blepharitis, and genital lesions [1, 17, 18]. In addition, MRS has shown comorbid associations with psoriasis, tobacco use, obesity, dyslipidemia, hypertension, diabetes mellitus, migraines, gastrointestinal symptoms, psychotic episodes, and obsessive-compulsive disorder [1, 19, 20]. Some complications with the chronification of the clinical profile have been noted, such as sinusitis, candidiasis, facial sun-rash, IgA nephropathy, vitiligo, and abnormalities in thyroid hormones [5].

The diagnosis of MRS is established during clinical suspicion. There do not exist any recognized diagnostic criteria nor a definitive clinical scoring guide. Some authors suggest that the presence of the classic symptom triad of recurring peripheral facial paralysis, orofacial edema, and a scrotal or fissured tongue is sufficient for a diagnosis [2, 7]. Also, it has been proposed that there must be a minimum of two symptoms in order to establish a clinical diagnosis, requiring a biopsy in monosymptomatic cases such as with Miescher cheilitis [4, 5]. A lip biopsy helps reinforce the diagnosis by confirming a noncaseating granulomatous inflammation [2, 11]. Other differential diagnoses are primarily related to granulomatous disorders, such as Crohn's disease and sarcoidosis, that can overlap with many of the classic triad of symptoms. Furthermore, diagnoses to consider that can imitate mono- or oligosymptomatic presentations are reactions to antibodies, recurring Bell paralysis, Wegener's vasculitis, amyloidosis, and infectious agents [21]. Complimentary exams should be conducted when the clinical profile is confusing, the patient's age is unusual in relation to the start of their symptoms, they have an autoimmune history, or a lymphoproliferative disease [2].

Some exams that we recommend are glucose readings, blood count, globular sedimentation rate, bran scan, brain MRI, thorax X-ray, serum levels of the angiotensin-converting enzyme, antibodies ANA and ANCA, and thyroid tests. Other exams that are more specific to the clinical profile are a colonoscopy, HLA for inflammatory bowel syndrome, C1 inhibitor, and genetic tests [5]. Also, electrodiagnostic tests, such as auditory evoked potentials, blink reflex, electromyography, and neuroconduction of the facial nerve, can complement the study. Some findings describe a global or partial rate loss of the facial nerve branches, an increase in distal latency, and a decrease of compound muscular action potentials, which correlates with entrapment neuropathy [22].

In the current case, immunological exams performed were negative. The only exam that resulted in an abnormal reading was the sickle cell trait. In the literature, there has not been a demonstrated association between MRS, sickle cell anemia, and sickle cell trait. A biopsy of the lip was not performed due to the presence of the classic clinical *t* associated to the characteristic clinical profile.

There does not exist a curative treatment. Pharmacological therapies are focused on modulating the immune response, making corticoids the mainstay treatment. There are not any clinical trials that suggest a type of corticoid or a dosage. Using corticoid therapy has been shown to cause a 50–80% improvement in patients. The treatment plan most utilized is a full dosage of oral corticoids for a week and a gradual reduction in the second week. In the most severe cases, intravenous methylprednisolone is given [5].

In cases of persistent orofacial edema, some authors suggest the use of intralesional corticoids, such as betamethasone and triamcinolone. Additionally, antibiotics with anti-inflammatory properties, such as doxycycline and minocycline, have been used as an adjuvant therapy [23, 24]. The main indicator to implement immunosuppressors is the comorbidity of an autoimmune system disease. Some case series have shown benefits of using monoclonal antibodies adalimumab and infliximab [5]. Other alternatives used are dietary changes, avoiding possible allergenics and nutraceuticals supplements [25]. Other medications such as anti-inflammatories, steroids, and antihistamines have been utilized to improve symptoms [26]. The effectivity of the pharmacological therapies is moderate and relapses occur frequently. The prognosis for permanent damage to the facial nerve when there is recurring paralysis is poor in the majority of the cases and is even worse in patients with recurring Bell paralysis [27]. Surgical treatment is reserved for patients with recurring facial paralysis and consists in the decompression of the facial nerve by means of a mastoidectomy. One study showed that none of the patients presented a recurrence of facial paralysis and about 90% of the patients recovered to an almost normal functioning level [28].

4. Conclusions

MRS is an infrequent disorder that is characterized by the classic symptom triad of orofacial edema, facial paralysis, and a fissured tongue but more commonly is mono- or oligosymptomatic. In the absence of other clinical information that points to another diagnosis, it is suggested that a clinical diagnosis can be established when two or three symptoms of the classic symptom triad are present. Occasionally, bilateral facial paralysis can initially manifest and should be considered in the broad range of the differential diagnosis.

References

[1] A. Basman, M. Gumusok, S. Degerli, M. Kaya, and M. Toraman Alkurt, "Melkersson-rosenthal syndrome: a case report," *Journal of Istanbul University Faculty of Dentistry*, vol. 51, no. 1, pp. 42–45, 2017.

[2] M. Cancian, S. Giovannini, A. Angelini et al., "Melkersson–Rosenthal syndrome: a case report of a rare disease with overlapping features," *Allergy, Asthma & Clinical Immunology*, vol. 15, no. 1, p. 1, 2019.

[3] S. Feng, J. Yin, J. Li, Z. Song, and G. Zhao, "Melkersson-Rosenthal syndrome: a retrospective study of 44 patients," *Acta Oto-Laryngologica*, vol. 134, no. 9, pp. 977–981, 2014.

[4] W. A. Critchlow and D. Chang, "Cheilitis granulomatosa: a review," *Head and Neck Pathology*, vol. 8, no. 2, pp. 209–213, 2014.

[5] S. R. Dhawan, A. G. Saini, and P. D. Singhi, "Management strategies of Melkersson-rosenthal syndrome," *A Review*, vol. 13, p. 61, 2020.

[6] S. Aydın, S. Öztürk, A. Faraşoğlu, T. Çakıl, and S. J. S. Çoruk, "Melkersson–Rosenthal syndrome," *A Case Report*, vol. 29, no. 2, 2018.

[7] O. B. Ozgursoy, S. Karatayli Ozgursoy, O. Tulunay, O. Kemal, A. Akyol, and G. Dursun, "Melkersson-Rosenthal syndrome revisited as a misdiagnosed disease," *American Journal of Otolaryngology*, vol. 30, no. 1, pp. 33–37, 2009.

[8] E. Brożek-Mądry, W. Jaremek-Ochniak, M. Straburzyński, and A. Krzeski, "Lower lip Oedema-Melkersson-Rosenthal Syndrome or Cheilitis Granulomatosa," *New American Journal of Otolaryngology Research*, vol. 1, pp. 1-2, 2019.

[9] X. Xu, L. Guan, Y. Lv et al., "Exome sequencing identifies FATP1 mutation in Melkersson-Rosenthal syndrome," vol. 31, no. 5, Article ID e230, 2017.

[10] Y. Pei, G. M. Beaman, D. Mansfield, J. Clayton-Smith, M. Stewart, and W. G. Newman, "Clinical and genetic heterogeneity in Melkersson-rosenthal syndrome," *European Journal of Medical Genetics*, vol. 62, no. 6, Article ID 103536, 2019.

[11] S. Bohra, P. B. Kariya, S. D. Bargale, and S. Kiran, "Clinicopathological significance of Melkersson-Rosenthal syndrome," *BMJ Case Reports*, vol. 2015, 2015.

[12] J.-J. Tang, X. Shen, J.-J. Xiao, and X.-P. Wang, "Retrospective analysis of 69 patients with Melkersson-Rosenthal syndrome in mainland China," vol. 9, no. 2, pp. 3901–3908, 2016.

[13] R. A. Gaudin, N. Jowett, C. A. Banks, C. J. Knox, and T. A. Hadlock, "Bilateral facial paralysis: a 13-year experience," *Plastic and Reconstructive Surgery*, vol. 138, no. 4, pp. 879–887, 2016.

[14] W. Zeng, S. Geng, X. Niu, and J. Yuan, "Complete Melkersson–Rosenthal syndrome with multiple cranial nerve palsies," vol. 35, no. 3, pp. 272–274, 2010.

[15] M. U. Aluclu, U. Keklikci, A. Guzel, K. Unlu, and M. Tatli, "Melkersson-Rosenthal syndrome with partial oculomotor nerve palsy," *Annals of Saudi Medicine*, vol. 28, no. 2, pp. 135–137, 2008.

[16] R. Liu and S. Yu, "Melkersson-Rosenthal syndrome: a review of seven patients," *Journal of Clinical Neuroscience*, vol. 20, no. 7, pp. 993–995, 2013.

[17] Z. Chu, Y. Liu, H. Zhang, W. Zeng, and S. Geng, "Melkersson-Rosenthal syndrome with genitalia involved in a 12-year-old boy," *Annals of Dermatology*, vol. 28, no. 2, pp. 232–236, 2016.

[18] T. Ogawa, M. N. Sotto, and M. P. Hoang, "Granulomatous dermatitis and others," in *Hospital-Based Dermatopathology: An Illustrated Diagnostic Guide*, M. P. Hoang and M. A. Selim, Eds., pp. 137–198, Springer International Publishing, Cham, Switzerland, 2020.

[19] G. Shalom, L. Bodner, and S. Halevy, "Melkersson-Rosenthal Syndrome: the possible role of comorbidities in the etiopathogenesis. Giornale italiano di dermatologia e venereologia: organo ufficiale, Societa italiana di dermatologia e sifilografia," vol. 154, no. 3, pp. 347–351, 2019.

[20] F. Kayhan, F. İlik, and A. Kayhan, "Obsessive–compulsive disorder concurrent with Melkersson-Rosenthal Syndrome: a case report," *General Hospital Psychiatry*, vol. 37, no. 5, p. 497, 2015.

[21] M. K. Elias, F. J. Mateen, and C. R. Weiler, "The Melkersson–Rosenthal syndrome: a retrospective study of biopsied cases," *Journal of Neurology*, vol. 260, no. 1, pp. 138–143, 2013.

[22] A. G. Saini, N. Sankhyan, H. Padmanabh, A. Das, and P. Singhi, "Recurrent facial palsy and electrophysiological findings in oligosymptomatic Melkersson rosenthal syndrome," *The Indian Journal of Pediatrics*, vol. 83, no. 10, pp. 1188–1190, 2016.

[23] L. Oudrhiri, S. Chiheb, F. Marnissi, S. Zamiati, and H. Benchikhi, "Successful treatment of Miescher's cheilitis in Melkersson-Rosenthal syndrome with betamethasone injections and doxycycline," vol. 13, 2012.

[24] C. Bacci and M. L. Valente, "Successful treatment of cheilitis granulomatosa with intralesional injection of triamcinolone," vol. 3, no. 24, pp. 363-364, 2010.

[25] I. Espinoza, J. Navarrete, J. Benedetto, A. Borzutzky, P. Roessler, and A. J. A. Ortega-Pinto, "Orofacial granulomatosis and diet therapy: a review of the literature and two clinical cases," vol. 93, no. 1, pp. 80–85, 2018.

[26] S. Rašković, J. Bolpačić, A. Perić-Popadić, Ž. Jovicić, R. Mišković, and M. Bogić, "Clinical characteristics and treatment of Melkersson-Rosenthal syndrome: overview of six patients," vol. 68, no. 11-12, pp. 401–404, 2015.

[27] J. Wang, P. Li, X. Jin, Y. Xu, and X. J. Zhang, "Outcomes of recurrent facial palsy in Melkersson Rosenthal syndrome," *Annals of Otology, Rhinology & Laryngology*, vol. 124, no. 3, pp. 232–234, 2015.

[28] Z. Tan, Y. Zhang, W. Chen, W. Gong, J. Zhao, and X. Xu, "Recurrent facial palsy in Melkersson Rosenthal syndrome: total facial nerve decompression is effective to prevent further recurrence," *American Journal of Otolaryngology*, vol. 36, no. 3, pp. 334–337, 2015.

Two Paediatric Patients with Encephalopathy and Concurrent COVID-19 Infection: Two Sides of the Same Coin?

Katerina Vraka ,[1] Dipak Ram ,[1] Siobhan West,[1] Wei Yen Evelyn Chia,[2] Praveen Kurup ,[2] Gayathri Subramanian,[2] and Hui Jeen Tan [1]

[1]*Department of Paediatric Neurology, Rotal Manchester Children's Hospital, Manchester M13 9WL, UK*
[2]*Department of Paediatric Intensive Care Unit, Rotal Manchester Children's Hospital, Manchester M13 9WL, UK*

Correspondence should be addressed to Katerina Vraka; katerina.vraka@mft.nhs.uk

Academic Editor: Mathias Toft

There is increasing evidence that SARS-CoV-2 has neurotropic potential. We report on two paediatric patients who presented with encephalopathy during COVID-19 illness. Both patients had ADEM-like changes in their neuroimaging, negative SARS-CoV-2 RNA PCR in CSF, and paucity of PIMS-TS laboratory findings. However, the first patient was positive for serum MOG antibodies with normal CSF analysis, and the second had negative MOG antibodies but showed significant CSF lymphocytic pleocytosis. We concluded that the first case was a typical case of demyelination, which could have been triggered by different cofactors. In the second case, however, we postulated that the encephalopathic process was triggered by SARS-CoV-2, as no other cause was identified. With these two contrasting cases, we provide evidence that SARS-CoV-2-associated encephalitis can show ADEM-like changes, which can present during the postinfectious phase of COVID-19 illness. As ADEM is a relatively common type of postinfectious encephalitis in children, the distinguishing line between the two conditions of encephalitis and ADEM can be relatively fine. The development of more reliable diagnostic tools (e.g., anti-SARS-CoV-2 antibodies in CSF) might play an assisting role in the differentiation of these encephalopathic processes.

1. Introduction

Although the primary target of SARS-CoV-2 is the respiratory system, neurological manifestations have been reported in affected patients [1]. The first case of SARS-CoV-2 meningoencephalitis was reported in March 2020 with a positive specific SARS-CoV-2 RNA in the cerebrospinal fluid (CSF). Since then, there have been multiple reports of SARS-CoV-2-associated encephalitis, with only few showing viral detection in the CSF. Here, we report two contrasting cases of neuroinflammatory involvement of SARS-COV-2 infection in children with absence of any respiratory symptoms.

2. Case 1

A previously healthy 13-month-old girl presented at a local hospital with altered consciousness, seizures, and a 3-day history of fever. She had received her MMR vaccination a month prior and had a febrile illness ten days before presentation. On admission, her pupils were equal and bilaterally reactive to light; she had no cranial nerve palsies, but she had decorticate posturing and a Glasgow Coma Scale of 5. She required intubation, intravenous antibiotics, aciclovir, fluid boluses, and levetiracetam and was transferred to our Critical Care Unit. She remained ventilated for 4 days and developed hypertension, needing treatment. Due to episodes of episodic right-hand twitching, she had an EEG, which showed diffuse slow-wave background activity, in keeping with encephalopathy, but no epileptiform discharges. Nasopharyngeal (NPA) PCR was initially positive for SARS-CoV-2 and adenovirus, but only SARS-CoV-2 remained positive for the following 2 weeks. CSF analysis showed 10/mm^3 white cells, being negative for SARS-CoV-2 RNA (Table 1). CT head showed bihemispheric white matter hypodensities, posteriorly more than anteriorly, and an

Table 1: Salient laboratory findings of presented cases.

	Case 1 Acute presentation	Case 2 Acute presentation	— 50 days later
CRP (max)	13	8	—
ESR (max)	—	37	—
Coagulation	Normal	Normal	—
Fibrinogen	4	3.5	—
d-Dimer	354	859	—
Troponin	—	Normal	—
Ferritin	172	209	—
Pro-BNP (max)	83	591	—
Vitamin D	155	31	—
Serum lactate (mmol/L)	1.5	1.2	1.7
Blood cultures	Negative	Negative	—
Viral serology (IgG/IgM)	—	EBV IgG positive/IgM negative CMV IgG positive/IgM negative	—
	CMV PCR negative	—	—
SARS-CoV-2 NPA PCR	Positive for 3 weeks	Positive for 4 weeks	Negative
Other NPA PCR virology	Adenovirus positive	No	—
Mycoplasma PCR	Negative	Negative	—
MOG IgG antibodies	Positive	Negative	Negative
NMDA rec. antibodies	—	Negative	Negative
VGKC antibodies	—	—	Negative
Vasculitis screen (including C3, C4, ANA, rheumatoid factor, IgG dsDNA, MPO and PR3, and cardiolipin profile)	—	Negative	—
Immunoglobulin profile	Normal	Normal	—
CSF WCC (cells/mm^3)	10	6075	—
93% lymphocytes	5	—	—
CSF RCC (cells/mm^3)	255	25	10
CSF protein (g/dL)	0.31	0.58	0.48
CSF glucose (mmol/L)	4.7	4.8	3
CSF lactate (mmol/L)	1.4	1.9	1.7
CSF organisms	No	No	No
CSF bacterial culture	Negative	Negative	Negative
CSF virology including SARS-CoV-2 RNA	Negative	Negative	Negative
CSF oligoclonal bands (paired with serum)	Normal	—	Normal

NPA: nasopharyngeal aspirate; MOG: myelin oligodendrocyte glycoprotein; WCC: white cell count; RCC: red cell count; CSF: cerebrospinal fluid.

initial suspicion of posterior reversible encephalopathy syndrome was raised. The subsequent MRI brain, on day 4 of admission, showed bilateral widespread white matter high-signal abnormalities, including the splenium of the corpus callosum with associated diffusion restriction and high signal in the thalami and pons (Figures 1(a) and 1(b)). This was initially felt to be consistent with COVID-19 encephalopathy, especially given the presence of the splenial lesion [2, 3]. Spinal MRI was normal. However, she was treated clinically with steroids for acute disseminated encephalomyelitis (ADEM). Her serum myelin oligodendrocyte glycoprotein (MOG) antibody result was subsequently detected (Table 1). She continued to respond well to the steroid therapy. She initially presented drowsy, with poor central tone and unsafe swallow. Progressively, she became increasingly alert and her tone improved. On discharge, she was able to sit, took a few steps, clapped with songs, recognised voices, and was able to eat and drink normally. However, she was not fixing and following consistently, and after a normal ophthalmic examination, it was presumed that she had cortical visual impairment. Four months following her presentation, her vision had improved, she was walking, and she showed good developmental progress, with no further seizures on levetiracetam.

3. Case 2

A previously healthy 10-year-old girl presented at a district hospital with vomiting, lethargy, and a 2-day history of pyrexia. Six days before, she had developed ageusia, headache, and malaise, and on day 3, she had a positive NPA PCR for SARS-CoV-2. On day 9, she developed fluctuating sensorium and urinary incontinence. On day 10, she stopped speaking, mobilising, and using her right arm, showing

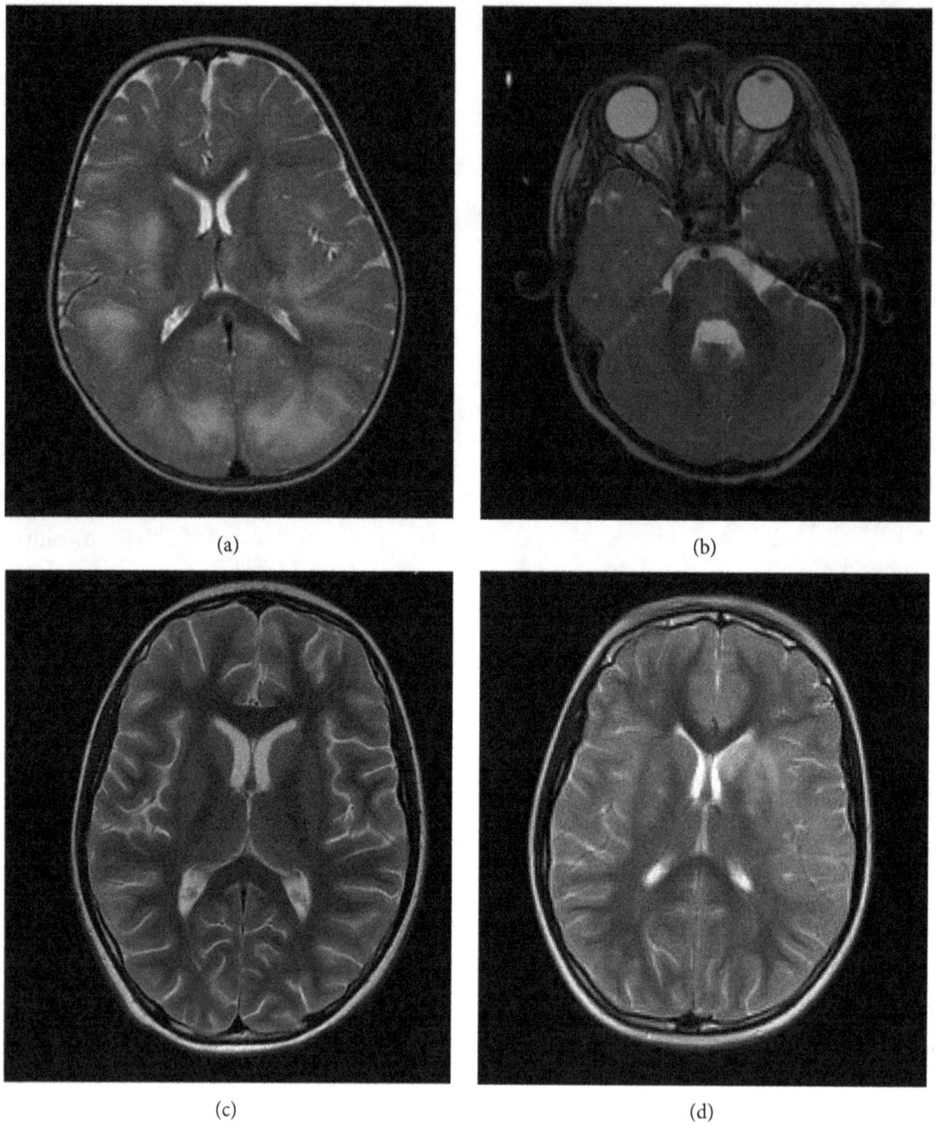

Figure 1: (a, b) MRI brain of Case 1 showing bilateral T2 hyperintensities of the subcortical white matter of all the brain and splenium of the corpus callosum with associated diffusion restriction and signal change in thalami and pons. (c) Case 2: normal MRI brain on acute presentation. (d) Repeat MRI brain 50 days later showing bilateral T2 hyperintensity of the basal ganglia and parasagittal frontal lobes, anterior limb of the left internal capsule, insula, and subcortical white matter regions.

hypertonia, brisk reflexes, right-sided Babinski, and sluggish pupils. She received intravenous aciclovir and antibiotics, had a normal CT head, and was transferred to our Critical Care Unit. On day 11, she was noted to have autonomic disturbance with hypertension and was intubated for neuroprotection for suspected raised intracranial pressure. MRI brain and spine, on day 12, were unremarkable (Figure 1(c)), but CSF analysis showed a markedly raised white cell count (WCC) of 6075/mm^3 with 93% lymphocytes and CSF protein of 0.58 g/L. CSF SARS-CoV-2 RNA test was negative. There were no clinical and laboratory findings in keeping with a diagnosis of paediatric inflammatory multisystem syndrome temporally associated with COVID-19 (PIMS-TS), i.e., absence of multisystem involvement clinically and no signs of inflammation on laboratory or radiological tests [4]. MOG, NMDA receptor, and VGKC antibodies were negative (Table 1). She was extubated on day 13 and, a week later, improved to her normal abilities apart from fatiguability and neglect of her right arm. SARS-CoV-2 NPA PCR remained positive for 30 days. She was discharged from the hospital, but due to her persistent right-arm neglect, MRI neuroaxis, lumbar puncture, EEG, and MOG antibody serology were repeated 50 days after her illness onset. Repeat MRI brain (Figure 1(d)) showed asymmetric bilateral high-signal lesions in the basal ganglia and the subcortical white matter in the frontal and temporal lobes, with involvement of the left internal capsule and left hippocampus. MRI orbits and spine, repeated CSF analysis, MOG antibodies (Table 1), and EEG were unremarkable. Two months later, she was well, with some neglect of her right upper limb, and concerned around her verbal memory, awaiting formal neurocognitive assessments.

4. Discussion

SARS-CoV-2 uses the angiotensin-converting enzyme 2 (ACE2) receptor for entry and the serine protease TMPRSS2 for S protein priming [5]. Recent studies demonstrate that SARS-CoV-2 exhibits neurotropic properties [6, 7]. A direct neuroinvasive effect of the virus could be explained by its retrograde movement along the olfactory or the peripheral lung nerves to the central nervous system (CNS) or via haematogenic migration through the CNS endothelia that express ACE2 receptors. An indirect effect can result from the leakage of inflammatory mediators through a permeable blood-brain barrier [8].

Neither of our patients, interestingly, had respiratory symptoms or signs of PIMS-TS. Case 1 had a splenial lesion, which appears to be a consistent finding in children with PIMS-TS [2]. ADEM is a rare immune-mediated demyelinating disease that can be triggered by viruses or vaccines and dominated by an encephalopathic picture. It is important to consider COVID-19 infection in children with ADEM-like illnesses, even in the absence of respiratory symptoms or signs of PIMS-TS.

The coexistence of encephalopathy, seizures, MOG antibodies, and the typical MRI findings in Case 1 supports the diagnosis of a demyelination process related to MOG antibodies. As this child had a concurrent adenovirus infection on presentation, with a recent history of MMR vaccination, it is difficult to establish whether the trigger that initiated the neuroinflammatory process was COVID-19 infection alone or a combination of these factors. The consequence of having MOG-positive antibodies is a risk of relapsing demyelination and may have different implications for long-term management.

The temporal sequence of signs of encephalopathy and neurological symptoms, in a known COVID-19 infection, along with the later MRI brain changes in Case 2, is in keeping with a neuroinflammatory process triggered by SARS-CoV-2. Lymphocytic pleocytosis (with a WCC of fewer than 100 cells/mm^3) is common in ADEM [9], but our case noted unusually high numbers. Higher cell counts have been reported in patients with PIMS-TS and encephalopathy [2]. For this reason, it was important to perform a full screen to exclude other causes.

Reported cases of COVID-19 acute encephalitis did not show such a marked pleocytosis in the CSF, and it was common to see MRI changes during the acute phase of the encephalopathic illness rather than during the recovery phase [1]. The absence of MOG antibodies, the lymphocytic pleocytosis, and the ADEM-like changes could suggest that SARS-CoV-2 may have triggered a neuroinflammatory process in this child.

The SARS-CoV-2 CSF RNA test was negative in both cases, but we acknowledge that this is not a validated test. The detection of anti-SARS-CoV-2 antibodies in CSF could support the diagnosis of patients with COVID-19 encephalitis, but this is currently unavailable in our centre [10].

In conclusion, although SARS-CoV-2 can trigger an inflammatory process mimicking ADEM, it is important to exhaust all means of investigations before labelling an encephalopathy as acute COVID-19 encephalitis.

Consent

Informed consent was obtained from the patients' parents for publication of this case report and accompanying medical image.

Acknowledgments

The authors would like to thank their neuroradiologists for their contribution in the prompt imaging and reporting of these cases.

References

[1] M. A. Ellul, L. Benjamin, B. Singh et al., "Neurological associations of COVID-19," *The Lancet Neurology*, vol. 19, no. 9, pp. 767–783, 2020.

[2] O. Abdel-Mannan, M. Eyre, U. Löbel et al., "Neurologic and radiographic findings associated with COVID-19 infection in children," *JAMA Neurology*, vol. 77, no. 11, pp. 1440–1445, 2020.

[3] C. E. Lindan, K. Mankad, D. Ram et al., "Neuroimaging manifestations in children with SARS-CoV-2 infection: a multinational, multicentre collaborative study," *Lancet Child Adolesc Health*, vol. 5, 2020.

[4] Royal College of Paediatrics and Child Health Guidance, *Paediatric Multisystem Inflammatory Syndrome Temporally Associated with COVID-19*, Royal College of Paediatrics and Child Health, London, UK, 2020, https://www.rcpch.ac.uk/sites/default/files/2020-05/COVID-19-Paediatric-multisystem-%20inflammatory%20syndrome-20200501.pdf.

[5] M. Hoffmann, H. Kleine-Weber, S. Schroeder et al., "SARS-CoV 2 cell entry depends on ACE2 and TMPRSS2 and is blocked by a clinically proven protease inhibitor," *Cell*, vol. 181, no. 2, pp. 271–280, Article ID e278, 2020.

[6] J. Meinhardt, J. Radke, C. Dittmayer et al., "Olfactory transmucosal SARS-CoV-2 invasion as a port of central nervous system entry in individuals with COVID-19," *Nature Neuroscience*, vol. 24, 2020.

[7] C. K. Bullen, H. T. Hogberg, A. Bahadirli-Talbott et al., "Infectability of human BrainSphere neurons suggests neurotropism of SARS-CoV-2," *ALTEX*, vol. 37, no. 4, pp. 665–671, 2020.

[8] Z. Zhou, H. Kang, S. Li, and X. Zhao, "Understanding the neurotropic characteristics of SARS-CoV-2: from neurological manifestations of COVID-19 to potential neurotropic mechanisms," *Journal of Neurology*, vol. 267, no. 8, pp. 2179–2184, 2020.

[9] A. C. Anilkumar, L. A. Foris, and P. Tadi, "Acute disseminated encephalomyelitis," in *StatPearls*, StatPearls Publishing LLC., Treasure Island, FL, USA, 2020.

[10] H. Alexopoulos, E. Magira, K. Bitzogli et al., "Anti-SARS-CoV-2 antibodies in the CSF, blood-brain barrier dysfunction, and neurological outcome: studies in 8 stuporous and comatose patients," *Neurol Neuroimmunol Neuroinflamm*, vol. 7, no. 6, 2020.

15

Optic Neuritis Presented as Syndrome of Inappropriate Antidiuretic Hormone Secretion in an 8 Year Old

T. G. M. Prasadani,[1] Kapila Panditha,[1] and D. Irugalbandara[2]

[1]*Pediatric Ward, District General Hospital Avissawella, Avissawella, Colombo, Sri Lanka*
[2]*Ophthalmology Unit, Lady Ridgeway Hospital for Children, Colombo, Sri Lanka*

Correspondence should be addressed to T. G. M. Prasadani; manoriprasadani@gmail.com

Academic Editor: Isabella Laura Simone

Optic neuritis is a rare demyelinating disorder, which involves the optic nerve. It can be a monophasic self-limiting illness due to postinfectious or postvaccination etiology. It can also be an initial presentation of a relapsing demyelinating disorder such as multiple sclerosis or neuromyelitis optica spectrum of disorders. It is characterized to aquaporin-4 antibody-rich areas in the brain, optic nerve, and spinal cord. The hypothalamus and periventricular area are also rich in specific antibodies and may lead to dysfunction in the hypothalamic-pituitary axis. Antidiuretic hormone (ADH) is synthesized in the hypothalamus and stored in the posterior pituitary and may secrete inappropriately due to this disturbance. This will impair water excretion from the kidney, leading to hyponatremia. When hyponatremia is significant, the patient will present with confusion, agitation, and convulsions. This case report discusses acute symptomatic hyponatremia as the initial presentation of optic neuritis due to syndrome of inappropriate ADH secretion (SIADH).

1. Introduction

Optic neuritis usually presents with eye-related symptoms. We present an 8-year-old girl, who presented with acute symptomatic hyponatremia due to SIADH. Within 12 hours, she developed acute loss of vision. Optic neuritis was confirmed with retrobulbar involvement in ophthalmologic examination and prolonged latency in visual evoked potential. MRI of the brain and optic tract was inconclusive due to the difficulty in performing postgadolinium enhancement.

The child dramatically improved with corticosteroids, but still, the left eye is having prolonged latency even after 8 weeks of the initial presentation. It could be evolving neuromyelitis optica spectrum of disorders, which may relapse later in the disease course.

2. Case History

An 8-year-old previously healthy girl presented to a base hospital in Sri Lanka, and she has had watery diarrhea for 2 days followed by several bouts of vomiting. There was a febrile proceeding upper respiratory illness in the recent past (2 weeks) noted.

There was no drug or toxin exposure to be noted.

On presentation, she developed a generalized tonic-clonic seizure, which lasted for 2 minutes. Following the convulsion, she was confused, agitated, and was difficult to control.

Her initial serum sodium was 125 mmol/l, serum osmolality was 256 mmol/l, urinary osmolality was 356 mmol/l, and urinary sodium was 55 mmol/l. Her hematocrit was normal. Serum albumin was 4.5 g/dl.

She was hemodynamically normal, and there were no features of dehydration. Her sodium was corrected with 3% NaCl 3 ml/kg as a bolus over 20 minutes followed by 0.9% NaCl maintenance. Her sodium took three days to normalize with sodium supplementation, and SIADH did not recur. Her serum electrolytes were monitored closely. She improved clinically with settlement of drowsiness, confusion, and agitation.

On first day afternoon, she lost her vision of bilateral eyes suddenly. There were no other neurological symptoms evident. Her complete neurological examination was normal, other than vision. Color vision was completely absent in both eyes (0/14). Bilateral pupillary reaction had relative afferent pupillary defect. Her visual acuity was impaired; in both eyes, it was 6/9.

Her ophthalmologic evaluation of the right and left eyes was normal as shown in Figures 1(a) and 1(b), respectively.

Her bilateral visual evoked potential was delayed. All these findings together clinically confirmed bilateral retrobulbar neuritis.

MRI of the brain, spine, and optic tracts was done, but gadolinium enhancement was not performed as her serum creatinine was high. The patient was given IV acyclovir assuming it to be meningoencephalitis initially, and the patient developed acute kidney injury secondary to acyclovir therapy.

The MRI findings of the brain (Figure 2(a)) and spine (Figure 2(b)) were normal.

Her complete blood count was normal, ESR was 61 mm/1st hour, and CRP was <5. Antinuclear antibodies (ANA) for CMV (cytomegalovirus), EBV (Epstein–Barr virus), VZV (varicella-zoster virus), and mycoplasma were negative. Rheumatoid factor was negative.

CSF full report was normal, protein level was 24 mg/dl, glucose level was 5 mg/dl, and no cells were detected. CSF HSV (herpes simplex virus) 1, 2 PCR, EBV, CMV, measles, mumps, and rubella were negative. CSF tuberculosis culture and GeneXpert study were negative. CSF oligoclonal bands were negative. Anti-aquaporin-4 antibody (AQP4-Ab) and anti-myelin oligodendrocyte antibody (MOG) were negative.

She was diagnosed with optic neuritis.

Intravenous methyl prednisolone 30 mg/kg/day was given for 3 days followed by oral prednisolone which was tapered gradually.

Her clinical symptoms improved dramatically with IV methyl prednisolone, and on day 3 of commencement, she regained her normal visual acuity. Her color vision was completely restored in one week time. Her ESR was 21/1st hour after 2 weeks.

However, the repeat visual evoked potential after 8 weeks still prolonged in the left eye and was normal in the right eye (Figure 3).

Throughout the illness up to now, she did not develop any other neurological manifestations.

3. Discussion

Optic neuritis is an acquired demyelinating disorder in the central nervous system [1, 2].

It has a postinfectious or postvaccination etiology most of the time, but it could be the first presentation of multiple sclerosis and neuromyelitis optica spectrum of disorders (NMOSD) [1–3].

It can be secondary to systemic inflammatory conditions (SLE and sarcoidosis), mitochondrial disorders (Leber hereditary optic neuropathy), toxins (etanercept), ischemia, and compressive neuropathy (primary tumors, metastasis, and tuberculoma) [1].

It is usually sudden in onset and presents as acute unilateral/bilateral blindness, color vision impairment (dyschromatopsia), impairment of unilateral/bilateral visual acuity, painful eye movements, and relative afferent pupillary defect [1, 3].

Acute hyponatremia due to syndrome of inappropriate secretion of antidiuretic hormone (SIADH) is a rare association of NMOSD and optic neuritis-associated NMOSD [4, 5].

SIADH is a disease entity where dysfunction of the hypothalamic-pituitary axis leads to excessive secretion of the antidiuretic hormone (ADH) or ADH-like substances [5].

AQP4-Ab is found in the brain throughout, but its expression is quite rich in the optic nerve and spinal cord, making patients more susceptible to develop optic neuritis and NMOSD [5].

Its expression is abundant in the hypothalamus and periventricular area also; hence, dysfunction of these brain structures can give rise to SIADH [5].

The presence of AQP4-Ab and MOG-Ab is supportive for the diagnosis of optic neuritis or evolving NMOSD, but mere absence does not disregard the diagnosis. There is an entity described as seronegative NMOSD, where the aforementioned antibodies are negative [6].

SIADH will lead to impaired water excretion. Therefore, the patient will have dilution of intravascular volume, resulting in hyponatremia. There will be an expansion of extracellular volume as a result of water retention. The kidney will attempt to excrete sodium, and urinary sodium will increase. Urine osmolality will be > 100 mosm/kg, serum osmolality will be < 280 mosm/kg, and urine sodium will be >30 mmol/l.

Since it is euvolemic hyponatremia, no features of dehydration or shock will be encountered.

In this case, it was a previously normal child presenting with symptomatic hyponatremia with generalized convulsion, confusion, and agitation, but was euvolemic.

After the correction of hyponatremia, her general condition improved, and acute visual loss developed in 12 hours. It was diagnosed to be optic neuritis, with suggestive ophthalmologic examination and VEP, but the MRI of the brain, spinal cord, and optic tracts was inconclusive without postgadolinium enhancement.

The patient improved dramatically with intravenous corticosteroids, and her subsequent serum sodium levels were also normal.

However, she still has prolonged latency of her left eye in her latest VEP (Figure 3).

It is difficult to comment at this stage whether this is monophasic optic neuritis or evolving NMOSD. She needs regular follow-up in the disease course.

There are very few published cases which discussed the association of SIADH and NMOSD. Reported pediatric cases are even rare.

This case highlights the possibility of optic neuritis or evolving NMOSD, presenting with an unusual presentation of acute symptomatic hyponatremia due to SIADH.

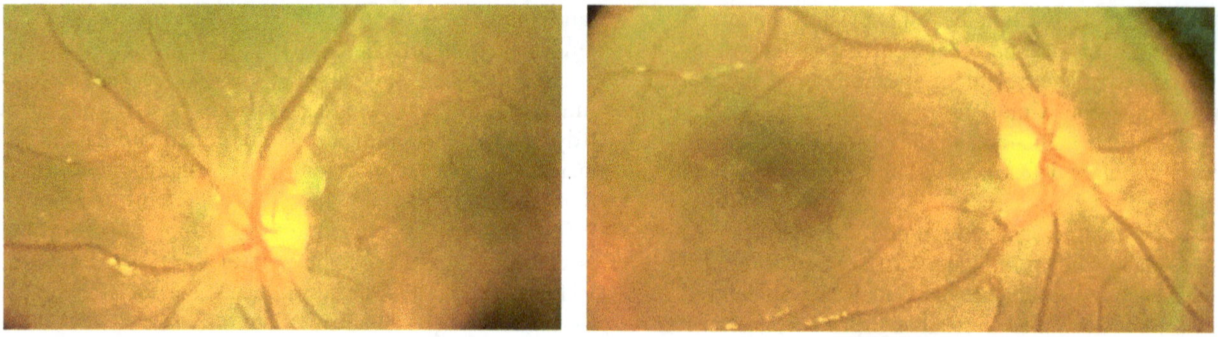

(a) (b)

FIGURE 1: Normal fundus photograph of the (a) right and (b) left eye.

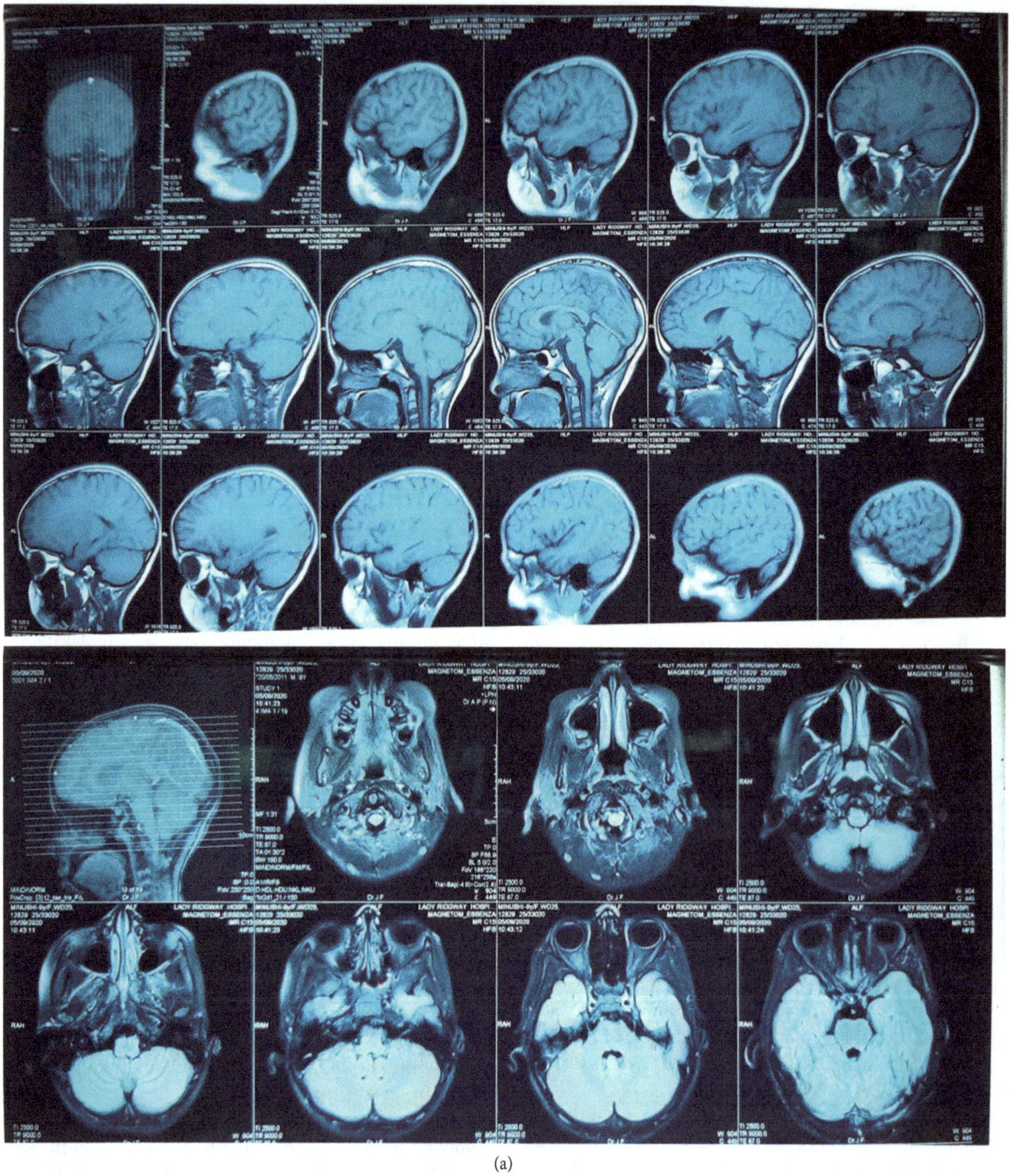

(a)

FIGURE 2: Continued.

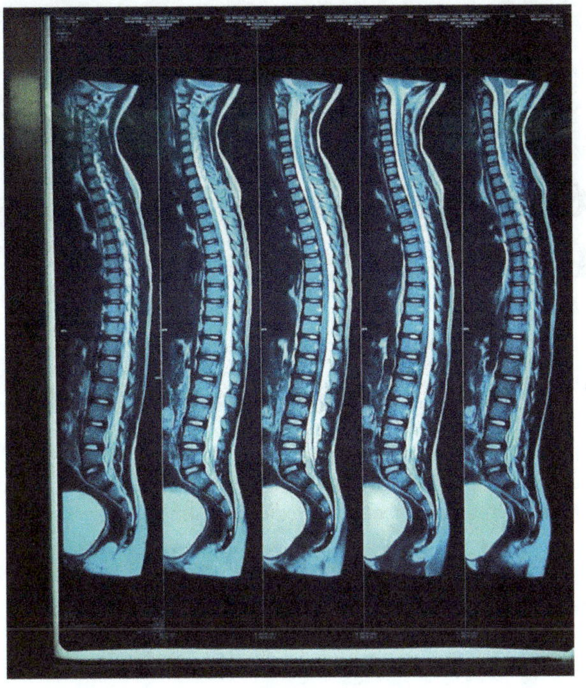

(b)

FIGURE 2: Normal MRI of the (a) brain and optic tract without gadolinium enhancement and (b) spine without postgadolinium enhancement.

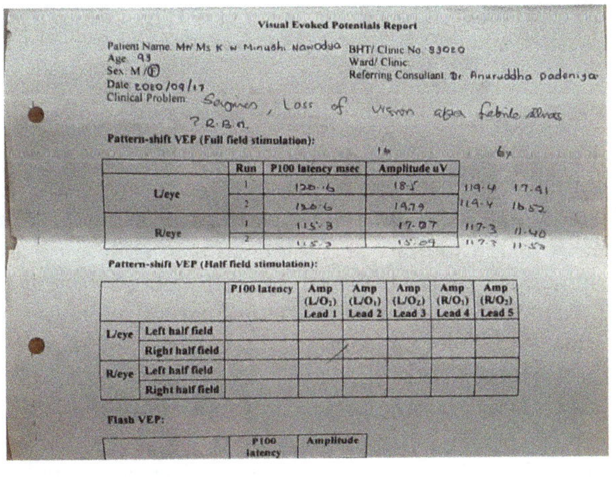

Visual Evoked Potentials Report

Patient Name: Mr/ Ms

Age:

Sex: M/F

Date:

Clinical Problem:

BHT/ Clinic No.

Ward/ Clinic

Referring Consultant

Pattern-shift VEP (Full field stimulation):

	Run	P100 latency msec	Amplitude uV
L/eye	1	120.6	18.5
	2	120.6	19.79
R/eye	1	115.8	17.07
	2	115.3	15.09

Pattern-shift VEP (Half field stimulation):

		P100 latency	Amp (L/O$_2$) Lead 1	Amp (L/O$_1$) Lead 2	Amp (L/O$_z$) Lead 3	Amp (R/O$_1$) Lead 4	Amp (R/O$_2$) Lead 5
L/eye	Left half field						
	Right half field						
R/eye	Left half field						
	Right half field						

Flash VEP:

	P100 latency	Amplitude

FIGURE 3: Visual evoked potential after 2 weeks of the acute event.

Consent

Written informed consent was obtained from the parents of the patient for publication of this case report.

Acknowledgments

The authors would like to acknowledge the neurology team of Lady Ridgeway Hospital, Colombo, Sri Lanka, for their contribution in management.

References

[1] S. M. Duignan and C. A. Hemingway, "Pediatric acquired demyelinating syndromes," *Pediatric and Child Health Journal*, vol. 29, no. 11, pp. 468–475, 2019.

[2] A. Gupta, "A case of unilateral optic neuritis in a 13 year old boy," *HSOA Journal of Ophthalmology & Clinical Research*, vol. 6, no. 2, pp. 1–4, 2019.

[3] S. Ramdas, D. Morrison, M. Absoud, and M. Lim, "Acute onset blindness: a case of optic neuritis & review of childhood optic neuritis," *BMJ Case Reports*, Article ID bcr2016214929, 2016.

[4] K. B. Holroyd, G. S. Manzano, and M. Levy, "Update on Nueromyelitis optica spectrum of disorder. Prime pubmed," *Current Opinion in Ophthalmology*, vol. 31, no. 6, pp. 462–468, 2020.

[5] H. Nakajima, Y. Fujiki, T. Ito, H. Kitaoka, and T. Takahashi, "Anti-aquaporin-4 antibody-positive neuromyelitis optica presenting with syndrome of inappropriate antidiuretic hormone secretion as an initial manifestation," *Case Reports in Neurology*, vol. 3, no. 3, pp. 263–267, 2011.

[6] S. J. Oh, C. G. Ihm, T. W. Lee et al., "Syndrome of inappropriate anti diuretic hormone secretion associated with seronegative Neuro myelitis optica spectrum disorder," *Kidney Research and Clinical Practice*, vol. 36, no. 1, pp. 100–104, 2017.

Demyelinating Changes Alike to Multiple Sclerosis: A Case Report of Rare Manifestations of COVID-19

Fatemeh Yavari,[1] **Sara Raji**,[2] **Fatemeh Moradi**,[2] **and Morteza Saeidi**[3]

[1]*Mashhad University of Medical Sciences, Mashhad, Iran*
[2]*Student Research Committee, Faculty of Medicine, Mashhad University of Medical Sciences, Mashhad, Iran*
[3]*Department of Neurology, Ghaem Hospital, Faculty of Medicine, Mashhad University of Medical Sciences, Mashhad, Iran*

Correspondence should be addressed to Sara Raji; rajis921@mums.ac.ir

Academic Editor: Tapas Kumar Banerjee

COVID-19, as a global concern and pivotal issue in the healthcare system, could have various presentations, leading to difficulty in diagnosis and management. Neuroinvasive potency, as claimed by preliminary studies, is a considerable pathogenesis. Serious neurological disorders like multiple sclerosis (MS) were out of the blue to be the first demonstration of COVID-19. This report highlights the representation of MS in a young woman, which resulted in a COVID-19 diagnosis.

1. Introduction

In the shadow of a global pandemic of COVID-19, researchers and clinicians recently identified neurological manifestations in some patients peculiarly who suffered from severe diseases and had older ages [1–5]. Regarding reports of cases with demyelinating lesions and encephalitis in the context of COVID-19, this disease might mimic known conditions such as multiple sclerosis [6]. MS is an unexpected presentation of COVID-19 which had not been reported as the first demonstration of this infection. This study aims to represent a young woman with an established diagnosis of COVID-19 appearing with multiple sclerosis manifestations.

2. Case Presentation

A former healthy 24-year-old woman with no family history of neurological problems presented to the neurology clinic complaining of sore throat, low-grade fever, and myalgia since last month. The patient displayed no respiratory symptoms, such as cough and dyspnea. Next, blurred vision and diplopia were added to her symptoms, and the severity of diplopia gradually increased within one day. Continuously, fever, sore throat, and myalgia persisted. Afterward, she developed anosmia, drooping at the corner of the left lip, paresthesia of the fingertips in both upper extremities, left eyelid drooping, and left eyebrow sagging of left facial nerve involvement. Despite the delay due to the phobia of confronting incurable diseases, she finally got the neurologist appointment.

On physical examination, the blood pressure was 110/75 mmHg, the heart rate 70 beats per minute, the temperature 37.7°C, the respiratory rate 12 breaths per minute, and the oxygen saturation 94%. The Mini-Mental State Examination (MMSE) was within the normal range. Her pupils reacted equally to the light. There was no evidence of poppy edema on fundoscopy, neither increased intracranial pressure nor meningeal irritation signs. Except for bilateral anosmia and left-sided nerve facial paresis, other cranial nerve examinations were unremarkable. The muscular strength was 5/5 in all four limbs; also, muscle tone was normal. The deep tendon reflexes and flexor plantar response were normal. We did not detect any sensory levels in the patient. Besides, there was no evidence of urinary or fecal incontinence.

Magnetic resonance imaging (MRI) was notable for multiple plaques in different brain areas with hypersignal intensity in T2 and fluid-attenuated inversion recovery (FLAIR) sequences. Subsequently, laboratory markers tests such as ANA profile (vasculitis test), tuberculin test (PPD), Coombs Wright & 2ME tests, and Venereal Disease Research Laboratory (VDRL) test were performed. Moreover, routine viral markers such as the varicella-zoster virus antibody (VZV-Ab), hepatitis B virus antigen and antibody (HBV-Ag and HBV-Ab), hepatitis C virus antibody (HCV-Ab), and human immunodeficiency virus (HIV) type 1 and type 2 antibodies, as well as human T-cell lymphotropic virus type 1 (HTLV-1) antibody, were checked which had no significant results. Also, erythrocyte sedimentation rate (ESR) was 10 mm/h.

Regarding multiple hypersignal plaques reported in MRI with the suspicion of demyelinating processes such as multiple sclerosis (MS), full-field pattern reversal visual evoked potential (PRVEP) test and brain and cervical MRI with and without gadolinium had been undertaken. The VEP did not indicate any abnormal visual pathways. The MRI again demonstrated multiple plaques with hypersignal intensity on T2-weighted and FLAIR images plus active plaques on T1 with contrast (Figure 1). According to the patient's clinical manifestations and the existence of reported plaques, the diagnosis of multiple sclerosis had been clinically suspected. Furthermore, the patient fits McDonald criteria, one clinical attack plus more than two lesions with objective clinical evidence and dissemination in time evident on MRI (appearance of active plaques in T1 with Gd and plaques in T2); hence, pulse therapy with 1 g methylprednisolone with dextrose 5% in water daily divided into two doses for four days was started. After initiating the treatment, fingertips paresthesia and facial nerve paresis improved, without any resolution of intermittent fever and anosmia. Concerning lack of improvement in myalgia, anosmia, and intermittent fever plus occasional dyspnea, as well as being in the era of COVID-19 pandemic, we retrograde re-evaluated MRI and hesitated to COVID-19. Following this, we discovered the atypical pattern of the plaques in MRI, which were larger than the routine plaques found in MS patients. In addition to common areas such as periventricular and juxtacortical, the plaques were established deeper and farther from periventricular and juxtacortical areas. Hence, a nasopharyngeal sample of the patient was taken for real-time polymerase chain reaction (RT-PCR) assay, which tested positive for SARS-CoV-2. This result prompted the lung high-resolution computed tomography (HRCT), which was notable for bilateral diffuse ground-glass opacities for SARS-CoV-2 pneumonia.

Due to the possible diagnosis of COVID-19 neurological complications, the treatment was started with azithromycin 500 mg daily (first day BID) and naproxen 500 mg BID for one week. About maintenance therapy, we decided to order a drug covering both MS and COVID-19 symptoms; thus, subcutaneous interferon-beta-1a (Resigen, continued for three months) three times a week was chosen consensually.

Furthermore, escitalopram 10 mg daily and clonazepam 0.5 mg daily were added to control the patient's anxiety. In the follow-up, the patient somewhat recovered except for an occasional nonproductive cough. After three months of therapy, we will evaluate the patient's status and take an MRI to decide appropriately for further long-term treatment.

3. Discussion

The widespread COVID-19 crisis, with its various manifestations, causes a striking burden in the health system since some patients do not represent typical symptoms and signs like fever or ground-glass opacity in CT scans [7]. Although SARS-CoV-2 mostly affects the respiratory tract, extra-respiratory involvements, including gastrointestinal, cardiac, renal, hepatic, hematological, dermatological, and neurological, can occur. Recently, plausible documents suggested the neurotropic feature of COVID-19 and its effects on the nervous system as a principal organ [3, 8, 9]. It is assumed that human coronaviruses' neurovirulence might contribute to short- and long-term neurological diseases such as encephalomyelitis and multiple sclerosis. As they longer persist in the CNS, the more long-term sequelae could develop [10]. There is mounting evidence that focused on similarities between coronaviruses and their neurotropism features, which could be applicable for SARS-CoV-2 [4]. Mindfully, to elucidate how COVID-19 acts as a neuropathogen, some authors blamed various mechanisms of neurotropism of COVID-19. The virus in blood circulation as a direct pathway might enhance the permeability of the blood-brain barrier via cytokines produced from macrophages, which promote it to penetrate the brain; however, the evidence is inadequate to prove this hypothesis.

Moreover, COVID-19 could directly invade the CNS through the olfactory tract and cause an altering sense of smell and demyelinating destruction. Indirectly, hypoxia can occur due to inflammatory exudate by virus proliferation in lung tissue cells and alveolar gas exchange, which puts patients at risk of cerebrovascular accidents. Also, COVID-19 elevates blood pressure by binding to angiotensin-converting enzyme 2 (ACE2) receptors that predispose the patients to develop ischemic stroke and cerebral hemorrhage and coagulopathic side effects. Lastly, cytokine storm syndrome, as a known consequence of COVID-19, might account for a hyperimmune response, which results in chronic inflammation and CNS damage [5, 9, 11, 12].

The most common brain lesions reported in COVID-19 patients were white matter hyperintensities on MRI and hypodensities on CT scan, specifically adjacent to ventricles. Nevertheless, a shortage of brain images on all patients might alter the results. Also, the deeper brain structures, cerebellum, and midline involvement were rarely reported [13].

Neurologic alterations in COVID-19 patients described in the literature included viral encephalitis, toxic encephalopathy, acute cerebrovascular disease, multiple sclerosis, Guillain–Barre syndrome, acute disseminated encephalomyelitis (ADEM), and peripheral nerve disease [5, 9, 12]. To clarify coronavirus's role, which may affect the autoimmune process in multiple sclerosis, some experimental studies had been done [5].

Duffy et al. believed Toll-like receptors might take part in MS pathophysiology via contributing to host defense and

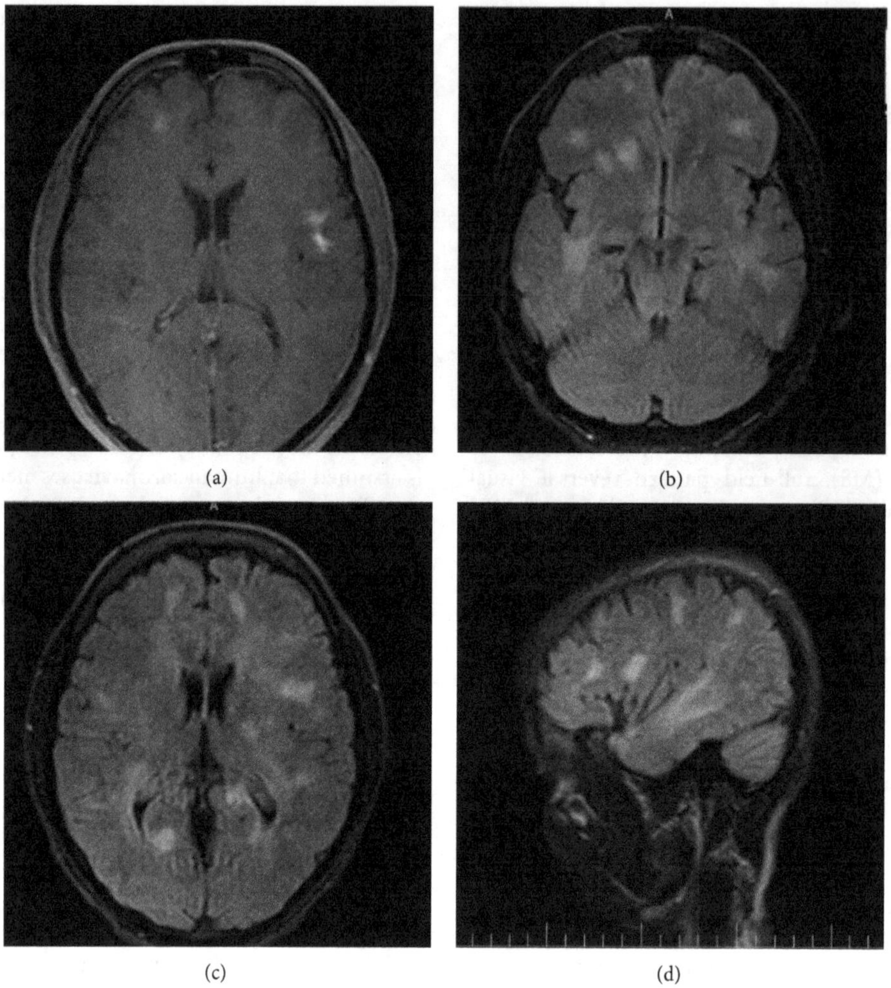

FIGURE 1: (a) Head-MRI T1 sequence with gadolinium demonstrates various hypersignal lesions in favor of active demyelinating plaques in left temporal and right frontal areas of the brain. (b, c) Axial and (d) sagittal FLAIR views show plaques with larger sizes in deeper areas of the brain.

identifying detrimental microorganisms. Likewise, these receptors were represented to recognize those viral pathogens to modify patients' immune response suffering from MS. For instance, some authors reported a notable prevalence of defined strains of coronavirus such as 229E and OC43 in brain samples of MS patients. Moreover, in some murine experimental research, inoculated mice with coronavirus developed acute encephalomyelitis through a chronic demyelinating process; also, macrophages and oligodendrocytes invasion by autoimmune triggering against myelin protein was detected. Of note, a correlation between SARS-CoV-2 and MS has not been determined [5, 14]. The demyelinating plaques in our patient's MRI, with suspicion of MS, have been represented atypically. They had two dominant features that distinguished them from routine plaques defined by McDonald criteria previously. First, the plaques were overall larger than typical plaques. Second, the places where the plaques have appeared were deeper and farther from juxtacortical, infratentorial, and periventricular areas than the typical plaques. Our study's potential limitation was lacking CSF analysis due to the patient's discontent to perform a lumbar puncture. Hence, concerning the patient's autonomy and ethical issues, we could not interpret CSF analysis.

Compatible findings with COVID-19 in CT scan and suggestive clinical manifestations with positive PCR strengthened our study to confirm COVID-19 diagnosis in the patient. COVID-19 pandemic leads scientists to consider drug repurposing of such antiviral options with potential effects to defeat SARS-CoV-2 quickly. Interferon (IFN) β-1a, which is known as a beneficial therapy in MS, could have a significant therapeutic impact in COVID-19 patients [15]. According to Clementi et al.'s study, IFN-β-1a could effectively have an inhibitor role in virus-contaminated cells [15]. Furthermore, it was recommended to use IFN-β-1a therapy to preserve functional B-cell-mediated humoral immunity in MS patients in the COVID-19 era [16]. As we utilize IFN-β-1a with a brand name of Resigen in the first-line therapy of MS patients, we initiated it in our patient, which resulted in a beneficial outcome [16]. Despite all these findings, further and strong surveys are necessary to investigate the correlation between MS and SARS-CoV-2 for possible pathophysiology and appropriate management. Eventually, considering COVID-19 in patients with such neurological manifestations is pivotal to avoid detrimental outcomes and complications.

4. Conclusion

COVID-19, with its neurotropism feature, might appear in the first place of some neurological disorders like multiple sclerosis which require further evidence to establish causality.

Consent

Written informed consent was obtained from the patient.

Acknowledgments

The authors would like to thank the Student Research Committee of Mashhad University of Medical Sciences for their support.

References

[1] M. Ellul, A. Varatharaj, T. R. Nicholson et al., *Defining Causality in COVID-19 and Neurological Disorders*, BMJ Publishing Group Ltd, London, UK, 2020.

[2] E. Beghi, V. Feigin, V. Caso, P. Santalucia, and G. Logroscino, "COVID-19 infection and neurological complications: present findings and future predictions," *Neuroepidemiology*, vol. 54, no. 4, pp. 1-6, 2020.

[3] A. O. Correia, P. W. G. Feitosa, J. L. de Sousa Moreira, S. ÁR. Nogueira, R. B. Fonseca, and M. E. P. Nobre, "Neurological manifestations of COVID-19 and other coronaviruses: a systematic review," *Neurology, Psychiatry and Brain Research*, vol. 37, pp. 27–32, 2020.

[4] K. C. N. K. Kwong, P. R. Mehta, G. Shukla, and A. R. Mehta, "COVID-19, SARS and MERS: a neurological perspective," *Journal of Clinical Neuroscience*, vol. 77, pp. 13–16, 2020.

[5] V. Montalvan, J. Lee, T. Bueso, J. De Toledo, and K. Rivas, "Neurological manifestations of COVID-19 and other coronavirus infections: a systematic review," *Clinical Neurology and Neurosurgery*, vol. 194, Article ID 105921, 2020.

[6] A. Zoghi, M. Ramezani, M. Roozbeh, I. A. Darazam, and M. A. Sahraian, "A case of possible atypical demyelinating event of the central nervous system following COVID-19," *Multiple Sclerosis and Related Disorders*, vol. 44, Article ID 102324, 2020.

[7] W.-j. Guan, Z.-y. Ni, Y. Hu et al., "Clinical characteristics of coronavirus disease 2019 in China," *New England Journal of Medicine*, vol. 382, no. 18, pp. 1708–1720, 2020.

[8] C.-C. Lai, W.-C. Ko, P.-I. Lee, S.-S. Jean, and P.-R. Hsueh, "Extra-respiratory manifestations of COVID-19," *International Journal of Antimicrobial Agents*, vol. 56, no. 2, Article ID 106024, 2020.

[9] H. Abboud, F. Z. Abboud, H. Kharbouch, Y. Arkha, N. El Abbadi, and A. El Ouahabi, *COVID-19 and SARS-Cov-2 Infection: Pathophysiology and Clinical Effects on the Nervous System*, World Neurosurgery, 2020.

[10] V. Kato and B. Laure, "Neurological manifestations of COVID-19, SARS and MERS," *Acta Neurologica Belgica*, vol. 120, no. 5, pp. 1051–1060, 2020.

[11] A. M. Baig, A. Khaleeq, U. Ali, and H. Syeda, "Evidence of the COVID-19 virus targeting the CNS: tissue distribution, host-virus interaction, and proposed neurotropic mechanisms," *ACS Chemical Neuroscience*, vol. 11, no. 7, pp. 995–998, 2020.

[12] Y. Wu, X. Xu, Z. Chen et al., "Nervous System Involvement after Infection with COVID-19 and Other coronaviruses," *Brain, Behavior, and Immunity*, vol. 87, pp. 18–22, 2020.

[13] A. R. Egbert, S. Cankurtaran, and S. Karpiak, "Brain Abnormalities in COVID-19 Acute/subacute Phase: A Rapid Systematic review," *Brain, Behavior, and Immunity*, vol. 89, pp. 543–554, 2020.

[14] L. Duffy and S. C. O'Reilly, "Toll-like receptors in the pathogenesis of autoimmune diseases: recent and emerging translational developments," *ImmunoTargets and Therapy*, vol. 5, p. 69, 2016.

[15] N. Clementi, R. Ferrarese, E. Criscuolo et al., "Interferon-β-1a inhibition of severe acute respiratory syndrome-coronavirus 2 in vitro when administered after virus infection," *The Journal of Infectious Diseases*, vol. 222, no. 5, pp. 722–725, 2020.

[16] M. Severa, C. Farina, M. Salvetti, and E. M. Coccia, "Three decades of interferon-β in multiple sclerosis: can we repurpose this information for the management of SARS-CoV2 infection?" *Frontiers in Immunology*, vol. 11, 2020.

17

Sinking Skin Flap Syndrome following Posttraumatic Hydrocephalus

Ashish Chugh, Prashant Punia, and Sarang Gotecha

Dr. D. Y. Patil Medical College and Hospital, Pimpri, Pune, Maharashtra, India

Correspondence should be addressed to Prashant Punia; getdrprashant@gmail.com

Academic Editor: Tapas Kumar Banerjee

Introduction. Complications following craniotomy are not uncommon and Sinking Skin Flap Syndrome (SSFS) constitutes a rare entity that may present after a large Decompressive Craniectomy. Although the entity is widely reported, the literature mostly consists of case reports. Authors present a case series of three patients with review of literature highlighting the various factors which can prove therapeutic and can help in avoidance of complications. *Materials and Methods.* The study was conducted over a period of 3 years, from 2016 to 2019, and included 212 patients who underwent unilateral Decompressive Craniectomy (DC) for trauma in our institute. All 212 patients underwent a similar DC following a strict institutional protocol and the craniectomies were performed by the same surgical team. At total of 160 patients survived and elective cranioplasty was planned at a 3-month interval. Out of a total of 160 patients who survived, 38 developed hydrocephalus, 3 patients presented with hydrocephalus acutely and had to be shunted before cranioplasty and underwent ventriculoperitoneal (VP) shunting on the opposite side of craniectomy. All 3 of these patients developed SSFS and were the focus of this case series wherein review of literature was done with emphasis being laid on the salient features towards management of SSFS in such precranioplasty shunted patients. These 3 patients were treated via rehydration using normal saline (NS) till the Central Venous Pressure (CVP) equaled 8–10 cm of water, nursing in Trendelenburg position and shunt occlusion using silk 3-0 round bodied suture tied over a "C"-loop of VP shunt tube over clavicle. This was followed by cranioplasty within 2 days of presentation using a flattened, nonconvex artificial Polymethyl Methacrylate (PMMA) bone flap with central hitch suture taken across the bone flap and release of shunt tie in immediate postoperative period. The PMMA bone flap was made intraoperatively after measuring the defect size accurately after exposure of defect. 3D printing option was not availed by any patient considering the high cost and patients' poor socioeconomic status. *Results.* Out of a total of 212 patients, thirty-eight patients (19%) developed posttraumatic hydrocephalus and out of 38, three presented with SSFS over the course of time. Two patients presented with hemiparesis of the side opposite to sunken flap while 1 other patient was brought by relatives in stuporous state. All 3 were subjected to VP shunt tie, rehydration, and cranioplasty using flattened artificial bone flap and showed gradual recovery in postoperative period without any complications. *Conclusion.* Various factors like nursing in Trendelenburg position, adequate rehydration, early cranioplasty after resolution of oedema, preoperative tying of VP shunt and its subsequent release in immediate postoperative period, use of flattened PMMA bone flaps, placement of a central dural hitch suture across the bone, and a preoperative central burr hole in the bone flap may accelerate healing and, in most cases, reversal of sensory-motor deficits along with reduction in complication rates.

1. Introduction

Complications following craniotomy are not uncommon and Sinking Skin Flap Syndrome (SSFS) constitutes a rare entity that may present after a large Decompressive Hemicraniectomy (DC) [1]. Also known by other names such as syndrome of the "trephined," it consists of sunken skin above the bone defect along with neurological symptoms which can be but are not limited to headaches, motor and sensory deficits, mental changes, and seizures. Although the entity is widely reported, the literature mostly consists of case reports. Authors present a case series of three patients with review of literature highlighting the various factors which can prove therapeutic and can help in avoidance of complications.

2. Materials and Methods

The study was conducted over a period of 3 years, from 2016 to 2019, and included 212 patients who underwent unilateral Decompressive Craniectomy (DC) for trauma in our institute. All 212 patients underwent a similar DC following a strict institutional protocol and the craniectomies were performed by the same surgical team. At total of 160 patients survived and elective cranioplasty was planned at a 3-month interval.

Out of a total of 160 patients who survived, 38 developed hydrocephalus and 17 of these 38 patients were managed perioperatively during cranioplasty with ventricular/lumbar drain, 6 other patients denied any further treatment and left against medical advice, and 5 patients developed hydrocephalus after cranioplasty and were shunted within 6 weeks from cranioplasty with no complications. A total of 7 patients were lost to follow-up while the remaining 3 patients presented with hydrocephalus acutely and had to be shunted before cranioplasty and underwent ventriculoperitoneal (VP) shunting on the opposite side of craniectomy. These 3 patients were shunted with a low pressure VP shunt after measuring the opening pressure of the ventricle tap. Cranioplasty was not chosen to be done alongside VP shunting to avoid the added risk of infection.

All 3 of these patients developed SSFS and were the focus of this case series wherein review of literature was done with emphasis being laid on the salient features towards management of SSFS in such precranioplasty shunted patients.

3. Procedures

3.1. Decompressive Craniectomy. On the affected side, a question mark/reverse question mark incision was made 2 cms from midline with a limb length of 15 cms reaching zygoma. Craniectomy was done in a standard and uniform fashion with 4 burr holes each at the apex of bony exposure. Burr holes were connected and temporal bone was nibbled away in the region of zygoma. The standard sized craniotomy provided a uniform and adequate decompression. Hemostasis was achieved and incision was closed in 2 layers.

3.2. Cranioplasty for SSFS. These 3 patients were treated via rehydration using normal saline (NS) till the Central Venous Pressure (CVP) equaled 8–10 cm of water, nursing in Trendelenburg position, and shunt occlusion using silk 3-0 round bodied suture tied over a "C"-loop of VP shunt tube over clavicle. This was followed by cranioplasty within 2 days of presentation using a flattened, nonconvex artificial Polymethyl Methacrylate (PMMA) bone flap with central hitch suture taken across the bone flap and release of shunt tie in immediate postoperative period. The PMMA bone flap was made intraoperatively after measuring the defect size accurately after exposure of defect. 3D printing option was not availed by any patient considering the high cost and patients' poor socioeconomic status.

4. Case Series

4.1. Case 1. A 55-year-old female patient who sustained head trauma in a Road Traffic Accident (RTA) and underwent left frontotemporoparietal decompression craniectomy was brought by relatives with deteriorated neurological status (GCS-9) after 2 months. Examination revealed a tense scalp skin flap at the craniectomy site and the patient was rushed to CT scan which revealed hydrocephalus. Ventriculoperitoneal shunt (VP shunt) on the right side was done in emergency setting and the patient gradually progressed to her preoperative neurological status and was discharged.

The patient again presented 2 months later with right side spastic hemiparesis and severely sunken skin flap on the operated site. A diagnosis of SSFS was made and cranioplasty was planned. The patient was positioned in Trendelenburg position and rehydrated using NS and shunt was tied at the level of clavicle using silk 3-0 round bodied suture after making a C-loop of shunt so that it can be safely removed after cranioplasty. In 2 days, the flap was spontaneously significantly elevated and cranioplasty was performed with a flattened, artificial PMMA bone flap. Shunt occlusion was released immediately postoperatively and the patient gradually fully recovered her hemiparesis and was discharged on the 7th postoperative day (Figure 1).

4.2. Case 2. A 22-year-old male patient who had undergone a decompression craniotomy on the right side for a RTA 1 month back presented with sudden deterioration on consciousness and headache. CT brain revealed hydrocephalus and patient underwent VP shunt procedure on the left side. Patient improved significantly after VP shunt and was discharged on the 7th postoperative day; however, 2 months later, he presented to us in a stuporous state (GCS-9) with a severely sunken skin flap over the right side of the skull. The patient was rehydrated and nursed in Trendelenburg position for 2 days along with tying his VP shunt tube at the level of clavicle. Two days later, he underwent cranioplasty using a flattened, nonconcave artificial PMMA bone flap. Shunt tube block was removed in immediate postoperative period and the patient started showing improvement to be discharged on the 11th postoperative day. Postoperative CT scan showed minimal subdural collection without any mass effect at the cranioplasty site which resolved on its own a few days later (Figure 2).

4.3. Case 3. A 59-year-old female who underwent left decompression craniotomy for acute Subdural Hematoma (SDH) following RTA 1 month back presented to us with complaints of headache. She was investigated and CT brain plain was suggestive of communicating hydrocephalus for which the patient was posted for VP shunting in the right side. The patient's headache gradually improved in the early postoperative period and she was discharged on the 7th postoperative day. Two months later, the patient was

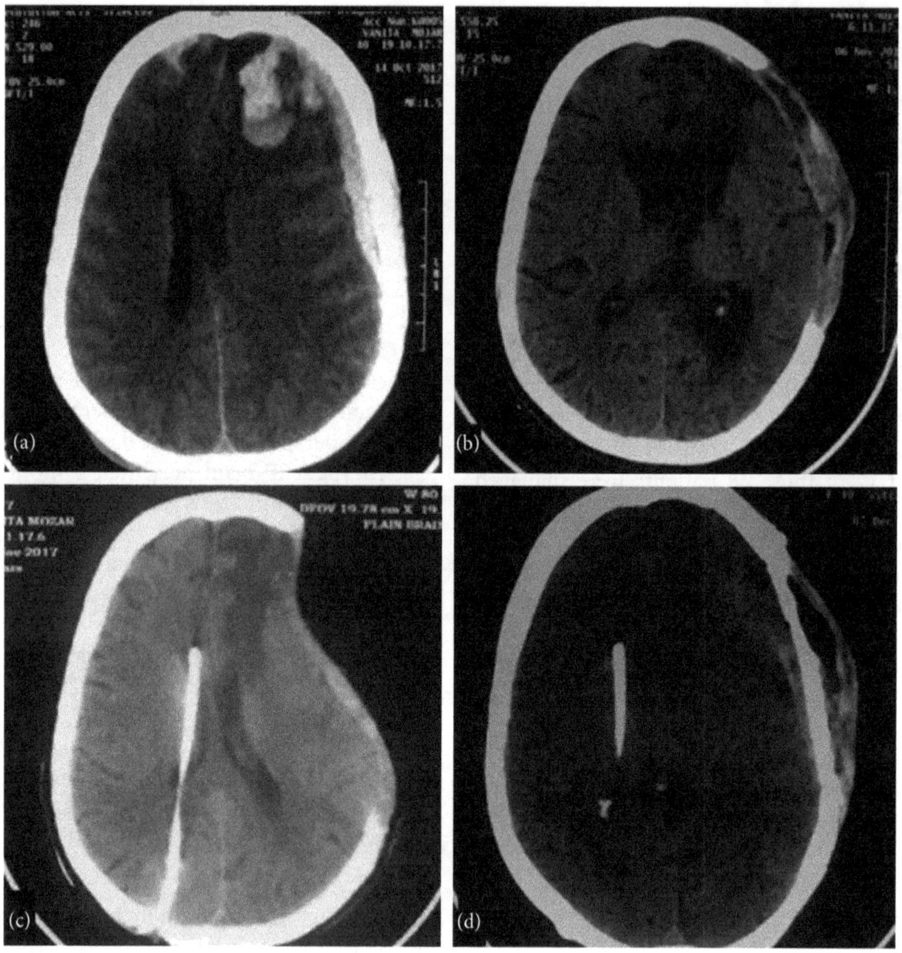

FIGURE 1: (a) Computed tomography (CT) plain brain, axial view showing hyperdense collection along left subdural plane extending across frontal, temporal, and parietal regions. (b) Computed tomography (CT) plain brain, axial view showing dilated ventricles and herniation of brain from craniectomy site. (c) Computed tomography (CT) plain brain, axial view showing VP shunt in situ and excessively sunken brain at craniectomy site causing midline shift to right side. (d) Computed tomography (CT) plain brain, axial view on postoperative day 1, showing cranioplasty using flattened bone. Also, partial resolution of midline shift can be seen.

brought by relatives with complaints of a severely sunken skin flap over the skull and right hemiparesis. A diagnosis of SSFS was made and the patient was rehydrated and nursed in Trendelenburg position for 2 days along with tying her VP shunt tube in the anterior chest wall, at the level of clavicle. Patient underwent cranioplasty using flattened, nonconcave artificial PMMA bone flap and a central hitch suture over dura. Shunt block was removed immediately postoperatively and the patient showed gradual recovery to full power in her postoperative period. Postoperative CT scan showed good expansion of brain and partial resolution of midline shift and the patient was discharged on 15th postoperative day with no deficits (Figure 3).

5. Discussion

Out of a total of 160 patients, thirty-eight patients (24%) developed posttraumatic hydrocephalus. The rate was slightly lower to 28% as observed by Nasi et al. [2] but was more than the rates reported by Yang et al. [3] who reported posttraumatic hydrocephalus in 17.6% of their patients. Rienzo et al. [4] in their prospective series of 269 patients of trauma reported an incidence of posttraumatic hydrocephalus in 34% of their patients which is comparable to our statistics.

A total of 21 out of 35 patients who developed hydrocephalus but did not progress to SSFS were males and 14 females whereas 2 out of 3 patients who developed SSFS were females. Across all major series, male predominance is seen and the reversal of this ratio in our series can be attributed to the limited size of 3 patients. All included patients in this series were operated on (DC) for trauma which has been seen as the leading cause for decompression craniotomy and is comparable with other larger studies [4]. In our series, in the non-SSFS group of 35 patients, 16 were operated on for Subdural Hematoma (SDH) alone while 11 others had SDH along with contusions. The remaining 8 patients were operated on for multiple contusions. In the SSFS group of 3 patients, 2 were diagnosed with SDH + contusions while 1 patient was operated on for SDH alone. Volume loss has been regarded as a potential causative factor towards SSFS and the same has been put across by Rienzo et al. [4] who

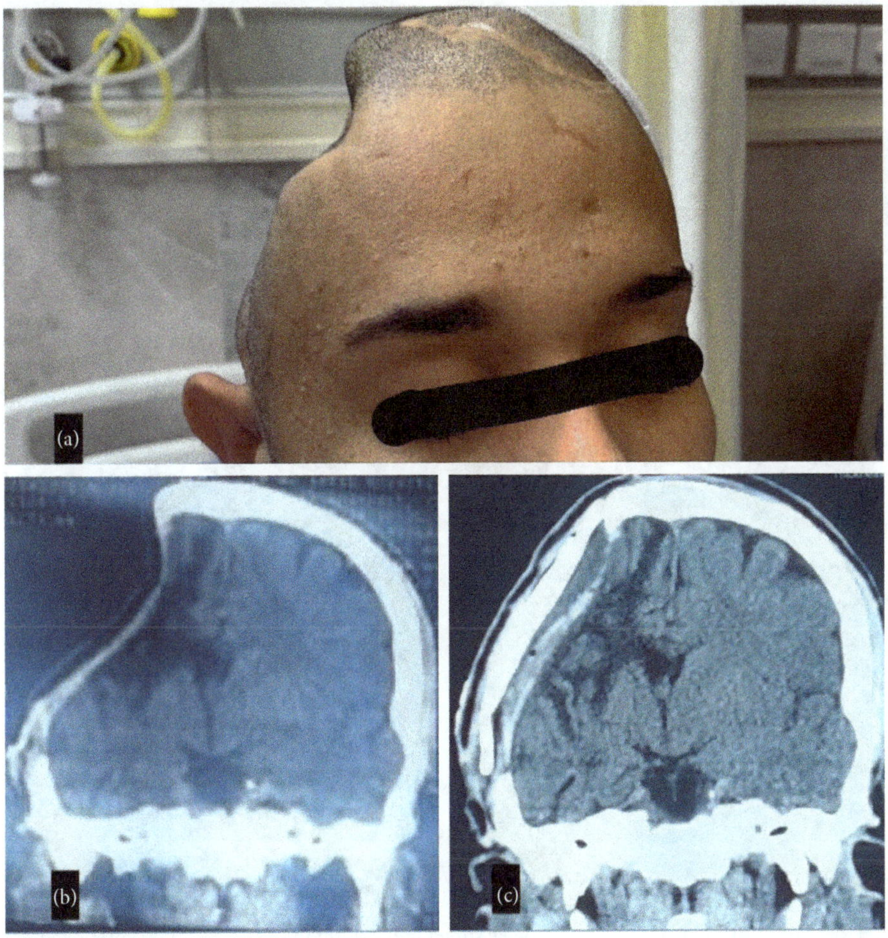

FIGURE 2: (a) Clinical photograph showing sunken skin flap 3 months after craniectomy. (b) Computed tomography (CT) plain brain, coronal view showing right-sided craniectomy with severely sunken hemisphere on the same side. (c) Computed tomography (CT) plain brain, coronal view on postoperative day 1, showing cranioplasty using flattened bone. Also, partial resolution of pressure effects can be seen.

stated that the brain's capacity to counterbalance the atmospheric pressure is significantly hampered when more brain tissue is lost [4].

As this case series is free of surgeon and surgery bias, the substantial difference between the patients not developing SSFS and those developing it remains preoperative VP shunting. It has been observed frequently that pre-cranioplasty shunting leads to development of SSFS. This theory has been supported by Ashayari et al. [5] who stated that an increased gradient between atmospheric and intracranial pressures caused by CSF flow contributes to the development of SSFS. Although the pathophysiology of SSFS has never been adequately elucidated and the sample size of our series is too less to derive conclusions based on statistical analysis, it resonates with the published findings and it can be safely reiterated that precranioplasty shunting and an injury causing volume loss can be proposed as causative mechanisms.

Decompression Craniectomy (DC) is a life-saving procedure for patients presenting with raised intracranial pressure (ICP) due to various reasons. It renders the brain only with a skin cover which is desirable in the given circumstances; however, large cranial defects lead to ex-vacuo/compensatory dilatation and subsequent shifting of ipsilateral lateral ventricle resulting frequently in shunt dependent hydrocephalus [6]. The pathophysiology for development of posttraumatic hydrocephalus is poorly understood and it is attributed to the failure of arachnoid villi to absorb CSF as the craniectomy defect may lead to loss of normal waveform pattern of intracranial pressure (ICP) which, in turn, leads to loss of gradient which is essential to keep the villi open to absorb CSF.

Decompressive Craniectomy status, thus, leads to disturbances in CSF circulation and the same coupled with VP shunting and gradual decrease in pressure from inside due to resolving brain oedema aids in manifestation of detrimental effects of atmospheric pressure on the unsupported scalp. This leads to disturbances in arterial flow and venous return and the subsequent lowering of cortical perfusion in comparison to noncraniectomy hemisphere thus contributing to brain metabolism disorders [6]. Ashayeri et al. [5] defined 4 major factors responsible for development of SSFS viz atmospheric pressure, cerebral blood flow, CSF flow, and cerebral metabolism. They further stated that decreases in cerebral blood flow (CBF) have been shown and attributed the same to both atmospheric pressure and impairment of

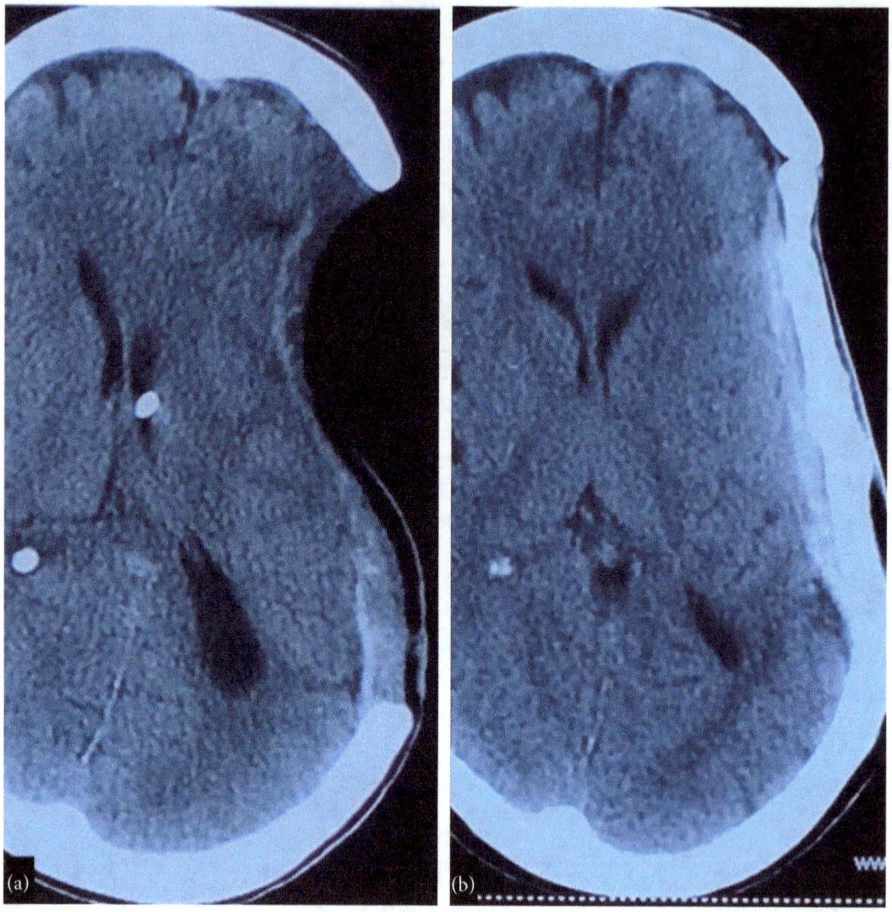

Figure 3: (a) Computed tomography (CT) plain brain, axial view showing VP shunt in situ and excessively sunken brain at craniectomy site causing midline shift to the right side. (b) Computed tomography (CT) plain brain, axial view on postoperative day 1, showing cranioplasty using flattened bone. Also, partial resolution of midline shift can be seen.

venous blood flow through the brain. These undesirable results may be compounded by posttraumatic brain atrophy or parenchymal volume loss on the affected side. This statement is further strengthened by the findings of Wee and Kuo [7], who stated that a VP shunt placement in patients with skull defect may lead to excessive sinking at the craniectomy site as a result of atmospheric pressure gradient, which can be aggravated by change in position.

Patients with SSFS who have a profound neurological deficit after DC have a favorable outcome after cranioplasty and the same has been observed across many case series and studies. Yamamura et al. [8] were one of the first to report clinical improvement after cranioplasty in patients with DC and depressed skin flap. Ashayeri et al. [5] in their series on SSFS stated that all of their patients showed some form of improvement with some patients showing improvement as early as 24 hours and at an average of 4 days. All 3 patients in our series started showing recovery in immediate postoperative phase and gradually recovered to preoperative status prior to discharge on the 7th day.

Timing of cranioplasty has been an issue of debate and many authors recommend an early cranioplasty. The same has been described in various studies as that occurring between 1 and 6 months following DC. Songara et al. [9] in their prospective study on early cranioplasty observed significant improvement in GCS, Glasgow Outcome Scale (GOS), and Mini Mental State Examination (MMSE). They concluded that cranioplasty, when done early, is likely to restore the cerebral perfusion and CSF dynamics and decrease the complications as compared to late cranioplasty. Yoshida et al. [10] studied dynamics of cerebral blood flow and metabolism in patients with cranioplasty via spectroscopy and observed that cranioplasty should be carried out as soon as cerebral oedema has decreased because the defect in the bone by itself may cause decreased blood flow and disturbed metabolism. This view was seconded by Winkler et al. [11] who observed that that cranioplasty appears to increase blood flow velocity and cerebrovascular reserve capacity of both ipsilateral middle cerebral artery and internal carotid artery. Yang et al. [3] in their study tried to determine the timing of the earliest possible cranioplasty and concluded that cranioplasty can be considered as early as 34 days following DC. In authors' opinion, performing cranioplasty at a 3-month interval on the one hand gives adequate time for wound healing and recovery and at the same time saves the patient from deleterious effects of a late cranioplasty including SSFS. Malcolm et al. [12] concluded that cranioplasty might improve neurological function regardless of timing, but earlier cranioplasty may enhance this effect.

Many a times across developing countries, the patients do not turn up for regular follow-ups and protocols for timely cranioplasty cannot be ubiquitously applied. A total of 7 patients were lost to follow-up in our series and another 6 patients refused any further treatment due to poor socioeconomic status.

Also, delay in cranioplasty is seen in a subset of patients who present acutely with symptoms of raised intracranial pressure and neurological deterioration due to hydrocephalus before the planned 3-month interval, as seen with 3 of our patients. These patients were subjected to a VP shunting in emergency setting and cranioplasty was postponed to a later date. However, literature has multiple accounts stating that cranioplasty can itself lead to hydrocephalus resolution but at times the same is not feasible due the poor neurological status and tense craniectomy flap at presentation due to hydrocephalus and the surgeon is left with no option. The authors chose not to perform cranioplasty in the same sitting to prevent the risk of exposure of both CSF and flap contamination. Our view is shared by Di Rienzo et al. [4] who advocated that this practice of precranioplasty shunting should not be banished but should be tailored. They also agree with the authors' view on the increased risk of infection by performing dual procedures involving a foreign body.

After treatment of hydrocephalus, all 3 patients in our series presented with SSFS within 3 months and considerable doubt still remains on the time taken for SSFS to develop after VP shunting as the literature is scarce on such patients and further studies with a bigger sample size are needed to ascertain the same. Di Rienzo et al. [4] did not find a significant statistical correlation between timing of cranioplasty among patients with and without SSFS and even reported cranioplasty after 6 months from craniectomy in 16 patients with SSFS. The authors' view is that once SSFS is recognized, care must be taken not to delay the cranioplasty to the point of development of new deficits. Literature strongly stresses the relation between the use of shunts and occurrence of sinking as seen with 3 of our patients and the recognition of onset of the same should be taught to the patient/patient's relatives for quick recognition and action. This is sometimes delayed as these patients are often neglected and severely sunken flap along with motor weakness are the easily recognizable signs as compared to cognitive deficits [4]. Two of our patients were brought by relatives with hemiparesis and 1 was brought with a severely sunken flap.

5.1. Treatment. Performing a cranioplasty in a patient with severely convex flap has its demerits as it provides a potential dead space for accumulation of blood and/or fluids. Liao and Kao [13] concur with the authors and stated that a procedure for expansion of this dead space would be prudent. Han et al. [14] overcame this difficulty by reprogramming the shunt valve and temporarily increasing the valve pressure thus allowing expansion. This method may not be always possible especially in a developing country and thus tying and subsequent release of VP shunt is a cheap alternative with similar benefits. The shunt tie has to be over a bony prominence (clavicle) for easy recognition via palpation and shunt tube must be looped into "C" shape for hassle-free release of the tie after cranioplasty. All three of our patients were managed using shunt tie and its release in immediate postoperative period without any complications and the authors strongly recommend the same wherever a programmable shunt is not in place. Kim et al. [15] used the same technique with comparable results and stated that, apart from being a simple procedure without complications, it has other benefits too, like it can be done in the ward under local anaesthesia which is especially helpful to medically compromised patients wherein it saves the patient from multiple surgeries of shunt removal and subsequent insertion if needed.

Other strategies for expansion of the dead space are rehydration and putting the patient in Trendelenburg position. Rehydration is particularly helpful as these patients are usually chronically dehydrated. Both these measures were used in conjunction with shunt tie in our study as the effect of Trendelenburg position in increasing intracranial blood volume is limited as stated by Liao et al.

The shape of bone flap plays an important role by itself in patients with SSFS as a convex/natural shaped flap provides extra potential dead space and thus, the authors used flattened bone flaps made with synthetic bone cement (PMMA) in all 3 of our patients. It was observed in late postoperative period that no appreciable change in skull shape was evident after full hair growth. The description on use of flattened bone flaps is limited in the available literature and because the current case series is limited to 3 cases, a detailed study is the need of the hour to prove the effectiveness of the same beyond doubt (Figure 4).

The material used for cranioplasty does not seem to play a role in postoperative complications and Lee et al. [16] demonstrated that the type of material used (PMMA vs. autologous) had no bearing on postoperative complications like extradural fluid collection (EFC). Moreover, Kim et al. [17] reported higher rates of EFC in autologous bone graft (61.1%) as compared to PMMA (43.2%). The authors, thus, used and recommend a flattened PMMA bone graft in patients with severely concave skin flaps, as in SSFS. This coupled with a central hitch suture put across the bone flap facilitated obliteration of extradural space and in turn decreases the chances of EFC.

Placement of a trephination burr hole Intra-operatively at the center of the cranioplasty flap has been recommended by a few [18] and although the authors were not aware of the entity during the study time period, they can safely assert the obvious importance of the same in cases where postoperative collection is expected. Extradural fluid collection, if present, can safely be aspirated via this burr hole and this small step can prove vital in avoiding a resurgery.

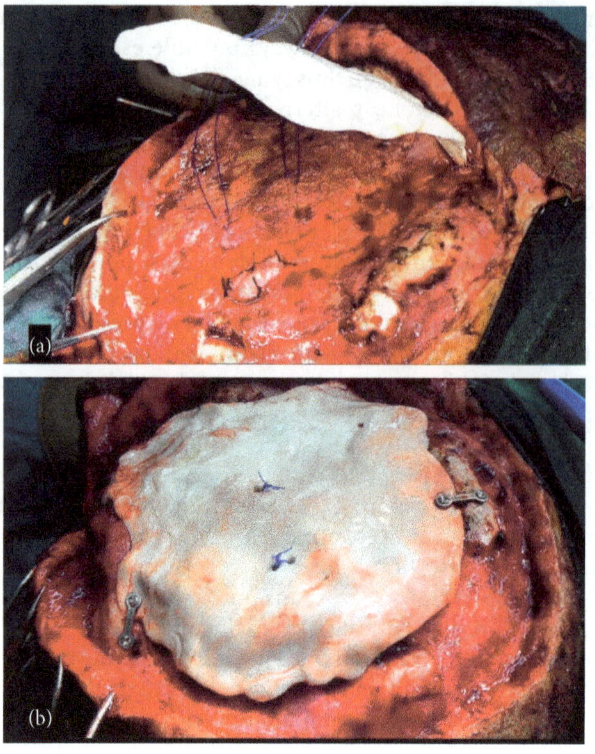

FIGURE 4: (a) Intraoperative photograph showing placement of central hitch suture across the flattened bone flap. (b) Intraoperative photograph after placement of central hitch suture across the bone flap.

6. Conclusion

Sinking Skin Flap Syndrome (SSFS) in patients after DC and VP shunting is not an uncommon entity in neurosurgical practice; yet, clear guidelines for treatment and avoidance of complications are not universal. The authors, with their own experience and after reviewing the relevant limited literature available, conclude that various factors like nursing in Trendelenburg position, adequate rehydration, early cranioplasty after resolution of oedema, preoperative tying of VP shunt and its subsequent release in immediate postoperative period, use of flattened PMMA bone flaps, placement of a central dural hitch suture across the bone, and a Intra-operatively central burr hole in the bone flap may accelerate healing and, in most cases, reversal of sensory-motor deficits along with reduction in complication rates. Neurosurgeons across the globe should be well versed with the entity the and above said factors and their role; being forewarned is being forearmed.

Consent

Informed consent was obtained from all individual participants included in the study.

Authors' Contributions

A. Chugh conceived and designed the study. P. Punia helped in drafting the manuscript. S. Gotecha contributed to collection of data and final review.

References

[1] M. Sarov, J.-P. Guichard, S. Chibarro et al., "Sinking skin flap syndrome and paradoxical herniation after hemicraniectomy for malignant hemispheric infarction," *Stroke*, vol. 41, no. 3, pp. 560–562, 2010.

[2] D. Nasi, M. Dobran, A. Di Rienzo et al., "Decompressive craniectomy for traumatic brain injury: the role of cranioplasty and hydrocephalus on outcome," *World Neurosurgery*, vol. 116, pp. e543–e549, 2018.

[3] N. R. Yang, J. Song, K. W. Yoon, and E. k. Seo, "How early can we perform cranioplasty for traumatic brain injury after decompressive craniotomy? A retrospective multi centre study," *World Neurosurgery*, vol. 110, pp. e160–e167, 2017.

[4] A. Di Rienzo, R. Colasanti, M. Gladi et al., "Sinking flap syndrome revisited: the who, when and why," *Neurosurgical Review*, vol. 43, no. 1, pp. 323–335, 2020.

[5] K. Ashayeri, E. M. Jackson, J. Huang, H. Brem, and C. R. Gordon, "Syndrome of the trephined," *Neurosurgery*, vol. 79, no. 4, pp. 525–534, 2016.

[6] X. J. Yang, G. L. Hong, S. B. Su, and S. Y. Yang, "Complications induced by decompressive craniectomies after traumatic brain injury," *Chinese Journal of Traumatology = Zhonghua Chuang Shang Za Zhi*, vol. 6, no. 2, pp. 99–103, 2003.

[7] H. Y. Wee and J. R. Kuo, "Never neglect the atmospheric pressure effect on a brain with a skull defect," *International Medical Case Reports Journal*, vol. 7, pp. 67–69, 2014.

[8] A. Yamamura, M. Sato, K. Meguro, T. Nakamura, and K. Uemura, "Cranioplasty following decompressive craniectomy- analysis of 300 cases," *No Shinkei Geka*, vol. 5, no. 4, pp. 345–353, 1977.

[9] A. Songara, R. Gupta, N. Jain, S. Rege, and R. Masand, "Early cranioplasty in patients with posttraumatic decompressive craniectomy and its correlation with changes in cerebral perfusion parameters and neurocognitive outcome," *World Neurosurgery*, vol. 94, pp. 303–308, 2016.

[10] K. Yoshida, M. Furuse, A. Izawa, N. Iizima, H. Kuchiwaki, and S. Inao, "Dynamics of cerebral blood flow and metabolism in patients with cranioplasty as evaluated by 133Xe CT and 31P magnetic resonance spectroscopy," *Journal of Neurology, Neurosurgery & Psychiatry*, vol. 61, no. 2, pp. 166–171, 1996.

[11] P. A. Winkler, W. Stummer, R. Linke, K. G. Krishnan, and K. Tatsch, "Influence of cranioplasty on postural blood flow regulation, cerebrovascular reserve capacity, and cerebral glucose metabolism," *Journal of Neurosurgery*, vol. 93, no. 1, pp. 53–61, 2000.

[12] J. G. Malcolm, R. S. Rindler, J. K. Chu et al., "Early cranioplasty is associated with greater neurological improvement: a systemic review and meta-analysis," *Neurosurgery*, vol. 82, no. 3, pp. 278–288, 2017.

[13] C.-C. Liao and M.-C. Kao, "Cranioplasty for patients with severe depressed skull bone defect after cerebrospinal fluid shunting," *Journal of Clinical Neuroscience*, vol. 9, no. 5, pp. 553–555, 2002.

[14] P. Y. Han, J. H. Kim, H. I. Kang, and J. S. Kim, ""Syndrome of the sinking skin-flap" secondary to the ventriculoperitoneal shunt after craniectomy," *Journal of Korean Neurosurgical Society*, vol. 43, no. 1, pp. 51–53, 2008.
[15] S.-Y. Kim, C.-H. Lee, I. S. Park, S. H. Hwang, and J. W. Han, "Sinking skin flap syndrome after craniectomy in a patient who previously underwent ventriculoperitoneal shunt," *Korean Journal of Neurotrauma*, vol. 8, no. 2, pp. 149–152, 2012.
[16] J. W. Lee, J. H. Kim, H. I. Kang, B. G. Moon, S. J. Lee, and J. S. Kim, "Epidural fluid collection after cranioplasty fate and predictive factors," *Journal of Korean Neurosurgical Society*, vol. 50, no. 3, pp. 231–234, 2011.
[17] S. p. Kim, D. S. Kang, J. H. Cheong, J. H. Kim, K. Y. Song, and M. H. Kong, "Clinical analysis of epidural fluid collection as a complication after cranioplasty," *Journal of Korean Neurosurgical Society*, vol. 56, no. 5, pp. 410–418, 2014.
[18] P. Jeyaraj, "Importance of early cranioplasty in reversing the "syndrome of the trephine/motor trephine syndrome/sinking skin flap syndrome"," *Journal of Maxillofacial and Oral Surgery*, vol. 14, no. 3, pp. 666–673, 2015.

18

Prolonged Postoperative Pyrexia and Transient Nonnephrogenic Vasopressin-Analogue-Resistant Polyuria following Endoscopic Transsphenoidal Resection of an Infundibular Epidermoid Cyst

Yuichiro Yoneoka,[1] **Yasuhiro Seki**,[1] **Katsuhiko Akiyama**,[1] **Yuki Sakurai**,[2] **Nobumasa Ohara**,[2] **and Go Hasegawa**[3]

[1]*Department of Neurosurgery, Uonuma Kikan Hospital, Uonuma Institute of Community Medicine, Niigata University Medical and Dental Hospital, Niigata 949-7302, Japan*
[2]*Department of Endocrine, Uonuma Kikan Hospital, Uonuma Institute of Community Medicine, Niigata University Medical and Dental Hospital, Niigata 949-7302, Japan*
[3]*Department of Pathology, Uonuma Kikan Hospital, Uonuma Institute of Community Medicine, Niigata University Medical and Dental Hospital, Niigata 949-7302, Japan*

Correspondence should be addressed to Yuichiro Yoneoka; yone@bri.niigata-u.ac.jp

Academic Editor: Peter Berlit

Prolonged postoperative pyrexia (PPP) due to Mollaret's meningitis following endoscopic transsphenoidal surgery (eTSS) for an intracranial epidermoid cyst can be confused with postoperative meningeal infection after transsphenoidal resection, especially in the middle of the COVID-19 pandemic. Anosmia, as well as dysgeusia, cannot be evaluated in patients of eTSS for a while after surgery. We report a case of an infundibular epidermoid cyst with post-eTSS Mollaret's meningitis (MM). The post-eTSS MM caused vasopressin-analogue-resistant polyuria (VARP) in synchronization with PPP. A 59-year-old man experiencing recurrent headaches and irregular bitemporal hemianopsia over three months was diagnosed with a suprasellar tumor. The suprasellar tumor was an infundibular cyst from the infundibular recess to the posterior lobe of the pituitary, which was gross-totally resected including the neurohypophysis via an extended eTSS. Since awakening from general anesthesia after the gross total resection (GTR) of the tumor, the patient continuously had suffered from headache until the 13th postoperative day (POD13). The patient took analgesics once a day before the surgery and three times a day after the surgery until POD11. Pyrexia (37.5–39.5 degree Celsius) in synchronization with nonnephrogenic VARP remitted on POD18. Intravenous antibiotics had little effect on changes of pyrexia. Serum procalcitonin values (reference range <0.5 ng/mL) are 0.07 ng/mL on POD12 and 0.06 ng/mL on POD18. His polyuria came to react with sublingual desmopressin after alleviation of pyrexia. He left the hospital under hormone replacement therapy without newly added neurological sequelae other than hypopituitarism. After GTR of an infundibular epidermoid cyst, based on values of serum procalcitonin, post-eTSS MM can be distinguished from infection and can be treated with symptomatic treatments. The postoperative transient nonnephrogenic VARP that differs from usual central diabetes insipidus can react with sublingual desmopressin after alleviation of PPP in the clinical course of post-eTSS MM. An infundibular epidermoid cyst should be sufficiently resected in one sitting to minimize comorbidities, its recurrence, or postoperative MM to the utmost.

1. Introduction

Mollaret's meningitis, a benign recurrent aseptic disease, is known to be associated with intracranial and intraspinal epidermoid cysts [1–7]. In practice, Mollaret's meningitis following resection of an intracranial epidermoid cyst can be confused with postoperative bacterial meningitis, especially after transsphenoidal surgery (TSS). We report a case of an infundibular epidermoid cyst with a hard-to-control polyuria in synchronization with prolonged postoperative pyrexia (PPP) during the postoperative course coincidentally in the middle of the coronavirus disease 2019 (COVID-19) pandemic. This report provides insight into the differential diagnosis of PPP from bacterial/viral meningitis and insight into coping to synchronized hard-to-control polyuria (vasopressin-analogue-resistant polyuria, which is described below) that differs from usual central diabetes insipidus (DI). For future reference, we describe these rare clinical manifestations in this report.

2. Case Report

A 59-year-old man presented with a three-month history of gradually progressive blurred vision with headaches (mainly retrobulbar pain). The headaches were frequently associated with coughs or sneezes. Magnetic resonance (MR) imaging demonstrated a sellar-suprasellar tumor compressing the optic chiasm superiorly (Figures 1(a)–1(f)). Postcontrast computed tomography (CT) showed the enhanced rim of the sellar-suprasellar tumor without apparent calcification (Figures 1(g) and 1(h)). Postcontrast MR images demonstrated the enhanced rim of the tumor, indicating that the tumor was a cystic lesion with some contents (Figure 1(b)). Reconstructed CT and MR images revealed that the cyst corresponded to the pituitary stalk (Figures 1(g)–1(j)). Goldmann perimeter (GP) revealed irregular bitemporal hemianopsia predominantly in the left eye (Figure 1(k)). A closed interview detected the patient's recent polyuria and polydipsia. His headaches were associated with visual blurring. These symptoms got worse, and he decided to undergo an endoscopic transsphenoidal surgery (eTSS) for resection of the cyst. Preoperative diagnosis was craniopharyngioma, Rathke's cleft cyst, or sellar-suprasellar epidermoid cyst. On admission, the patient's body temperature was 36.4 degree Celsius (°C). A chest CT scan did not show pneumonia, pneumonitis, nor ground glass opacities, but clear lung fields. Complete blood count revealed neither lymphocytopenia nor thrombocytopenia. The patient had not experienced anosmia nor dysgeusia. He did not have any high-risk contact with COVID-19-infected persons.

Under general anesthesia, an endoscopic transsphenoidal surgery was performed. The sellar floor and the adjacent tuberculum sellae were removed to expose the dura around the sella turcica. The dura was opened (Figure 2(a)) to expose the tumor and the pituitary gland (Figures 2(b) and 2(c)). Prior to the resection, the cyst was punctured with a long needle (Figure 2(d)). Some of the orange-xanthochromic mucus were aspirated. After the cyst aspiration (Figure 2(e)), not to disseminate the cyst contents for prevention of chemical meningitis, the cyst was opened and dissected (Figure 2(f)). The solid cyst contents appeared as tissue debris, keratin, and solid cholesterol, and their mixtures were meticulously removed. The cyst wall was carefully detached from the optic chiasm. Since the cyst wall was the tumorized pituitary stalk, the cyst was gross-totally removed from the intrasellar part to the infundibular part (Figure 2(g)). The opened skull base (Figure 2(h)) was reconstructed with a fat-on-fascia graft plug [8]. Corticosteroid (hydrocortisone) was administrated continuously because of total hypophysectomy after operation. Since awakening from general anesthesia after the gross total resection (GTR) of the tumor, the patient continuously suffered from headaches until the 13th postoperative day (POD13). The patient took analgesics once a day before the surgery and three times a day after the surgery until POD11. The patient's diabetes insipidus (DI) became stronger after the eTSS. This DI was controlled with sublingual desmopressin tablets until POD11. Pyrexia did not emerge until the patient's peroral analgesic dose decreased on POD11. This pyrexia (37.5–39.5°C) continued until POD18. This prolonged postoperative pyrexia (PPP) could be controlled with peroral nonsteroidal antiinflammatory drugs (NSAIDs). In addition, hard-to-control polyuria (4730 ± 1361 ml, mean ± SD), in other words, vasopressin-analogue-resistant polyuria (VARP), emerged in synchronization with PPP and continued with some alterations until POD35. This PPP was unresponsive to intravenous pitressin or sublingual desmopressin tablets. The plasma natrium fluctuated from 123 mEq/L to 135 mEq/L, which was below the normal range (138 mEq/L–145 mEq/L), during the VARP. Water supply and sodium correction were performed on the basis of laboratory data. Although his nuchal stiffness was not observed, his neck was not supple retrospectively. Although anosmia and dysgeusia could not be estimated because of postoperative nasal packing, leukocytopenia was not found in the patient [9]. Intravenous antibiotics had little effect on changes of pyrexia. Serum procalcitonin values (reference range < 0.5 ng/mL) were 0.07 ng/mL on POD12 and 0.06 ng/mL on POD18. Based on values of serum procalcitonin, we provided him with symptomatic treatments in addition to prophylactic antibiotics: piperacillin and amikacin. His pyrexia remitted on POD18. After POD18, he did not suffer from headaches. His polyuria began to react with sublingual desmopressin after alleviation of pyrexia and turned into usual DI after 5 weeks of the eTSS. The plasma natrium was normalized. His corrected vision was 20/16 in both eyes despite his bitemporal hemianopsia not improving sufficiently. The patient left the hospital without new sequalae except for postoperative panhypopituitarism under hormone replacement therapy including peroral hydrocortisone, levothyroxine, and desmopressin. Histopathological analysis confirmed the cyst as an epidermoid cyst (Figure 3). In fact, we had encountered a dearth of coronavirus testing kits during his perioperative care in the middle of the COVID-19 pandemic. MR imaging at 4 months (19 weeks) after surgery showed that the displaced optic chiasm (Figures 4(a)–4(d)) had been successfully decompressed and the infundibular dermoid cyst was totally resected (Figures 4(e)–4(h)).

3. Discussion

Only six cases of infundibular epidermoid cysts were reported prior to this report (Table 1) [10–15]. In fact, infundibular epidermoid cysts are rare, and surgical experiences are valued.

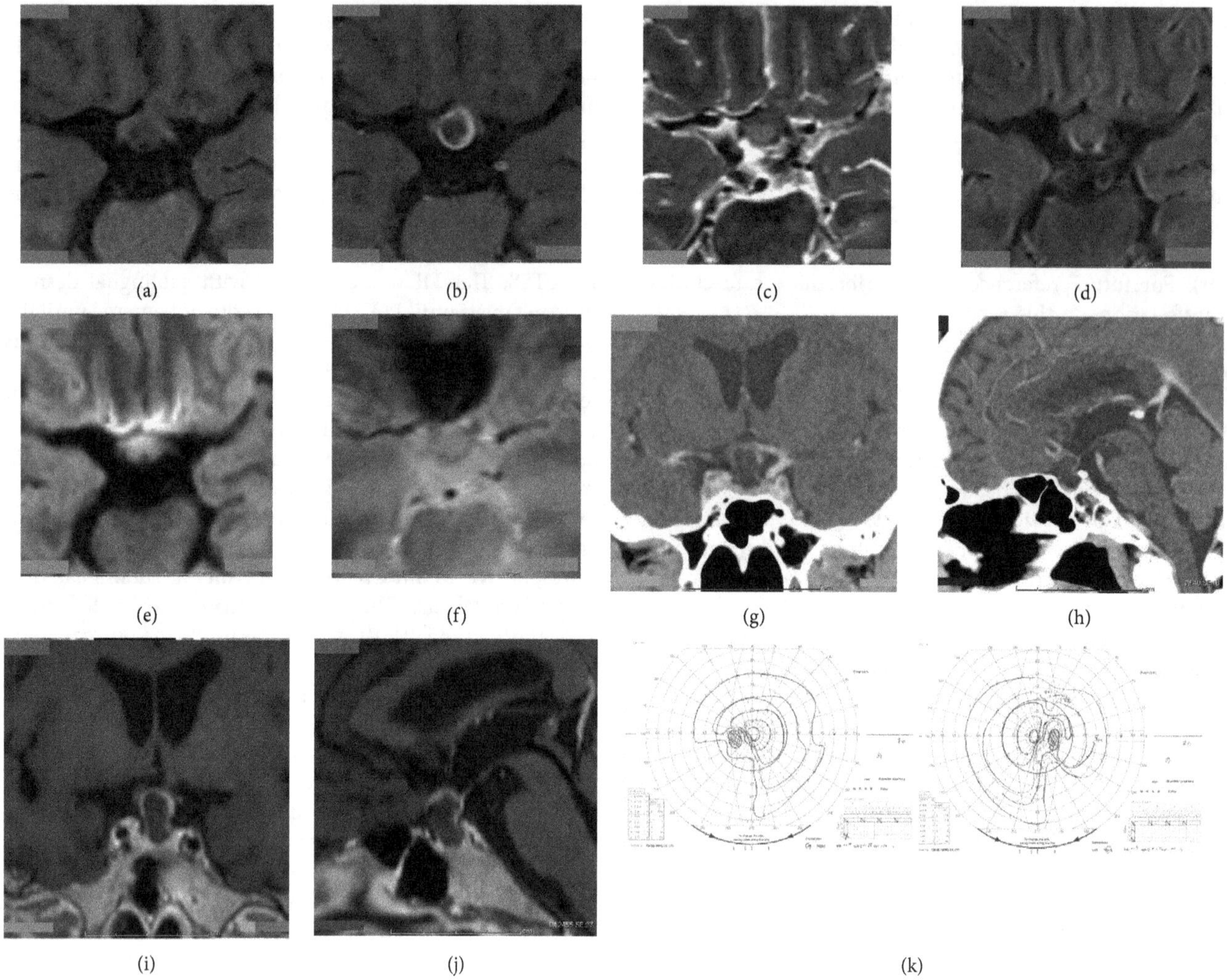

FIGURE 1: Precontrast T1-weighted axial image showing a suprasellar tumor compressing the optic pathway (a). Gadolinium-enhanced axial image showing an enhanced rim of the tumor (b). The contents of the tumor are of low signal intensity on the T1-weighted image (a) and Gadolinium-enhanced image (b), slightly high on T2-weighted image (c), iso on fluid-attenuated inversion recovery image (d), and relatively high on diffusion-weighted image (e) and T2∗-weighted image (f). Contrast-enhanced computed tomography showing a cystic lesion (g) from the sella turcia to the suprasellar space (h). Calcified components are not found in it. Postcontrast magnetic resonance imaging shows the enhanced cystic wall displacing the optic chiasm upward (i). This cystic lesion occupies the suprasellar region but not the third ventricle (h), (j). Goldmann perimeter reveals irregular bitemporal hemianopsia (k). Constriction of the visual field is more predominant in the right eye than in the left eye (k).

From this case, we have found two things that the previous reports did not refer to [10–15]; the first is postoperative prolonged pyrexia (PPP), and the second is postoperative transient vasopressin-analogue-resistant polyuria (VARP).

3.1. Postoperative Prolonged Pyrexia (PPP). The PPP should be distinguished from a symptom of postoperative bacterial meningitis. Because healthcare-associated meningitis or ventriculitis is a serious complication in different neurosurgical procedures and is associated with significant morbidity and mortality [16], in the middle of the COVID-19 pandemic, the PPP should also be distinguished from COVID-19 infection [17].

Fever is a relatively common occurrence among patients in the intensive care setting. Although the most obvious and concerning etiology is sepsis, drug reactions, venous thromboembolism, and postsurgical fevers are all on the differential diagnosis [18]. In the middle of the COVID-19 pandemic, not only sepsis but also COVID-19 infection is a nonnegligible differential diagnosis [19], as well as postoperative meningitis. There is abundant evidence that fever is detrimental in acute neurologic injury [18]. Raised temperature may be due to a regulated readjustment in the hypothalamic "set point" in response to inflammation and infection, or it may occur as a consequence of damage to the hypothalamus and/or its pathways [20]. This primarily occurs in SAH and TBI, with hypothalamic injury being the proposed mechanism.

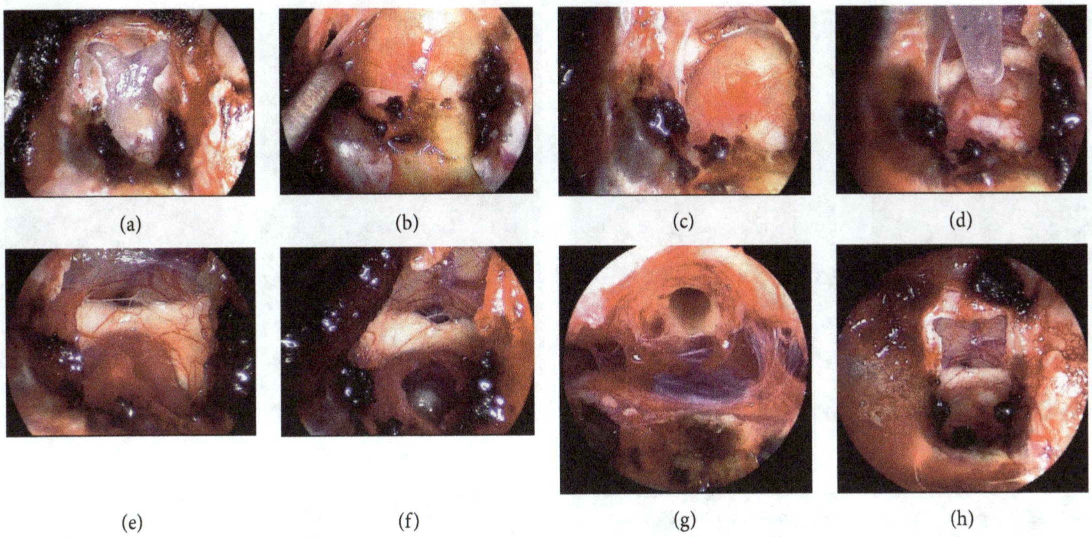

Figure 2: The intercavernous sinus has been cut after cauterization (a). A Y-shaped dural incision is made (a). The cyst wall is found above the pituitary gland (b). Vascular streaks are found on the cyst wall, indicating the pituitary stalk is tumorized (b). The cyst is displacing the optic chiasm (c). The cyst contents are aspirated via a long needle (d). After the aspiration (d), the cyst is shrunken so that the working space in this tumor resection is secured. An indentation is observed in the inferior surface of the decompressed optic chiasm (e). The solid cyst contents appeared as tissue debris, keratin, solid cholesterol, and their mixtures, which were meticulously removed (f). Since the cyst wall is the tumorized pituitary stalk, the cyst was gross-totally removed from the intrasellar part to the infundibular part (g). The opened skull base (h) is reconstructed with a fat-on-fascia graft plug [8].

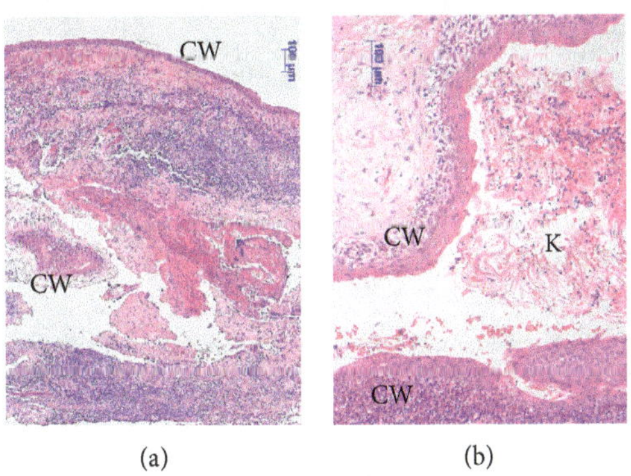

Figure 3: Histopathological examination shows features of the dermoid cyst. The lining is typically a squamous epithelium adjacent to glial tissues with inflammation (a). The cyst lumen contains keratin (b). CW: cyst wall and K: keratin.

Paroxysmal sympathetic hyperactivity is another source of hyperthermia commonly seen in the population with traumatic brain injury [18]. In the brain, the preoptic area and the paraventricular hypothalamus are part of a neuronal network mediating sympathetic activation underlying fever [21]. Thus, it is no wonder that infundibular epidermoid cysts cause central hyperthermia following chemical meningitis that is known as Mollaret's meningitis [1–7]. Ganko et al. reported level II evidence that establishes the efficacy of prophylactic steroids utilized in patients undergoing surgery for epidermoid cysts to prevent postoperative chemical meningitis [22].

Serum procalcitonin levels seem to be the best marker in differentiating between bacterial and viral meningitis in adults [23]. In addition, serum procalcitonin might be able to discriminate between bacterial and chemical causes of meningitis in postmyelographic meningitis [24]. In our case, after GTR of the infundibular epidermoid cyst, the patient's pyrexia with headaches was diagnosed as postoperative Mollaret's meningitis following the infundibular epidermoid cyst that was treated with symptomatic treatments based on values of serum procalcitonin [24, 25]. The patient's serum procalcitonin values (reference range < 0.5 ng/mL) were 0.07 ng/mL on POD12 and 0.06 ng/mL on POD18. In addition, a nuchal rigidity (stiff neck) was unobserved as well as nausea in the patient, and his level of consciousness was 15 on the Glasgow Coma Scale even with a fever greater than 38°C [26–28]. Serum procalcitonin is a useful tool in the evaluation of patients with a known or suspected central nervous system infection [25].

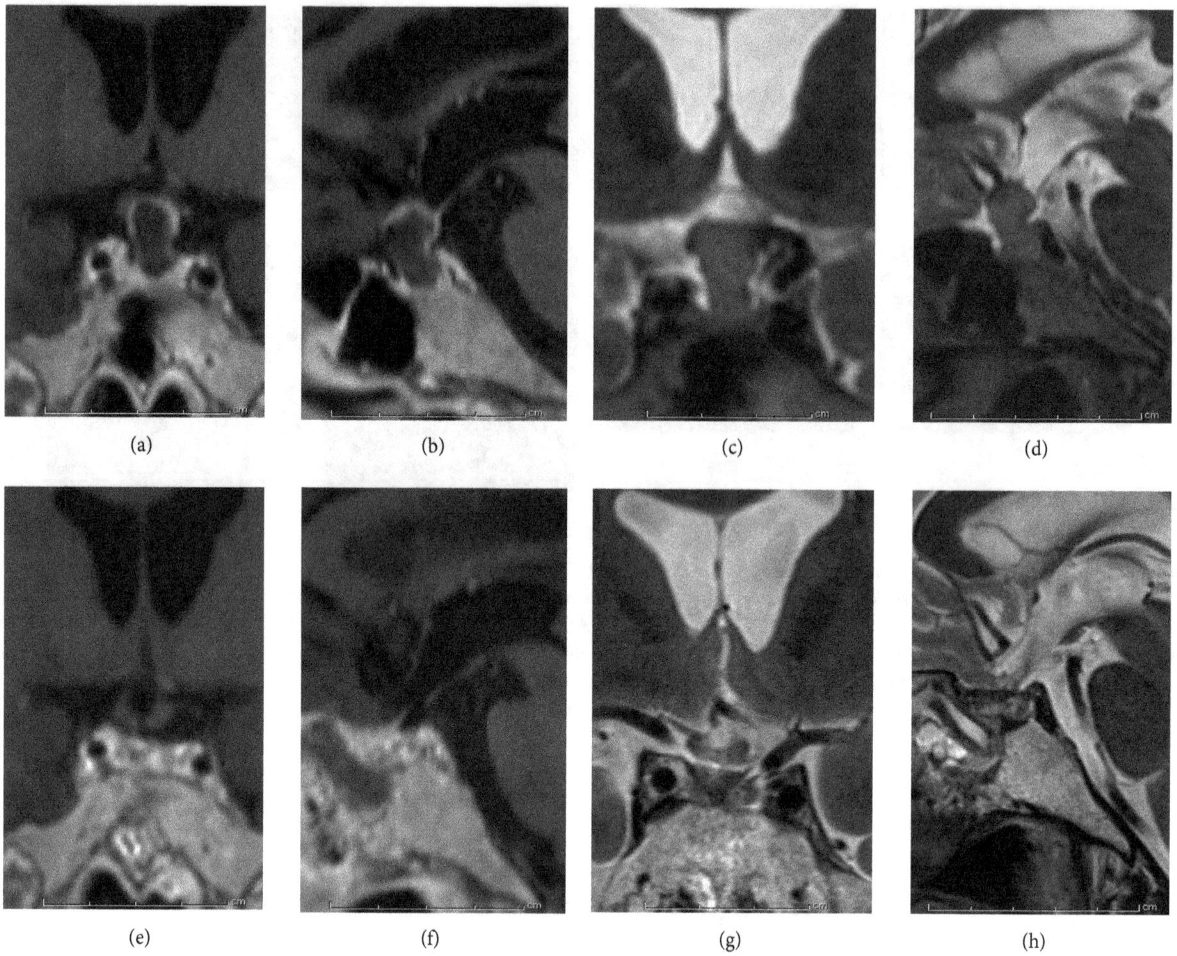

FIGURE 4: The displaced optic chiasm (a, b, c, and d) is successfully decompressed, and the cyst is totally resected (e, f, g, and h) on MR imaging at 4 months (19 weeks) weeks after surgery.

TABLE 1: Characteristics of previous and current case reports of pituitary stalk epidermoid cysts.

Paper	Age/sex	Presentation	Imaging characteristics	Operative approach	Postoperative status
Costa et al., 2013 [10]	27-year-old female	Amenorrhea, galactorrhea, polyuria, and polydipsia	Mixed signal, bilobed rim and enhancing cystic lesion	Endoscopic endonasal extended transsphenoidal	Not reported
Nakassa et al., 2017 [11]	54-year-old female	Headache, visual disturbance, polyuria, and polydipsia	Mixed signal and nonenhancing cystic lesion	Endoscopic endonasal	Persistent DI and subjective visual fields improvement
McCormack et al., 2018 [12]	36-year-old female	Headache and visual disturbance	Multilocular T1 hypointense, T2 hyperintense, and rim-enhancing lesion	Endoscopic endonasal extended transsphenoidal	Transient DI
Montaser et al., 2018 [13]	49-year-old female	Headache	Mixed signal and nonenhancing sellar/suprasellar cyst extending into the third ventricle	Endoscopic endonasal extended transsphenoidal	Persistent DI
Khan et al., 2019 [14]	55-year-old male	Decreased visual acuity	Mixed signal and rim-enhancing cystic lesion	Endoscopic endonasal extended transsphenoidal	Panhypopituitarism and subjective visual fields improvement
Lee et al., 2020 [15]	63-year-old male	Polydipsia and polyuria	T2 hyperintense and rim-enhancing cystic lesion	Pretemporal craniotomy	Persistent DI
Current case	59-year-old male	Headache and visual disturbance	Rim-enhancing cystic lesion	Endoscopic endonasal extended transsphenoidal	Panhypopituitarism, persistent DI, and visual fields improvement

3.2. Postoperative Hard-To-Control Polyuria: Vasopressin-Analogue-Resistant Polyuria. The postoperative hard-to-control polyuria: pitressin/desmopressin-resistant polyuria, which should instead be called vasopressin-analogue-resistant polyuria (VARP), differs from usual central diabetes insipidus (DI). VARP came to react with sublingual desmopressin after alleviation of pyrexia in the clinical course of post-eTSS Mollaret's meningitis in our case. The postoperative VARP is something different from usual DI: hypernatremia associating polyuria was not observed, indicating excessive excreted urinary natrium quantity during VARP. The VARP interacts with central hyperthermia (PPP), which suggests an involvement of the above-mentioned hypothalamic dysfunction during the transient VARP. This VARP may belong to the category of cerebral salt wasting syndrome coexisting with DI [29], or is VARP a new clinical entity? Further studies are warranted to answer this question.

3.3. Transient Hypothalamic Dysfunction Is Inflammation-Induced or Trauma-Induced? PPP in this case was linked with the patient intake of NSAIDs. The VARP settled as the PPP remitted. Based on these findings and the clinical course, transient hypothalamic dysfunction (HD) is probably inflammation-induced. If so, NSAIDs and corticosteroids might be effective for HD after resection of infundibular epidermoid cysts.

3.4. Resection of Infundibular Epidermoid, Gross Total, or Partial? This case is the first report of transient nonnephrogenic VARP synchronizing with PPP during Mollaret's meningitis after resection of an infundibular epidermoid cyst. As a similar mechanism, Rathke's cleft cysts (RCCs) sometimes present with acute onset, and the presentation is consistent with the features of pituitary apoplexy caused by pituitary adenoma [30]. As well, RCCs may cause Mollaret's meningitis and pituitary failure [31]. Because the infundibular epidermoid is close to the pituitary gland and hypothalamus, the infundibular epidermoid cyst and its contents should be sufficiently resected in one sitting, as much as possible within safe limits. According to a meta-analysis by Shear et al. [32], subtotal resection is the primary risk factor for cyst recurrence, which can occur many years after the initial surgery. In the meta-analysis of observational studies in 691 patients, the pooled rates of recurrence after gross total and subtotal resection were 3 and 21%, respectively [32]. The average recurrence rate for studies with longer follow-up durations (≥4.4 years) (17.4%) was significantly higher than the average recurrence rate for studies with shorter follow-up durations (<4.4 years) (5.7%) [32]. A recurrence rate of 21% in subtotal resection of an epidermoid should not be ignored. Thus, gross total resection is the primary treatment goal of an intracranial epidermoid, if possible. Among the previous reports of infundibular epidermoid cysts [10–15], not all epidermoid cysts were resected gross-totally. Based on the recurrence rate of 21% in subtotal resection of epidermoid [32], careful and long-term follow-up is necessary even after subtotal resection.

In our case, even under GTR of an infundibular epidermoid cyst, a post-eTSS Mollaret's meningitis continued until POD18 and had settled after POD19. If the eTSS resulted in insufficient resection, the Mollaret's meningitis would not have settled and been long lasting. Thus, surgical gross total resection remains the mainstay for treatment of intracranial epidermoid cysts [29, 33]. Here, again, an infundibular epidermoid cyst should be sufficiently resected in one sitting, as much as possible within safe limits.

In the middle of the COVID-19 pandemic, prolonged pyrexia should be appropriately diagnosed and distinguished from coronavirus infection or other diseases. Physicians need to correctly approach this new disease in daily clinical practice, often representing a challenge in terms of differential diagnosis [34].

4. Conclusions

After GTR of the infundibular epidermoid cyst, based on values of serum procalcitonin, post-eTSS Mollaret's meningitis can be distinguished from infection and can be treated with symptomatic treatments despite PPP. The postoperative VARP differs from usual central DI and can react with sublingual desmopressin after alleviation of PPP in the clinical course of post-eTSS Mollaret's meningitis. An infundibular epidermoid cyst should be sufficiently resected in one sitting on the basis of its recurrence rate.

Consent

Informed consent was obtained from the patient.

Acknowledgments

The authors would like to thank all laboratory medical technologists in Uonuma Kikan Hospital.

References

[1] J.-P. D. Chadarévian and W. J. Becker, "Mollaret's recurrent aseptic meningitis," *Journal of Neuropathology and Experimental Neurology*, vol. 39, no. 6, pp. 661–669, 1980.

[2] M. Szabó, C. Majtényi, and A. Guseo, "Contribution to the background of Mollaret's meningitis," *Acta Neuropathologica* vol. 59, no. 2, pp. 115–118, 1983.

[3] W. J. Becker, G. V. Watters, J.-P. d. Chadarevian, and M. Vanasse, "Recurrent aseptic meningitis secondary to intracranial epidermoids," *Canadian Journal of Neurological Sciences/Journal Canadien des Sciences Neurologiques*, vol. 11, no. 3, pp. 387–389, 1984.

[4] G. H. Crossley and W. E. Dismukes, "Central nervous system epidermoid cyst: a probable etiology of Mollaret's meningitis," *The American Journal of Medicine*, vol. 89, no. 6, pp. 805-806, 1990.

[5] J.-M. Achard, P.-Y. Lallement, and P. Veyssier, "Recurrent aseptic meningitis secondary to intracranial epidermoid cyst and Mollaret's meningitis: two distinct entities or a single disease? a case report and a nosologic discussion," *The American Journal of Medicine*, vol. 89, no. 6, pp. 807–810, 1990.

[6] F. J. Aristegui, R. A. Delgado, Z. L. Oleaga, and C. C. Hermosa, "Mollaret's recurrent aseptic meningitis and cerebral epidermoid cyst," *Pediatric Neurology*, vol. 18, no. 2, pp. 156–159, 1998.

[7] B. Gao, J. Yang, S. Zhuang et al., "Mollaret meningitis associated with an intraspinal epidermoid cyst," *Pediatrics*, vol. 120, no. 1, p. e220, 2007.

[8] Y. Yoneoka, N. Aizawa, Y. Nonomura, M. Ogi, Y. Seki, and K. Akiyama, "Traumatic nonmissile penetrating transnasal anterior skull base fracture and brain injury with cerebrospinal fluid leak: intraoperative leak detection and an effective reconstruction procedure for a localized skull base defect especially after coronavirus disease 2019 outbreak," *World Neurosurgery*, vol. 140, pp. 166–172, 2020.

[9] X. Meng, Y. Deng, Z. Dai, and Z. Meng, "COVID-19 and anosmia: a review based on up-to-date knowledge," *American Journal of Otolaryngology*, vol. 41, no. 5, p. 102581, 2020.

[10] F. Costa, M. Fornari, G. Felisati, A. Maccari, D. Bauer, and G. Lasio, "Epidermoid cyst of the pituitary stalk," *Neurosurgery Quarterly*, vol. 23, no. 2, pp. 108–111, 2013.

[11] A. C. I. Nakassa, J. D. Chabot, C. H. Snyderman, E. W. Wang, P. A. Gardner, and J. C. Fernandez-Miranda, "Complete endoscopic resection of a pituitary stalk epidermoid cyst using a combined infrasellar interpituitary and suprasellar endonasal approach: case report," *Journal of Neurosurgery*, vol. 128, no. 2, pp. 437–443, 2017.

[12] E. P. McCormack, J. M. Cappuzzo, Z. Litvack, M. I. Almira-Suarez, and J. S. Sherman, "Suprasellar epidermoid cyst originating from the infundibulum: case report and literature review," *Cureus*, vol. 10, Article ID e3226, 2018.

[13] A. Montaser, J. Revuelta Barbero, M. Shahein et al., "Endoscopic endonasal transtuberculum sellae approach for the resection of suprasellar intrainfundibular epidermoid cyst," *Journal of Neurological Surgery Part B: Skull Base*, vol. 79, no. S 03, pp. S279–S280, 2018.

[14] A. B. Khan, E. A. Goethe, C. C. Hadley et al., "Infundibular epidermoid cyst: case report and systematic review," *World Neurosurgery*, vol. 130, pp. 110–114, 2019.

[15] P. Lee, K. M. Krisht, P. Mukunyadzi, and A. F. Krisht, "Resection of an isolated pituitary stalk epidermoid cyst through a pretemporal approach: case report and review of the literature," *World Neurosurgery*, vol. 146, pp. 26–30, 2021.

[16] Y. Li, R. Wang, P.-X. Song et al., "Impact of an educational program on reducing health care-associated meningitis or ventriculitis in the neurosurgical intensive care unit," *American Journal of Infection Control*, vol. 48, no. 6, pp. 621–625, 2020.

[17] M. Fleseriu, M. Buchfelder, J. S. Cetas et al., "Pituitary society guidance: pituitary disease management and patient care recommendations during the COVID-19 pandemic-an international perspective," *Pituitary*, vol. 23, no. 4, pp. 327–337, 2020.

[18] K. Meier and K. Lee, "Neurogenic fever," *Journal of Intensive Care Medicine*, vol. 32, no. 2, pp. 124–129, 2017.

[19] H. Hasani, S. Mardi, S. Shakerian, N. Taherzadeh-Ghahfarokhi, and P. Mardi, "The novel coronavirus disease (COVID-19): a PRISMA systematic review and meta-analysis of clinical and paraclinical characteristics," *BioMed Research International*, vol. 2020, Article ID 3149020, 2020.

[20] C. Childs, "Human brain temperature: regulation, measurement and relationship with cerebral trauma: part 1," *British Journal of Neurosurgery*, vol. 22, no. 4, pp. 486–496, 2008.

[21] M. Griton and J. P. Konsman, "Neural pathways involved in infection-induced inflammation: recent insights and clinical implications," *Clinical Autonomic Research*, vol. 28, no. 3, pp. 289–299, 2018.

[22] R. Ganko, M. Rodriguez, J. Magnussen, M. Simons, E. Myint, and N. Assaad, "Do prophylactic steroids prevent chemical meningitis in surgery for epidermoid cysts? case report and literature review," *Surgical Neurology International*, vol. 11, no. 11, p. 472, 2020.

[23] A. Viallon, F. Zeni, C. Lambert et al., "High sensitivity and specificity of serum procalcitonin levels in adults with bacterial meningitis," *Clinical Infectious Diseases*, vol. 28, no. 6, pp. 1313–1316, 1999.

[24] A. Bender, M. Elstner, R. Paul, and A. Straube, "Severe symptomatic aseptic chemical meningitis following myelography: the role of procalcitonin," *Neurology*, vol. 63, no. 7, pp. 1311–1313, 2004.

[25] D. Velissaris, M. Pintea, N. Pantzaris et al., "The role of procalcitonin in the diagnosis of meningitis: a literature review," *Journal of Clinical Medicine*, vol. 7, no. 6, p. 148, 2018.

[26] M. W. Bijlsma, M. C. Brouwer, E. S. Kasanmoentalib et al., "Community-acquired bacterial meningitis in adults in The Netherlands, 2006-14: a prospective cohort study," *The Lancet Infectious Diseases*, vol. 16, no. 3, pp. 339–347, 2016.

[27] D. van de Beek, J. de Gans, L. Spanjaard, M. Weisfelt, J. B. Reitsma, and M. Vermeulen, "Clinical features and prognostic factors in adults with bacterial meningitis," *New England Journal of Medicine*, vol. 351, no. 18, pp. 1849–1859, 2004.

[28] S. I. Aronin, P. Peduzzi, and V. J. Quagliarello, "Community-acquired bacterial meningitis: risk stratification for adverse clinical outcome and effect of antibiotic timing," *Annals of Internal Medicine*, vol. 129, no. 11, pp. 862–869, 1998.

[29] J. S. Lee, H. J. Baek, C. J. Kim, and E. M. Yang, "Coexistence of central diabetes insipidus and prolonged cerebral salt wasting syndrome after brain tumor surgery: a case report," *Childhood Kidney Diseases*, vol. 24, no. 1, pp. 42–46, 2020.

[30] F. Komatsu, H. Tsugu, M. Komatsu et al., "Clinicopathological characteristics in patients presenting with acute onset of symptoms caused by Rathke's cleft cysts," *Acta Neurochirurgica*, vol. 152, no. 10, pp. 1673–1678, 2010.

[31] C. M. Dancer, M. L. Woods, R. D. Henderson, T. Robertson, M. Mungomery, and A. Allworth, "Mollaret's meningitis and pituitary failure associated with a Rathke's cleft cyst," *Internal Medicine Journal*, vol. 38, no. 7, pp. 609–611, 2008.

[32] B. M. Shear, L. Jin, Y. Zhang et al., "Extent of resection of epidermoid tumors and risk of recurrence: case report and meta-analysis," *Journal of Neurosurgery*, vol. 133, no. 2, pp. 291–301, 2020.

[33] L. Rehman, I. Bokhari, S. U. Siddiqi, V. Bagga, and M. M. Hussain, "Intracranial epidermoid lesions: our experience of 38 cases," *Turkish Neurosurgery*, vol. 28, no. 5, pp. 763–767, 2018.

[34] L. Bertolino, M. Vitrone, and E. Durante-Mangoni, "Does this patient have COVID-19? a practical guide for the internist," *Internal and Emergency Medicine*, vol. 15, no. 5, pp. 791–800, 2020.

19

Lighting Strikes Twice: Recurrent Guillain–Barré Syndrome (GBS) after Influenza Vaccination

Gregory Griffin,[1] Brittany Cunningham,[1] Jonathan M. Beary,[2] Yonatan Spolter,[1] Richard Gandee,[1,2] and Christopher R. Newey[1,3]

[1]*Cleveland Clinic Akron General, Neurological Institute, Akron General Avenue, Akron, OH 44307, USA*
[2]*AT Still University-Missouri Campus, Neurobehavioral Sciences, 800 West Jefferson Avenue, Kirksville, MO 63501, USA*
[3]*Cleveland Clinic, Neurological Institute, 9500 Euclid Avenue, Cleveland, OH 44195, USA*

Correspondence should be addressed to Christopher R. Newey; crnewey@gmail.com

Academic Editor: Roberto Massa

Guillain–Barré syndrome (GBS) is a rare acute demyelinating syndrome of the peripheral nervous system that is commonly preceded by infection. Vaccinations have also been associated with an increased incidence of GBS, though the risk is low. Caution with revaccination is recommended in patients with a history of GBS. Risks of revaccination compared with the risks of influenza complications should be considered. Patients who experience GBS after vaccination have not been shown to have an increased incidence of recurrent GBS after the influenza vaccine, though evidence is limited. We report a case of recurrent GBS in a patient following the influenza vaccine.

1. Introduction

Guillain–Barré syndrome (GBS) is a rare acute demyelinating syndrome of the peripheral nervous system [1]. It is classically characterized by ascending muscle weakness with loss of reflexes that progresses on average over five to ten days. Cerebrospinal fluid (CSF) analysis typically demonstrates an albuminocytologic dissociation (i.e., high CSF protein and normal cell counts) [2]. In severe cases, respiratory failure may occur requiring mechanical ventilation. Annually, there are 0.4–4.0 cases of GBS per 100,000 people. The incidence increases throughout adulthood being the highest in persons older than 75 years of age [3].

GBS is typically preceded by a nonspecific viral prodrome. Often, the offending pathogen is not identified. It has been shown to be associated with *Campylobacter jejuni.* Influenza infection and other upper respiratory tract infections have also been associated with an increased risk of GBS. The association between GBS and the influenza vaccine was first noted during the 1976 swine influenza season [3]. During this season, the cited risk of GBS was one additional case per 100,000 persons vaccinated [3]. The risk was highest within two to three weeks after receiving the vaccine. More recently, the 2009 pH1N1 vaccine was evaluated due to its swine origin [3]. Analysis suggests that with this strain of vaccine, the risk of GBS was 1–3 cases per 1 million persons vaccinated [3]. Overall, the association is approximated at 1-2 additional cases of GBS per 1 million persons vaccinated [3].

We present a case of recurrent GBS in a patient who received the influenza vaccination with a prior history of GBS following influenza vaccination five years prior.

2. Case

A 64-year-old male with a history of remote right middle cerebral artery (MCA) stroke and left hemiplegia was transferred from an outside hospital for ascending weakness of the right hemibody, areflexia, and acute respiratory failure requiring intubation. In 2015, he required 18 days of mechanical ventilation for GBS following influenza vaccination. At that time, he was treated with intravenous immunoglobulin (IVIG) and plasma exchange (PLEX) and made full recovery. He was eventually discharged to a long-term acute care hospital.

The patient received the 2020 influenza vaccine approximately five weeks prior to admission to an outside hospital. He developed paresthesias of the right hemibody and weakness that progressed to inability to feed himself and ultimately respiratory failure 48 hours later. Imaging of the neuraxis showed the prior right MCA stroke (Figure 1). Initial evaluation in the neurosciences intensive care unit found him to be alert. His negative inspiratory pressure (NIF) was −5 cm H_2O (normal > 60 cm H_2O) and right upper and lower extremity power 0/5 with 0/4 reflexes. He was on apixaban for atrial fibrillation; thus, initial lumbar puncture was deferred while waiting for clearance of the medication. Given his history and examination, PLEX was started. He received 5 sessions over a period of 8 days. Lumbar puncture was performed and showed normal cell counts with elevated protein (108 mg/dl (normal 15–45 mg/dl)). Nerve conduction study (NCS) showed prolonged motor distal latencies and severely slowed conduction velocities with reduced compound motor action potential (CMAP; Figure 2). Sural sensory response was normal. *F* waves were absent. Electromyography (EMG) showed fibrillation potentials (+1) in the right deltoid along with severely decreased recruitment in the right triceps and right tibialis anterior. These diagnostic tests were consistent with GBS. He continued to improve clinically. By day seven, right upper extremity strength had improved to 3+/5 and lower extremity at least 3−/5 in proximal muscle groups. Patellar muscle stretch reflex improved to 1+/4 but Achilles reflex remained 0/4. He was successfully extubated and eventually transferred to a long-term acute care hospital for anticipated long-term rehabilitation and treatment.

3. Discussion

We report a case of recurrent GBS. In both incidences, separated by approximately five years, the influenza vaccine was given within 6 weeks prior to symptom onset. GBS is suspected to be immune-mediated in which antibodies respond to antigens and cross-react with nerve ending antigens, resulting in ascending weakness, areflexia, and in serious cases such as respiratory failure, autonomic instability, and death. Infection prior to onset of GBS is common; however, the specific preceding infection is unknown in up to 60% of cases. Data supporting this molecular mimicry hypothesis with specific infectious causes are limited [3]. The prognosis following GBS can be poor with up to 20% of patients remaining severely disabled and mortality in up to 5% of patients. If a patient is unable to walk without assistance, immunotherapy is recommended. Treatment with intravenous immune globulin (IVIG) within 2 weeks of onset is as effective as plasma exchange. IVIG is typically given at 0.4 g/kg bodyweight daily for 5 days or at 2 g/kg bodyweight given in 2 days. PLEX is often performed with a total of 5 exchanges over seven to ten days. The use of PLEX after IVIG is not superior to either therapy alone [2]. There is no role for steroids in treating patients with GBS [4].

There may be an increased risk for developing GBS from pandemic influenza vaccinations (such as H1N1) compared to seasonal vaccination [3, 5]. In several GBS variants, autoantibodies to gangliosides and related glycolipids, including GM1, GD1a, GD1b, and GQ1b, have been described. It is theorized that there is a pathogenetic role involving antibodies to gangliosides after vaccination [6].

Another review aimed to describe vaccination and GBS recurrence in patients with a history of GBS [7]. A total of 550 patients with a history of GBS were identified. Eighteen of these patients initially had onset after influenza vaccine. Two of these patients were revaccinated with the influenza vaccine and did not experience recurrence. In this cohort, 989 vaccines were given to 279 patients. The most common vaccine administered was the influenza vaccine ($n = 107$). Of 550 patients with GBS, 6 individuals had recurrent GBS symptoms. However, there were no episodes of recurrent GBS after influenza vaccine [7]. This information has been recently disputed. In a large, nested case-control study over 4 years in three Chinese cities, the occurrence of GBS following vaccination of any kind was studied [8]. It was found that the odds ratio (OR) for GBS occurrence to be 1.09 (95% CI 0.88–1.32) in adult patients within 180 days following vaccination [8]. The odds ratio for the recurrence of GBS after vaccination was found to be 1.18 (95% CI 0.49–2.65) [8]. In other words, the authors highlight that there was no evidence of an increased risk of GBS and its recurrence within 180 days following vaccination of any kind, including influenza vaccination [8]. If there is recurrence of GBS, neurological symptoms in subsequent episodes are often similar, while the severity of the symptoms and the nature of the preceding infections can differ in individual patients [9].

A case series of patients with recurrent GBS sought to determine if symptoms or proceeding infection was similar in patients with recurrent GBS [9]. Thirty-two patients had a total of 81 episodes of GBS [9]. Clinical symptoms were similar in recurrent episodes in individual patients [9]. However, there was noted variability in preceding infection and severity of symptoms [9]. Patients with recurrent GBS were younger at a mean age of 34.2 years vs. nonrecurrent patients of 46.9 years ($p = 0.001$). Additionally, patients with recurrent GBS more often had Miller Fisher syndrome with the classic clinical triad of ataxia, ophthalmoplegia, and areflexia [9]. Notably, the patient described in our case did not meet all of these characteristics. He was older and had a classic GBS presentation. His presentation, however, was milder than his initial GBS. There likely is a genetic or immunologic host susceptibility that plays a role in recurrent GBS [9].

The Advisory Committee on Immunization Practices currently notes a precaution for revaccination in patients with a history of GBS after an influenza vaccine [4]. The committee also states that influenza vaccination may outweigh the possible risk for certain patients who have a history of GBS within six weeks of influenza vaccine if they are at higher risk for severe complications from influenza [4]. Although recurrence risk is documented to be low, clear risk factors for recurrent GBS have not been consistently defined in the literature. Further studies are needed to determine which patients are at the highest risk for recurrent GBS.

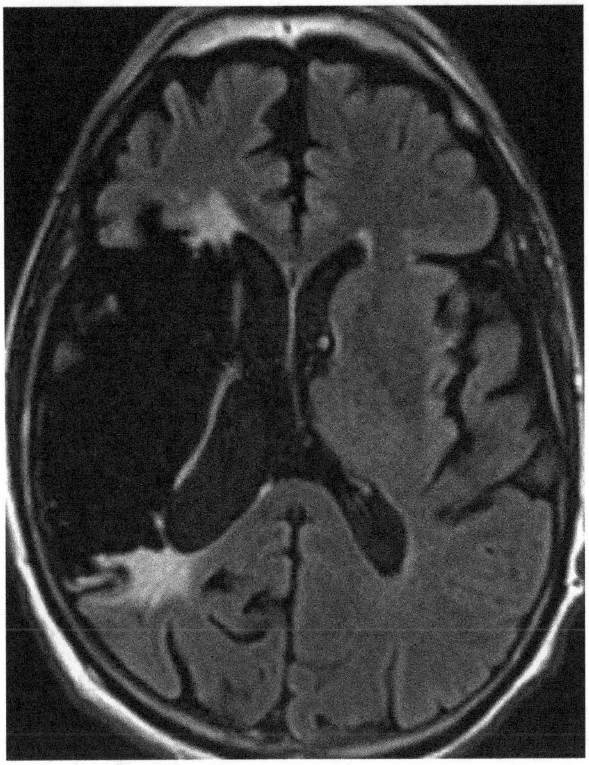

FIGURE 1: Magnetic resonance imaging (MRI). Fluid-attenuated inversion recovery (FLAIR) sequence shows the encephalomalacia from the right middle cerebral artery (MCA) infarct.

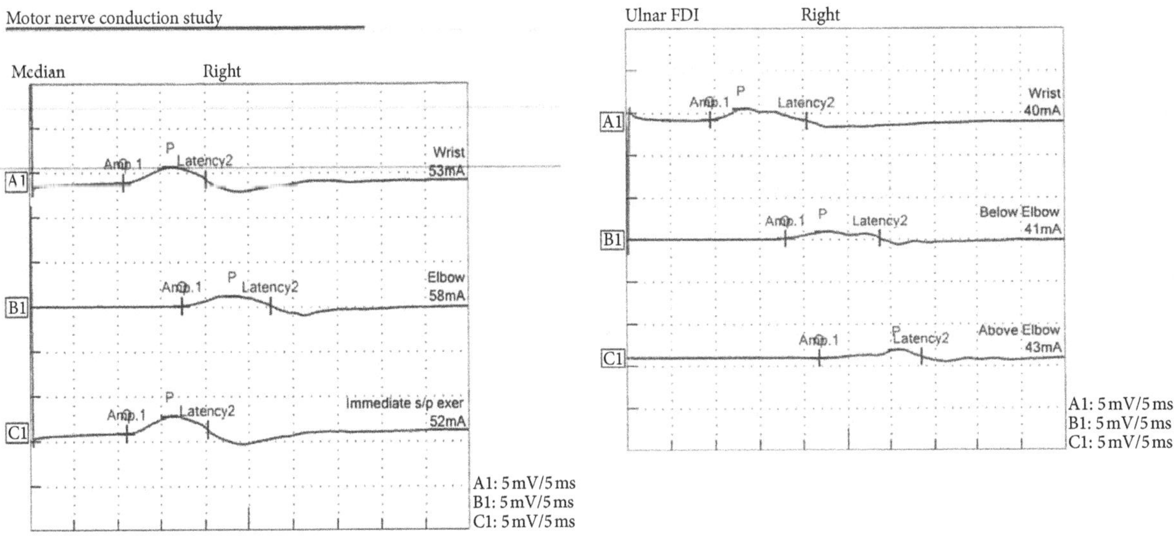

(a) (b)

FIGURE 2: Continued.

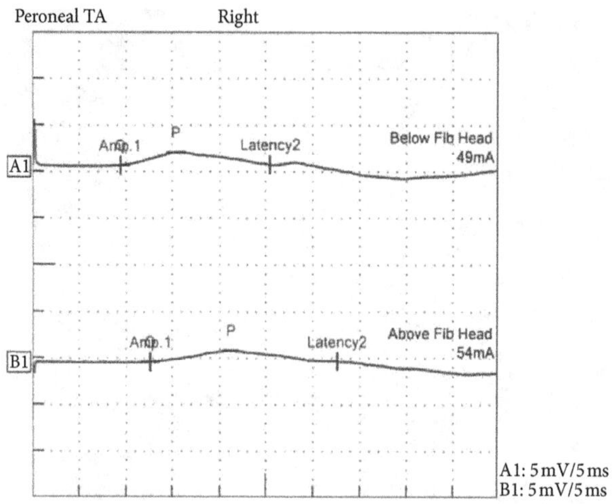

(c)

FIGURE 2: Nerve conduction study (NCS). Prolonged motor latency and reduced compound motor action potential (CMAP) amplitudes are noted and are shown in the median (a), ulnar (b), and peroneal (c) nerves.

4. Conclusion

The risk of GBS following vaccination is low at one to three cases per million patients vaccinated. Additionally, the incidence of GBS recurrence after vaccines appears low but has not been well described. However, despite the low incidence, it is important to carefully weigh risks and benefits of revaccination.

References

[1] H. J. Willison, B. C. Jacobs, and P. A. van Doorn, "Guillain-Barré syndrome," *The Lancet*, vol. 388, pp. 717–727, Article ID 10045, 2016.
[2] N. Yuki and H.-P. Hartung, "Guillain-barré syndrome," *New England Journal of Medicine*, vol. 366, no. 24, pp. 2294–2304, 2012.
[3] C. Vellozzi, S. Iqbal, and K. Broder, "Guillain-barre syndrome, influenza, and influenza vaccination: the epidemiologic evidence," *Clinical Infectious Diseases*, vol. 58, no. 8, pp. 1149–1155, 2014.
[4] L. A. Grohskopf, E. Alyanak, K. R. Broder et al., "Prevention and control of seasonal influenza with vaccines: recommendations of the advisory committee on immunization practices-United States, 2020-21 influenza season," *MMWR. Recommendations and Reports*, vol. 69, no. 8, pp. 1–24, 2020.
[5] L. H. Martín Arias, R. Sanz, M. Sáinz, C. Treceño, and A. Carvajal, "Guillain-Barré syndrome and influenza vaccines: a meta-analysis," *Vaccine*, vol. 33, no. 31, pp. 3773–3778, 2015.
[6] H. C. Lehmann, H.-P. Hartung, B. C. Kieseier, and R. A. Hughes, "Guillain-Barré syndrome after exposure to influenza virus," *The Lancet Infectious Diseases*, vol. 10, no. 9, pp. 643–651, 2010.
[7] R. Baxter, N. Lewis, N. Bakshi, C. Vellozzi, N. P. Klein, and CISA Network, "Recurrent Guillain-Barre syndrome following vaccination," *Clinical Infectious Diseases*, vol. 54, no. 6, pp. 800–804, 2012.
[8] Y. Chen, J. Zhang, X. Chu, Y. Xu, and F. Ma, "Vaccines and the risk of Guillain-Barré syndrome," *European Journal of Epidemiology*, vol. 35, no. 4, pp. 363–370, 2020.
[9] K. Kuitwaard, R. van Koningsveld, L. Ruts, B. C. Jacobs, and P. A. van Doorn, "Recurrent Guillain-Barré syndrome," *Journal of Neurology, Neurosurgery, and Psychiatry*, vol. 80, pp. 6–9, 2009.

20

Clinical Features of Painful Ophthalmoplegia with a High-Intensity Ring Appearance around the Optic Nerve on MRI: A Case Series

Yasunobu Nosaki, Ken Ohyama, Maki Watanabe, Takamasa Yokoi, and Katsushige Iwai

Department of Neurology, Toyohashi Municipal Hospital, Toyohashi, Japan

Correspondence should be addressed to Yasunobu Nosaki; nozaki-yasunobu@toyohashi-mh.jp

Academic Editor: Dennis J. Rivet

Objective. Painful ophthalmoplegia includes nonspecific magnetic resonance imaging (MRI) manifestations and various clinical features including orbital pain and cranial nerve palsies. Treatment for painful ophthalmoplegia remains controversial. The aim of this report was to describe detailed clinical features, MRI findings, treatments, and prognosis of patients with painful ophthalmoplegia. *Patients and Methods.* We retrospectively investigated four cases of patients with painful ophthalmoplegia diagnosed using the International Classification of Headache Disorders, 3rd edition. *Results.* All patients experienced unilateral orbital pain and oculomotor nerve palsy with diplopia but no vision loss. One of the four patients was diagnosed with Tolosa–Hunt syndrome based on the appearance of a granulomatous inflammation of the cavernous sinus on MRI. No specific lesions were detected on brain MRI for the other three patients; therefore, their headaches were attributed to ischaemic ocular motor nerve palsy. In all patients, a high-intensity ring appearance around the ipsilateral optic nerve was observed on MRI. Steroid therapy was administered to these patients, and good prognoses were anticipated. *Conclusion.* These results indicate that prednisolone is a useful treatment for painful ophthalmoplegia that displays ipsilateral hyperintense ring lesions around the optic nerve on MRI, regardless of the presence of granulomatous inflammation of the cavernous sinus.

1. Introduction

Painful ophthalmoplegia is a pathologic condition caused by nonspecific inflammation of the cavernous sinus due to tumors, vasculitis, basal meningitis, neurosarcoidosis, or diabetes [1]. It consists of periorbital or hemicranial pain with ipsilateral ocular motor nerve palsy and other cranial nerve palsies [1]. Due to the nonspecific nature of the inflammation, strategies for diagnosis, classifications, and treatment for painful ophthalmoplegia remain controversial. The International Classification of Headache Disorders, 3rd edition (ICHD-3), published in 2018, describes the diagnostic criteria of diseases applicable to painful ophthalmoplegia, including Tolosa–Hunt syndrome (THS), headache attributed to ischaemic ocular motor nerve palsy, and recurrent painful ophthalmoplegic neuropathy [2]. Brain magnetic resonance imaging (MRI) manifestations of painful ophthalmoplegia frequently reveal nonspecific findings, whereas some cases with normal brain MRI findings have been reported [3]. Herein, we present the cases of four patients with painful ophthalmoplegia diagnosed using ICHD-3 and describe the clinical features, MRI findings, and prognosis following considerable treatment.

2. Patients and Methods

We retrospectively investigated four patients with painful ophthalmoplegia who were referred to the Toyohashi Municipal Hospital between October 2014 and April 2019. The diagnosis of painful ophthalmoplegia was based on the ICHD-3 criteria. All patients underwent clinical and neurologic assessments, brain MRI, and treatment for painful ophthalmoplegia. Patient characteristics and clinical courses are described below and summarized in Table 1 and Figure 1.

Table 1: Clinical characteristics and MRI findings of our cases.

Case	Age/Sex	Diagnosis	Side	Underlying disease	Involvement of the cranial nerves	Visual disturbance	MRI findings: Granulomatous inflammation of the cavernous	MRI findings: High-intensity ring appearance around the optic nerve	Response to steroid therapy	Recurrence
1	39/M	T	Left	–	III, VI	–	+ (left)	+ (left)	+	–
2	68/F	H	Left	Diabetes mellitus	III	–	–	+ (left)	+	–
3	76/M	H	Right	Hypertension	III	–	–	+ (right)	+	–
4	67/M	H	Right	Hypertension	III, VI	–	–	+ (right)	+	–

+, present; –, absent; MRI, magnetic resonance imaging; III, oculomotor nerve; VI, abducens nerve; T, Tolosa–Hunt syndrome; H, headache attributed to ischaemic ocular motor nerve palsy.

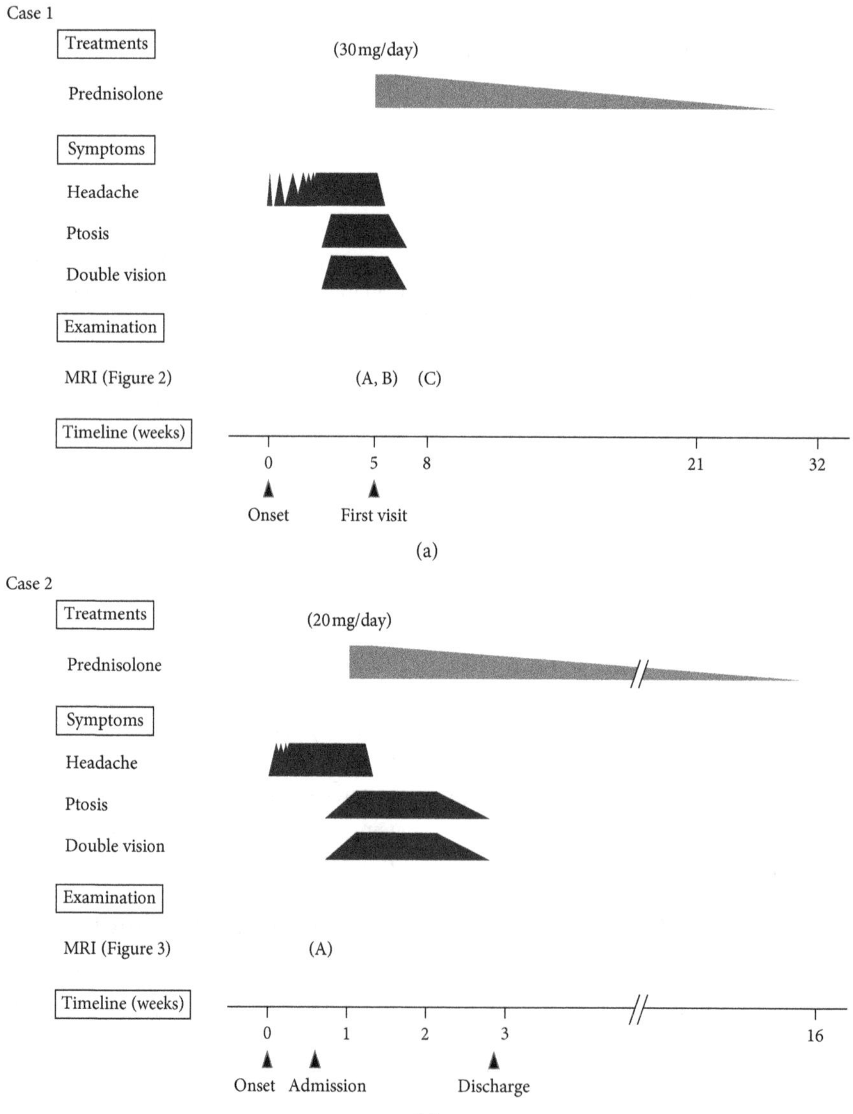

Figure 1: Continued.

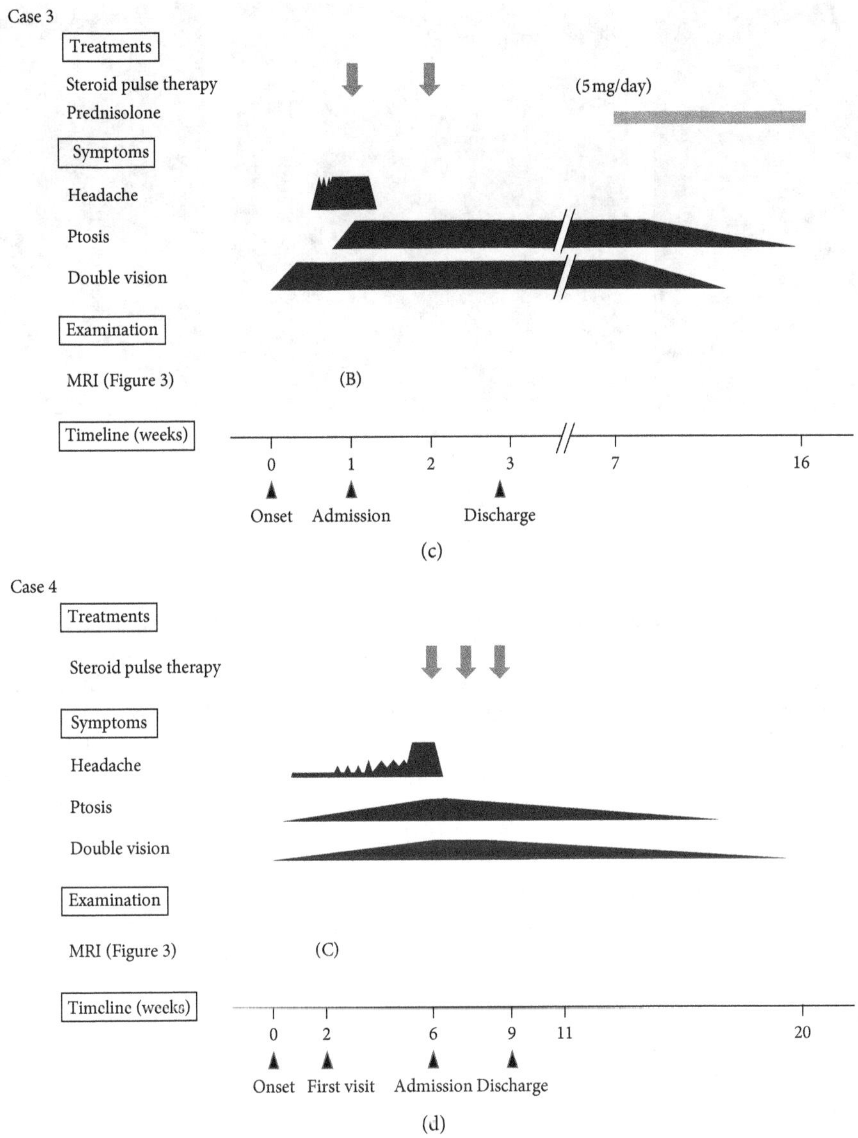

FIGURE 1: Clinical courses of patients with painful ophthalmoplegia during steroid therapy.

3. Report of Cases

3.1. Case 1. A 39-year-old man was referred for diplopia and left ptosis with severe headache persisting five weeks prior to the visit. Initially, he experienced recurring, abrupt, throbbing pain around his left cheek. The pain became more frequent and acquired a stabbing quality in the left peri-orbital and retro-orbital regions. Two weeks following onset of left unilateral pain, he developed left ptosis and his diplopia worsened with leftward gaze. At the time of the first visit to our department, he was alert, well-oriented, and afebrile. Although the neurological examination revealed third and sixth cranial nerve palsies, there were no visual field defects or visual disturbances. Conjunctival injection, chemosis, and periorbital edema were not observed in either eye. Funduscopic examination revealed no abnormalities in either eye, including the optic nerves. There were no neurological defects in other cranial nerve functions, the trunk of the patient, or his extremities.

Blood cell counts and blood chemistry tests were unremarkable. His C-reactive protein and β-D-glucan levels were normal. Tests for antineutrophil cytoplasmic autoantibody, myeloperoxidase antineutrophil cytoplasmic autoantibody, and Aspergillus and Cryptococcus antigens were negative. His brain MRI showed a mass lesion in the left cavernous sinus. The lesion was enhanced on the T1-weighted image and was observed to have extended into the superior orbital fissure (Figure 2(a)). Moreover, a high-intensity ring appearance around the left optic nerve was observed on short tau inversion recovery (STIR) MRI (Figure 2(b)).

This patient was diagnosed with THS and was treated with prednisolone (30 mg/day). Four days after treatment initiation, his headache improved. His diplopia and ptosis improved gradually after one week of steroid therapy. The patient fully recovered after oral prednisolone treatment which was subsequently tapered off over six months.

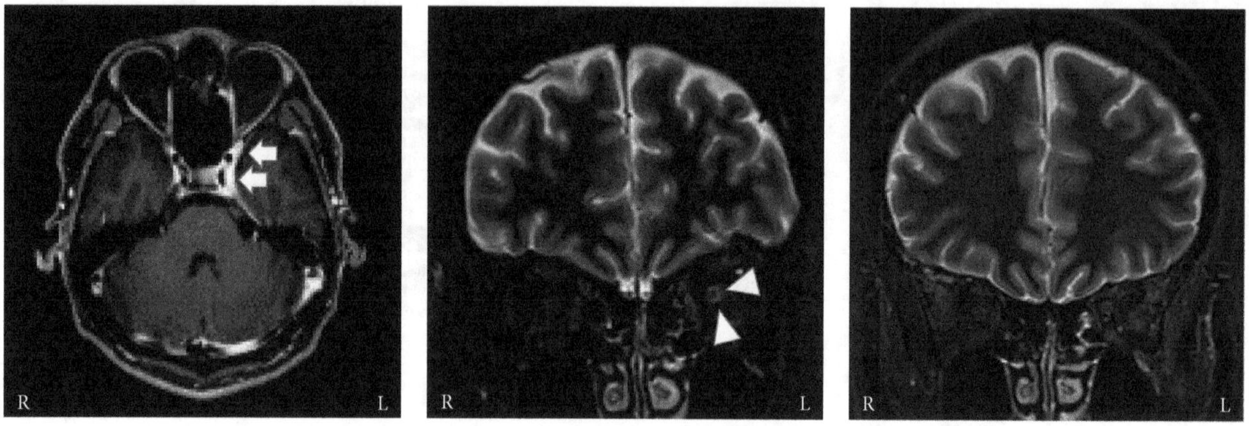

(a) (b) (c)

FIGURE 2: .Brain MRI of case 1. (a) The lesion (arrows) is enhanced on T1-weighted image and extends into the superior orbital fissure. (b) The high-intensity ring appearance (arrowheads) around the left optic nerve is seen on short tau inversion recovery (STIR) MRI. (c) The high-intensity ring appearance has disappeared on day 21 after initiating treatment.

His follow-up brain MRI three weeks after starting treatment revealed a reduction of the asymmetrical high-intensity ring appearance around the optic nerve (Figure 2(c)). He experienced no recurrence of his symptoms after discontinuing prednisolone although MRI images indicated that the lesion in the cavernous sinus remained until eight months after the onset.

3.2. Case 2. A 68-year-old woman was admitted to our hospital with severe headache. Her headache had emerged successively from three days prior and deteriorated gradually. She felt persistent pinprick retro-orbital pain on the left side. On day two of hospitalization, diplopia developed. She had a history of non-insulin-dependent diabetes mellitus with preproliferative diabetic retinopathy and had been treated with metformin, pioglitazone, and glimepiride for 20 years.

She was alert and well-oriented. Her pupils and light reflex were normal, and ptosis was not observed. She presented with oculomotor palsy with limited adduction ability on the left side, indicating incomplete left cranial nerve III palsy. No other neurological abnormalities or visual disturbances were observed. Conjunctival injection, chemosis, and periorbital edema were not observed upon ophthalmological examination. Funduscopic examination revealed preproliferative diabetic retinopathy in both eyes. Central critical flicker fusion frequency (CFF) was 38 Hz in the right eye and 36 Hz in the left eye (reference >35 Hz).

Her laboratory examinations, including cerebrospinal fluid (CSF) study, were unremarkable other than hemoglobin A1c (HbA1c) level of 7.6% (reference, 4.6–6.2%). Her MRI revealed no abnormalities in the brain and cavernous sinus, while a high-intensity ring appearance around the left optic nerve was observed on STIR MRI (Figure 3(a)). Using ICHD-3, we diagnosed her with headache attributed to ischaemic ocular motor nerve palsy due to diabetes mellitus. An effective treatment for painful ophthalmoplegia in diabetes mellitus has not been determined. As we considered the existence of inflammation around the orbital lesion to be due to the high-intensity ring appearance on MRI, prednisolone was administered, in a manner similar to the management of THS. Two days after initiation of prednisolone (20 mg/day) her headache gradually improved. She was discharged with improvement of diplopia 10 days after admission. Prednisolone was tapered and discontinued after four months, and she remained symptom-free for four years.

3.3. Case 3. A 76-year-old man was admitted to our hospital with diplopia, right ptosis, and right retro-orbital severe pain which began one week prior to the visit. Initially, he experienced diplopia without pain. Three days later, he developed persistent throbbing pain around the right periorbital and retro-orbital regions. Six days after the onset of diplopia, he developed right ptosis. He had a history of hypertension, controlled with medication, and left branch retinal vein occlusion at 73 years of age.

At the time of visit, he was alert and well-oriented. His pupils and photopupillary reflex were normal, but ptosis was observed on the right side, indicating right cranial nerve III palsy. There were no other neurological abnormalities or visual field defects. Although he had slight visual disturbances in the left eye because of previous left retinal vein occlusion, he had no visual disturbances in the right eye. No abnormalities were observed in either eye upon further ophthalmological examinations, with the exception of left retinal branch vein occlusion.

Blood cell counts and blood chemistry tests were unremarkable. Although no abnormalities or mass lesions in the cavernous and paranasal sinus were observed in MRI, a high-intensity ring appearance around the right optic nerve was observed in fat-suppressed T2-weighted MRI (Figure 3(b)).

He was diagnosed with headache attributed to ischaemic ocular motor nerve palsy based on ICHD-3 due to risk factors for microvascular ischemia. As we considered the existence of inflammation around the orbital lesion to be due

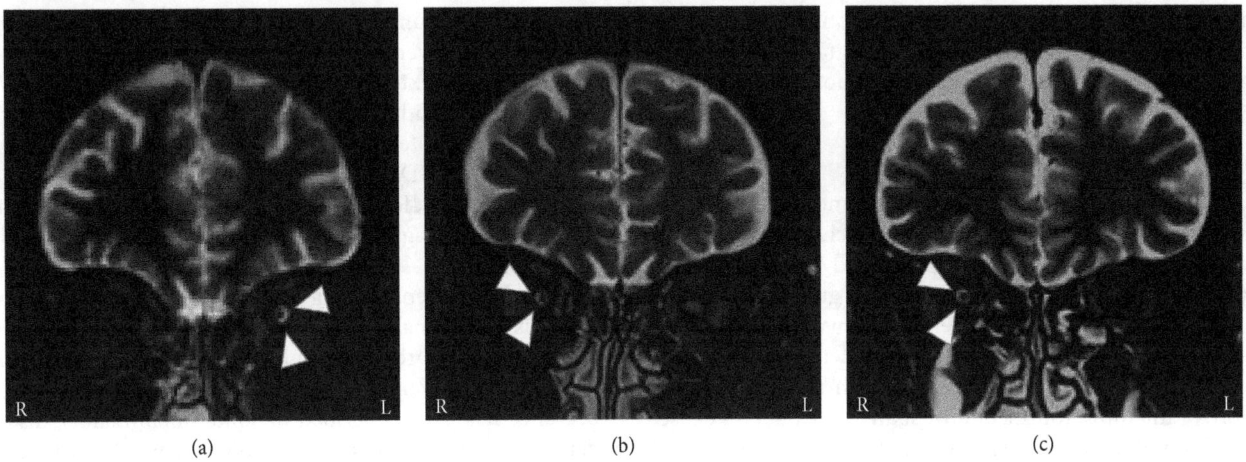

FIGURE 3: Brain MRI of cases 2–4. In case 2 (a), the high-intensity ring appearance (arrowheads) around the left optic nerve is found on STIR MRI. In cases 3 (b) and 4 (c), the high-intensity ring appearance (arrowheads) around the right optic nerve is found on fat-suppressed T2-weighted MRI.

to the high-intensity ring appearance on MRI, prednisolone was administered, in a manner similar to the management of THS. On the following initiation of steroid pulse therapy (intravenous methylprednisolone 1000 mg/day for three days), his headache improved. A second steroid pulse therapy was initiated one week later due to gradual improvements in diplopia and right ptosis in response to prednisolone. He was discharged on day 18. Because of persistent ptosis, oral prednisolone (5 mg/day) was prescribed. His symptoms fully recovered after four months; therefore, prednisolone was discontinued. There was no recurrence of his symptoms for over six months.

3.4. Case 4. A 67-year-old man with a history of mild hypertension was referred to our hospital because of headache, right ptosis, and diplopia. He noticed diplopia 11 days before his first visit. Three days after developing diplopia, he experienced right ptosis and dull pain in the right periorbital region. He was admitted one month after his first visit because his headache, ptosis, and diplopia progressively deteriorated. On admission, he complained of continuous severe headaches in the right periorbital area. He was alert and well-oriented. The diameter of his pupil was 4 mm in the right eye and 2 mm in the left eye in a bright room. Pupil responses to light were dull in the right eye. Divergent squint and outward and downward displacement of the right eye were observed. No abnormalities in the visual field or visual acuity were observed. The conjunctival injection, chemosis, and periorbital edema were not detected upon an ophthalmological examination. Funduscopic examination revealed no abnormalities in either eye, including the optic nerves. Further, no neurological abnormalities of other cranial nerve functions, the trunk of the patient, and his extremities were observed.

Blood cell counts, blood chemistry, and cerebrospinal fluid tests were unremarkable. While no mass lesion in the cavernous sinus was detected by brain MRI, a high-intensity ring appearance around the right optic nerve was observed in fat-suppressed T2-weighted MRI (Figure 3(c)).

There was no evidence of infectious diseases or tumors. Given the patient's history of mild hypertension, which is a risk factor for microvascular ischemia, we diagnosed him with headache attributed to ischaemic ocular motor nerve palsy according to ICHD-3. We considered the existence of inflammation around the orbital lesion to be due to the high-intensity ring appearance on MRI. Therefore, prednisolone was administered, in a manner similar to the management of THS. Steroid pulse therapy (intravenous methylprednisolone 1000 mg/day for 3 days) was initiated, and his headache improved immediately on day two of therapy. As ptosis and diplopia persisted, steroid pulse therapy was three times the duration. These symptoms gradually improved, and he was discharged three weeks after admission with no prescription for oral prednisolone. He fully recovered six months after the onset, with no recurrence of symptoms for over 10 months.

4. Results

All patients had unilateral orbital pain and oculomotor nerve palsy, and two patients also showed cranial nerve VI palsy. They had no visual field defects or visual loss upon examinations by the ophthalmologist.

All patients underwent MRI examinations during the acute stage. MRI findings are summarized in Table 1. One patient was diagnosed with THS based on the appearance of granulomatous inflammation of the cavernous sinus on MRI. The other three patients had no abnormal lesions of the cavernous sinus and were diagnosed with headache attributed to ischaemic ocular motor nerve palsy due to the existence of risk factors for microvascular ischemia based on ICHD-3. All patients' MRIs revealed high-intensity ring appearance around the optic nerve of the ipsilateral lesion in brain MRI.

All patients were treated with prednisolone and responded well, particularly in terms of immediate headache improvement. Follow-up MRI was available for only one patient, which indicated the disappearance of the high-intensity ring appearance around the optic nerve. None of the patients experienced relapse of orbital pain and ophthalmoplegia after discounting prednisolone.

5. Discussion

Painful ophthalmoplegia is classified under three groups according to ICHD-3: THS, headache attributed to ischaemic ocular motor nerve palsy, and recurrent painful ophthalmoplegic neuropathy. THS is a granulomatous inflammatory disease of the cavernous sinus, superior orbital fissure, or the orbit [4, 5] and has been defined as unilateral orbit or periorbital pain associated with palsies of one or more of the third, fourth, and/or sixth cranial nerves caused by a granulomatous inflammation [2]. Diagnosis of THS requires the presence of the granulomatous inflammation of these lesions demonstrated by either MRI or biopsy. For the treatment of THS, prednisolone is recognized as standard therapy with positive outcomes. Headache attributed to ischaemic ocular motor nerve palsy is described as unilateral frontal and/or periorbital pain and is caused by, and associated with, clinical signs of ischaemic paresis of the ipsilateral third, fourth, and/or sixth cranial nerves [2]. Patients with headache attributed to ischaemic ocular motor nerve palsy tend to have one or more vasculopathic risk factors, including diabetes, hypertension, and hypercholesterolemia [6] with no specific abnormalities on MRI [7]. Management and effective treatment of headache attributed to ischaemic ocular motor nerve palsy, despite the history of diabetes mellitus, have not been established. Recurrent painful ophthalmoplegic neuropathy, previously known as ophthalmoplegic migraine, is described by repeated attacks of one or more ocular cranial nerves (commonly the third cranial nerve) with ipsilateral headache [2, 8]. To diagnose recurrent painful ophthalmoplegic neuropathy, recurrences of the typical symptoms and exclusion of orbital, parasellar, or posterior fossa lesions are necessary [2]. Although no granulomatous inflammation was observed on MRI, it has been reported that brain MRI can detect the gadolinium enhancement or nerve thickening of cranial nerves [2]. In our study, cases 2, 3, and 4 had no typical MRI findings of THS, and no relapse of orbital pain and ophthalmoplegia; therefore, we diagnosed these patients with headache attributed to ischaemic ocular motor nerve palsy.

MRI findings are necessary for the diagnosis of painful ophthalmoplegia. Specifically, THS and recurrent painful ophthalmoplegic neuropathy are described in terms of their typical MRI abnormalities. In this study, all patients presented with the high-intensity ring appearance around the optic nerve on STIR or fat-suppressed T2-weighted MRI without presenting with visual disturbances. Although this MRI finding has been reported in a few other studies [9, 10], its clinical utility has not been evaluated in patients with painful ophthalmoplegia. The high-intensity ring appearance around the optic nerve on fat-suppressed T2-weighted MRI was also reported in patients with THS. It has been suggested that the presence of intracranial pressure elevation or peripheral circulatory insufficiency is due to compression caused by granulomatous lesions [9]. In patients with THS, optic nerve dysfunction occurs because the inflammatory lesions in the cavernous sinus involve the orbital apex and optic nerve, and extensive lesions were observed in MRI [10]. In the present study, cases 2, 3, and 4 were diagnosed with headaches attributed to ischaemic ocular motor nerve palsy according to ICHD-3 because there were no granulomatous lesions on brain MRI. However, there is no description of the high-intensity ring appearance around the optic nerve in ICHD-3.

The high-intensity ring appearance around the optic nerve is occasionally observed with all forms of inflammation or compression, which are not disease specific changes. Moreover, the unilateral high-intensity ring appearance has been described in some inflammatory disorders such as dysthyroid optic neuropathy, optic neuritis, and inflammatory optic neuropathies [11]. Therefore, we considered the high-intensity ring appearance around the optic nerve as a significant indicator for the existence of inflammation around the orbital lesion.

To investigate the etiology of the lesion, biopsy is the gold standard. However, biopsy of the lesion is challenging unless the patient complains of visual loss. We suggest that the appearance of the high-intensity ring around the optic nerve seems to be reflected in some minor inflammation without visual disturbance, and there is some possibility of visual dysfunction being caused by the progression of the disease. When the symptoms include either a high-intensity ring appearance showing ipsilateral to headache or ophthalmoplegia, clinicians should be attentive to the patient's visual function and consider the prompt initiation of treatment.

Focusing on the prognosis of painful ophthalmoplegia, the response to steroid therapy is different in each disease diagnosed by ICHD-3. Though THS and recurrent painful ophthalmoplegic neuropathy improved well with steroid therapy due to their inflammatory pathogenesis, headaches attributed to ischaemic ocular motor nerve palsy, particularly with diabetes, do not respond similarly [3]. In this report, we administered steroid therapy to all patients because of the existence of inflammation suspected by the high-intensity ring appearance. Although cases 2, 3, and 4 were diagnosed with headaches attributed to ischaemic ocular motor nerve palsy, all patients had a positive response and excellent prognosis to steroid therapy. We supposed that the high-intensity ring appearance was caused by inflammation given the improvement following steroid therapy. Therefore, the high-intensity ring appearance may be considered as a radiological hallmark for administering steroids to patients with painful ophthalmoplegia. Additional information about the high-intensity ring appearance is needed for the diagnostic criteria of painful ophthalmoplegia.

6. Conclusion

Despite the absence of visual disturbances in patients with painful ophthalmoplegia, attention should be paid to potential ipsilateral high-intensity ring appearance around the optic nerve on MRI. If this is detected, the existence of inflammation in the orbital apex or cavernous sinus should be suspected. Moreover, steroid therapy should be considered for improving these symptoms.

References

[1] L. B. Kline and W. F. Hoyt, "Nosological entities? The Tolosa-Hunt syndrome," *Journal of Neurology, Neurosurgery & Psychiatry*, vol. 71, no. 5, pp. 577–582, 2001.

[2] ICHD-3, "Headache classification committee of the international headache society, "the international classification of headache disorders, 3rd edition," *Cephalalgia*, vol. 38, no. 1, pp. 1–211, 2018.

[3] C. H. Hung, K. H. Chang, C. C. Chu et al., "Painful ophthalmoplegia with normal cranial imaging," *BMC Neurology*, vol. 14, no. 1, pp. 1–7, 2014.

[4] E. Tolosa, "Periarteritic lesions of the carotid siphon with the clinical features of a carotid infraclinoidal aneurysm," *Journal of Neurology, Neurosurgery & Psychiatry*, vol. 17, no. 4, pp. 300–302, 1954.

[5] W. E. Hunt, J. N. Meagher, H. E. Lefever, and W. Zeman, "Painful ophthalmoplegia: its relation to indolent inflammation of the cavernous sinus," *Neurology*, vol. 11, no. 1, p. 56, 1961.

[6] M. A. Tamhankar, V. Biousse, G.-S. Ying et al., "Isolated third, fourth, and sixth cranial nerve palsies from presumed microvascular versus other causes," *Ophthalmology*, vol. 120, no. 11, pp. 2264–2269, 2013.

[7] A. P. Murchison, M. E. Gilbert, and P. J. Savino, "Neuroimaging and acute ocular motor mononeuropathies," *Archives of Ophthalmology*, vol. 129, no. 3, pp. 301–305, 2011.

[8] ICHD, "Headache classification subcommittee of the international headache society, "the international classification of headache disorders: 2nd edition," *Cephalalgia*, vol. 24, no. Suppl 1, pp. 9–160, 2004.

[9] A. Tamura, A. Taniguchi, N. Ochiai, R. Sasaki, Y. Narita, and S. Kuzuhara, ""Tram-track" sign and "donut configuration" in Tolosa-Hunt syndrome," *Rinsho Shinkeigaku*, vol. 48, no. 4, pp. 271–274, 2008, in Japanese.

[10] C.-H. Hung, K.-H. Chang, Y.-M. Wu et al., "A comparison of benign and inflammatory manifestations of Tolosa-Hunt syndrome," *Cephalalgia*, vol. 33, no. 10, pp. 842–852, 2013.

[11] J. Selhorst and Y. Chen, "The optic nerve," *Seminars in Neurology*, vol. 29, no. 1, pp. 029–035, 2009.

21

Rasmussen's Encephalitis: A Report of a Tunisian Pediatric Case and Literature Review

Hedia Klaa,[1,2] Thouraya Ben Younes,[1,2] Hanene Benrhouma,[1,2] Sonia Nagi,[2,3] Aida Rouissi,[1,2] Ichraf Kraoua,[1,2] and Ilhem Ben Youssef-Turki[1,2]

[1]*Department of Child and Adolescent Neurology, Research Laboratory LR18SP04, National Institute Mongi Ben Hmida of Neurology, Tunis, Tunisia*
[2]*University of Tunis El Manar, Faculty of Medicine of Tunis, Tunis 1007, Tunisia*
[3]*Department of Neuroradiology, National Institute Mongi Ben Hmida of Neurology, Tunis, Tunisia*

Correspondence should be addressed to Thouraya Ben Younes; bythouraya@yahoo.fr

Academic Editor: Peter Berlit

Rasmussen's encephalitis (RE) is a rare progressive inflammatory disease of the central nervous system. It is characterized by unilateral hemispheric atrophy, pharmacoresistant focal seizures, and progressive neurological deficit. The exact etiopathogenesis still remains unknown. Brain imaging plays an important role in diagnosis and follow-up. Fluctuation of lesions in brain imaging was reported in few cases. Herein, we report an additional pediatric case of Rasmussen encephalitis with fluctuating changes in brain MRI.

1. Introduction

Rasmussen's encephalitis (RE) was first described in the late 1950s. It is a rare neurological disease of childhood characterized by unilateral hemispheric atrophy, pharmacoresistant focal seizures, and progressive neurological deficits. The exact etiopathogenesis still remains unknown. Brain imaging plays a pivotal role in diagnosis and control of disease progression. Few cases with atypical MRI features of RE represented by improvement and reoccurrence of signal abnormalities were reported.

We report on the clinical, electrophysiological, and imaging data of an additional pediatric case of RE with atypical MRI features.

2. Case Study

An 11-year-old boy was born to nonconsanguineous parents. He had a family history of febrile seizures in his sister, epilepsy in 2 cousins, and ulcerative colitis in his mother. He had no significant antenatal and perinatal history. Psychomotor development was normal. He was treated for adrenal insufficiency and dysthyroïdism. On August 2014, he was referred to our department, at the age of 11, with focal clonic right-sided seizures, which were preceded by gastroenteritis 1 month ago. Neurological examination showed right hemidystonia, myoclonia, right pyramidal syndrome, and right hemihypoesthesia. Interictal electroencephalogram (EEG) showed left frontotemporal discharge persisting during sleep (Figure 1). Brain magnetic resonance imaging (MRI) showed cortical and subcortical hyperintensity on T2-weighted (T2) and fluid-attenuated inversion recovery (FLAIR) images in the left frontoinsular region, homolateral lenticular, and caudate nuclei (Figure 2(a)). Spine MRI was normal. Initially, the diagnosis of acute disseminated encephalomyelitis (ADEM) was suspected. Routine blood and cerebrospinal fluid investigations were normal. Infectious serologies (HSV, CMV, EBV, HIV, VZV, HVC, HVB, syphilis, and Lyme) and immunological assessment (ANA, anti-DNA, ANCA, APL, ACL, anti-B2GP1, and anti-ENA) were negative. The patient received a pulse of steroids (1 g/day) during 5 days and, then, relay per os at the dose of 1 mg/kg/day for 10 days. Valproic acid and clobazam were prescribed with clinical improvement and partial seizure

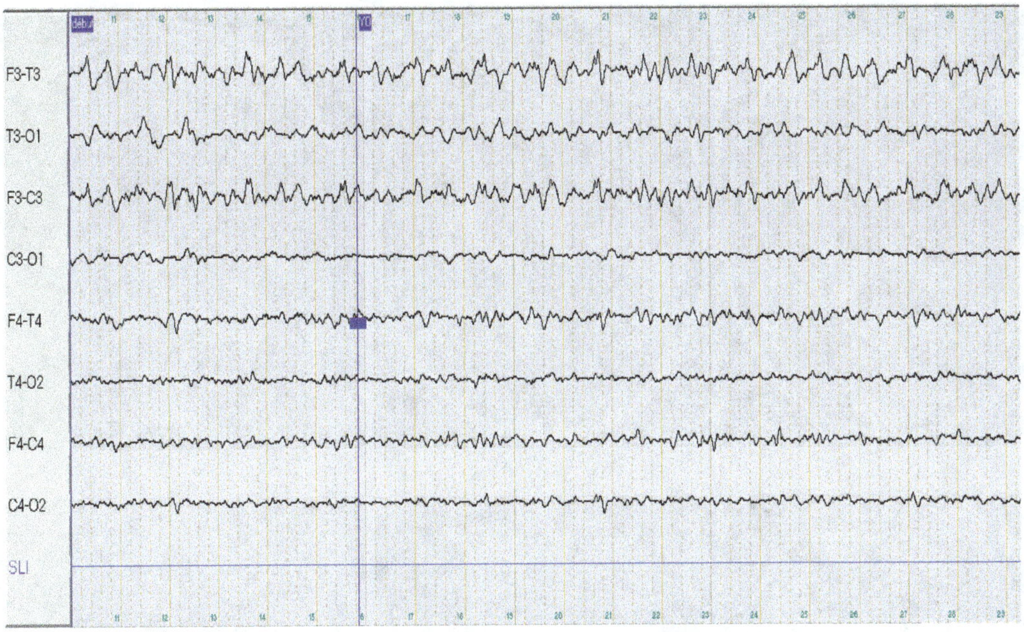

Figure 1: EEG showing asymmetric background activity with the left frontotemporal intercritical discharges.

control. A second brain MRI performed after 3 weeks was normal. On April 2015, he presented with intractable focal right seizures, progressive impairment of language abilities, and behavioral disorders with irritability, eating disorders (polyphagia), and worsening school performance with working memory problems. Neurological examination showed right hemiparesis and dystonia of the right upper limb. Given the fluctuating subacute course, seizures, behavioral disturbances, and progressive cognitive impairment, autoimmune encephalitis was suspected. Serum and CSF screening for an anti-N-methyl-D-aspartate (NMDA) receptor, anti-leucine-rich glioma-inactivated protein1 (LGi1), anti-contactin-associated protein-2 (Caspr2), anti-2-amino-3-(3-hydroxy-5-methylisoxazol-4-yl), propanoic acid (anti-AMPA), anti-GABAa and anti-GABAb, anti-glycine, anti-amphiphysin, anti-Hu, anti-Yo, anti-Ri, anti-CV2, anti-Ma1, and anti-GAD were negative. The brain MRI showed cortical hyperintensity on T2 and FLAIR images in left frontoinsular, left frontoinsular cortical atrophy with homolateral striatum atrophy, and dilatation of the ipsilateral ventricular system (Figure 2(b)). Given the clinical course and MRI finding, the diagnosis of RE was performed. Numerous regimens of antiepileptic drugs were prescribed (valproic acid 2 g/day, carbamazepine 1400 mg/day, levetiracetam 2500 mg/day, clonazepam 4 mg/day, and piracetam 1600 mg/day). A monthly steroid pulse at a dose of 1 g/day for 3 days was administered during 12 months. Azathioprine was prescribed on January 2017 at the dose of 100 mg/day. Partial control of seizures was obtained. Nevertheless, he presented with several status epilepticus concomitant to infectious episodes. The motor function improved mildly. A control of the brain MRI was performed on September 2017 and showed an increase of the left hemispheric atrophy (Figure 2(c)).

3. Discussion

We report the case of an 11-year-old boy presenting with focal seizures. The diagnosis of Rasmussen's encephalitis (RE) was made due to the clinical and radiological findings. Our patient illustrates a rare case of RE with fluctuating signal abnormalities on brain MRI.

RE is a progressive chronic inflammatory disease of the central nervous system. It was first reported by Theodore Rasmussen in 1958 [1]. The disorder is rare and affects mostly children. The median age of onset is 6 years. Our patient had a late-onset RE. Both sexes are equally affected [2, 3]. It is characterized by focal intractable seizures, progressive neurological deficit, and cognitive decline, with unihemispheric brain atrophy, found in our patient [2]. The etiopathogenesis of RE is unknown. Suggested etiologies include viral infections, an autoimmune phenomenon involving circulating antibodies against glutamate receptors, and cytotoxic T cells [3, 4]. Diagnosis of RE is based on characteristic clinical, radiological, and pathological features. Diagnostic criteria were established by Bien et al. in 2005 [5]. Three stages have been proposed. The prodromal stage is manifested with mild signs (low seizure frequency and mild hemiparesis). The acute stage is characterized by frequent focal seizures, progressive hemiparesis, and cognitive deterioration. The residual stage is characterized by stabilization of neurological deficits and continuation of seizures, but less frequent than in the acute stage [6]. In some cases, less common presentations such as unilateral movement disorders, including hemiathetosis and hemidystonia, have been reported [7]. Our patient had right hemidystonia.

Brain MRI is an important tool for diagnostic assessment and follow-up in RE [2, 5]. The majority of patients show, at an earlier stage, unilateral enlargement of the ventricular system which is accentuated in the insular and periinsular

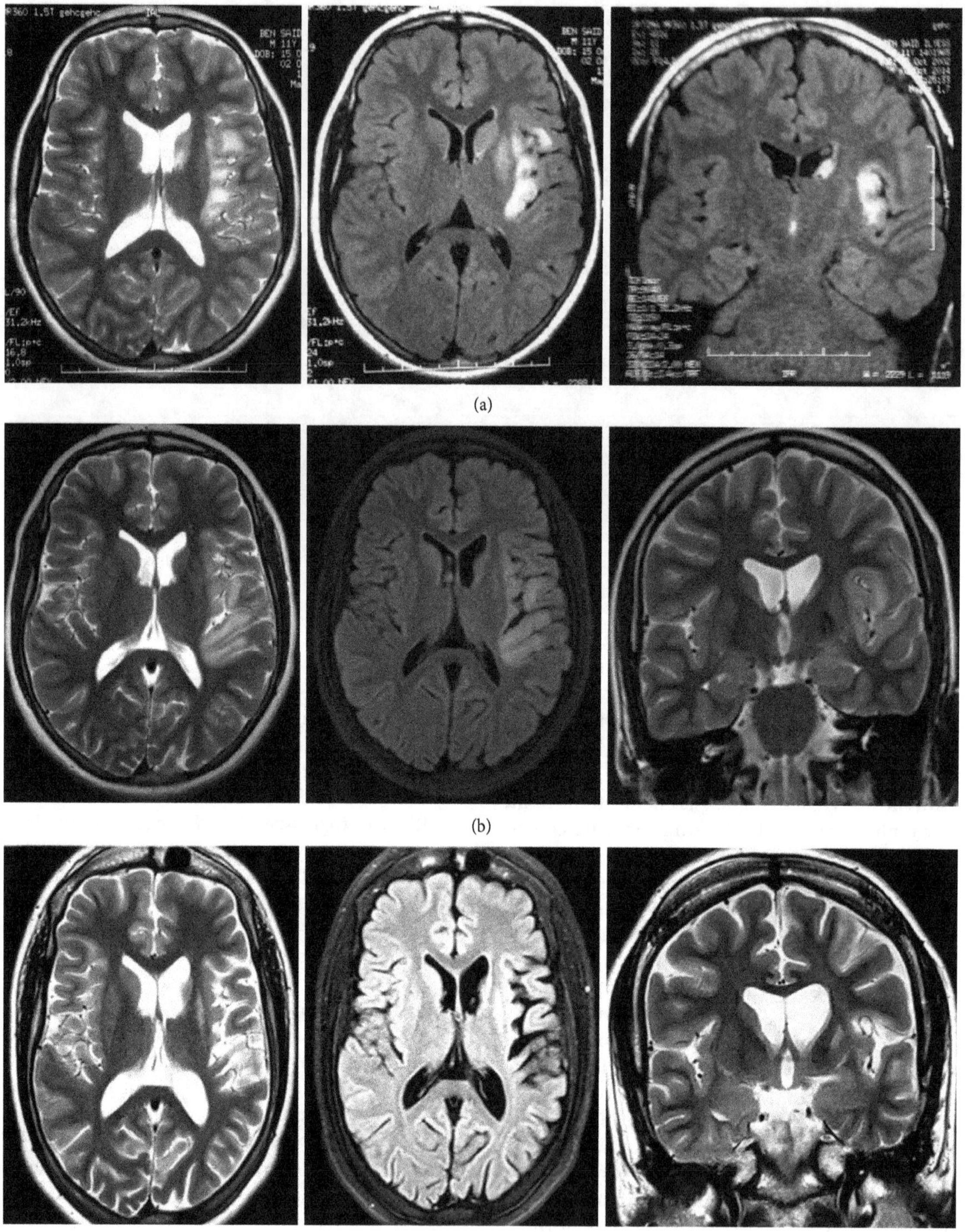

(a)

(b)

(c)

FIGURE 2: Serial MRIs in T2 and FLAIR sequences showing hyperintensity in the left frontoinsular region, lenticular, and caudate nuclei (a). Seven months after the first MRI, persistence of hyperintensity, left fronto-insular cortical and homolateral striatum atrophy, and dilatation of the ipsilateral ventricular system (b). After 3 years and 9 months from the first MRI, we noticed an increase of the left hemispheric atrophy (c).

regions. A T2/FLAIR hyperintense signal is often present in the cortical or subcortical regions. Afterwards, unihemispheric atrophy sets in and predominates typically in the perisylvian region, as in our case. Most of the tissue loss happens during the first 12 months after the onset of symptoms in the majority of patients. Atrophy of the ipsilateral head of the caudate nucleus is a typical feature. Gadolinium enhancement is very rare in RE [5]. Serial MRIs demonstrate progression of signal change and atrophy. Improvement and one reoccurrence of signal abnormalities represent an atypical MRI feature of RE. Reappearance of high signal intensity was associated with clinical seizure aggravation, as observed in our case. This fluctuation is indicative of the inflammatory process [8]. In the literature, 9 cases of RE showed regression followed by reappearance of lesions on serial MRIs [4, 8–10]. Only 3 of them had high signal intensity lesions at initial examination, similar to our observation [8]. In line with the fluctuating nature of the MRI changes, we evoked, initially, the diagnosis of ADEM.

In early disease stages, electroencephalograms (EEG) may contribute to the diagnosis of RE. Various abnormalities are seen in patients with RE. Some unihemispheric findings such as impairment of background activity with persistent polymorphic delta waves and sleep spindles, focal slow activity, subclinical ictal discharges, and multifocal ictal discharges are strongly suggestive of RE [2, 3]. The EEG of our patient showed intercritical left frontotemporal discharge persisting during sleep.

Brain biopsy can also help the diagnosis, but it is not required in all RE cases. The characteristic histopathological features are microglial and lymphocytic nodules, neuronal loss, neuronophagia, and perivascular cuffing, confined to one cerebral hemisphere with frontoinsular predilection [2, 5].

RE can be treated by antiepileptic drugs, immunosuppressive and immunomodulator regimens, and surgery. The aim of these treatments is to reduce seizure severity and improve the motor and cognitive performance [2, 5]. Frequently, seizures are resistant to antiepileptic drugs [11]. Patients receiving immunotherapy had a beneficial effect on seizure frequency and delayed deterioration [12]. Steroids, prescribed in our case, are the most effective treatment and the most widely used. Pulses of high-dose methylprednisolone have been reported to be effective to stop disease progression [11].

Intravenous immunoglobulin (IVIG) was used in some patients having RE with good results. The recommended dose is 2 g/kg monthly. The association of steroids and IVIG may be indicated when the two treatments alone are ineffective [13].

Plasmapheresis has good effects on seizures and neurological functions. It contributes to assessing the mental and residual motor function before surgery. The frequency was three to six single volume exchanges on consecutive or alternate days every 2 to 8 weeks [13].

Other medical treatments, such as using tacrolimus, rituximab, cyclophosphamide, azathioprine, and interferon, have been reported [11]. Our patient was treated by azathioprine.

Surgery (anatomic hemispherectomy, functional hemispherectomy, perisylvian hemispherotomy, trans-sylvian hemispherotomy, and central/vertical hemispherotomy) seems to be the only cure for the seizures and to improve cognitive outcome. However, inevitable sequelae (hemianopia, hemiparesis, and aphasia in the dominant hemisphere) should be considered [2]. Rehabilitation approach should be considered. It may improve the quality of life of RE patients.

4. Conclusions

Rasmussen's encephalitis is a progressive inflammatory disease of one cerebral hemisphere characterized by frequent focal seizures, hemiparesis, and mental deterioration. Brain imaging findings, associated with electroencephalogram and clinical data, may indicate early diagnosis and could be an indicative of prognosis. Knowledge of atypical radiological aspects is necessary in order to establish the right diagnosis. Rapid diagnosis and management can modify the progression of disease.

Authors' Contributions

All authors revised the manuscript critically and gave final approval of the version to be published.

References

[1] T. Rasmussen, J. Olszewski, and D. Lloyd-Smith, "Focal seizures due to chronic localized encephalitis," *Neurology*, vol. 8, no. 6, p. 435, 1958.

[2] S. Varadkar, C. G. Bien, C. A. Kruse et al., "Rasmussen's encephalitis: clinical features, pathobiology, and treatment advances," *The Lancet Neurology*, vol. 13, no. 2, pp. 195–205, 2014.

[3] B. Varghese, M. Aneesh, N. Singh, and P. Gilwaz, "A case of Rasmussen encephalitis: the differential diagnoses and role of diagnostic imaging," *Oman Medical Journal*, vol. 29, no. 1, pp. 67–70, 2014.

[4] K. Pradeep, S. Sinha, A. Mahadevan et al., "Clinical, electrophysiological, imaging, pathological and therapeutic observations among 18 patients with Rasmussen's encephalitis," *Journal of Clinical Neuroscience*, vol. 25, pp. 96–104, 2016.

[5] C. G. Bien, T. Granata, C. Antozzi et al., "Pathogenesis, diagnosis and treatment of Rasmussen encephalitis: a European consensus statement," *Brain*, vol. 128, no. 3, pp. 454–471, 2005.

[6] H. E. Olson, M. Lechpammer, S. P. Prabhu et al., "Clinical application and evaluation of the Bien diagnostic criteria for Rasmussen encephalitis," *Epilepsia*, vol. 54, no. 10, pp. 1753–1760, 2013.

[7] S. Frucht, "Dystonia, athetosis, and epilepsia partialis continua in a patient with late-onset Rasmussen's encephalitis," *Movement Disorders*, vol. 17, no. 3, pp. 609–612, 2002.

[8] E. Yamazaki, Y. Takahashi, N. Akasaka, T. Fujiwara, and Y. Inoue, "Temporal changes in brain MRI findings in Rasmussen syndrome," *Epileptic Disorders*, vol. 13, no. 3, pp. 229–239, 2011.

[9] S. Nakasu, T. Isozumi, A. Yamamoto, K. Okada, T. Takano, and Y. Nakasu, "Serial magnetic resonance imaging findings of Rasmussen's encephalitis," *Neurologia Medico-Chirurgica*, vol. 37, no. 12, pp. 924–928, 1997.

[10] A. Avberšek, A. Miserocchi, A. W. McEvoy et al., "Multiphasic presentation of Rasmussen's encephalitis," *Epileptic Disorders*, vol. 17, no. 3, pp. 315–320, 2015.
[11] R. H. Caraballo, S. Fortini, R. Cersósimo et al., "Rasmussen syndrome: an argentinean experience in 32 patients," *Seizure*, vol. 22, no. 5, pp. 360–367, 2013.
[12] C. G. Bien, H. Tiemeier, R. Sassen et al., "Rasmussen encephalitis: incidence and course under randomized therapy with tacrolimus or intravenous immunoglobulins," *Epilepsia*, vol. 54, no. 3, pp. 543–550, 2013.
[13] T. Granata, L. Fusco, G. Gobbi et al., "Experience with immunomodulatory treatments in Rasmussen's encephalitis," *Neurology*, vol. 61, no. 12, pp. 1807–1810, 2003.

22

Guillain–Barré Syndrome Associated with COVID-19 in a Japanese Male

Yoshiki Esa,[1] Yuta Kajiyama,[1] Misako Kaido,[1,2] Yushi Watanabe,[1] Harutoshi Fujimura,[1] Iwao Gohma,[3] Kenichi Takahashi,[4] and Junya Kobayashi[1]

[1]*Department of Neurology, Sakai City Medical Center, Sakai, Japan*
[2]*Department of Clinical Genetics, Sakai City Medical Center, Sakai, Japan*
[3]*Department of Respiratory Medicine, Sakai City Medical Center, Sakai, Japan*
[4]*Department of Respiratory Medicine, Kishiwada City Hospital, Kishiwada, Japan*

Correspondence should be addressed to Yuta Kajiyama; kajiyama@neurol.med.osaka-u.ac.jp

Academic Editor: Isabella Laura Simone

April 2021 saw a widespread outbreak of severe acute respiratory syndrome coronavirus 2 (SARS-CoV-2) in Osaka, Japan. We encountered the case of a 52-year-old man who had Guillain–Barré syndrome associated with coronavirus disease 2019 (COVID-19). After the relief of the respiratory symptoms owing to COVID-19, the patient experienced muscle weakness, which spread from his fingers to his extremities, and was unable to walk. Further examinations revealed mild protein elevation in the cerebrospinal fluid. In addition, nerve conduction studies showed demyelinating polyneuropathy, leading to the diagnosis of Guillain–Barré syndrome. After the administration of intravenous immunoglobulin and intravenous methylprednisolone, his symptoms drastically improved, and he was able to walk unaided 21 days after the onset of symptoms. On day 40, the patient was discharged with minimal muscle fatigue. Because Guillain–Barré syndrome associated with COVID-19 is expected to have a good prognosis, early diagnosis and treatment are important. Therefore, Guillain–Barré syndrome should be considered as a possible factor for muscle weakness during and after COVID-19 treatment.

1. Introduction

April 2021 saw a major outbreak of severe acute respiratory syndrome coronavirus 2 (SARS-CoV-2) in Osaka, Japan. From March to June 2021, there were more than 50,000 patients with coronavirus disease 2019 (COVID-19) in Osaka prefecture, which was the highest number of cases reported in Japan during that period. COVID-19 is widely recognized to present not only with respiratory symptoms but also with various neuromuscular complications. Several polyneuropathies such as Guillain–Barré syndrome and Miller-Fisher syndrome have been reported as neurological complications of COVID-19 [1]. In 2020, numerous case reports of Guillain–Barré syndrome during or after COVID-19 treatment were reported worldwide, and the rate of occurrence was assumed to be 15 per 100,000 patients [2]. It was also known that Guillain–Barré syndrome had regional variations in clinical features and outcomes [3]. Nevertheless, only a few cases of Guillain–Barré syndrome associated with COVID-19 were reported in Japan. Here, we report a case of Guillain–Barré syndrome after COVID-19, in which the clinical symptoms progressed very rapidly but drastically improved after immunological treatment.

2. Case Presentation

A 52-year-old man with a medical history of allergic rhinitis, reflux esophagitis, and asthma maintained on a combination of inhaled salmeterol xinafoate and fluticasone propionate, was admitted to our hospital with symptoms of Guillain–Barré syndrome after being treated for COVID-19. He worked as frontline healthcare professional for the COVID-19 response in his hospital. He received his first tozinameran (Pfizer-BioNTech COVID-19 Vaccine;

Comirnaty) vaccination at the end of March 2021. In early April, he developed a fever, olfactory disturbance, and dyspnea. Two days after the onset of these symptoms, he was diagnosed with COVID-19 via SARS-CoV-2 ribonucleic acid (RNA) detection in a nasopharyngeal swab. He then began experiencing respiratory impairment with decreased oxygenation and was admitted to a hospital, where he was treated with Remdesivir and dexamethasone, which resolved his fever and dyspnea. However, 10 days after the onset of COVID-19 (when the first symptoms presented), he experienced weakness in his fingers. His muscle weakness progressed rapidly to both of his lower limbs during the following 2 days, and he had difficulty in standing and walking. He was then transferred to the COVID-19 isolation ward in our hospital. On admission (day 2), he had no fever or respiratory difficulties. However, he showed symmetrical muscle weakness in the neck and extremities; specifically of grade 3 in his upper limbs and grade 4 in his lower limbs, according to the Medical Research Council (MRC) scale. The tendon reflexes of the extremities were also decreased. No abnormality was found in the cranial nerves testing, including the gag reflex. No sensory or autonomic disturbances were present, except for hyperhidrosis. Hematological tests showed a positive inflammatory reaction (CRP 1.56 mg/ml), but no other abnormalities were detected in the blood counts or biochemistry. The anti-ganglioside antibody test measured by ELISA showed a mildly positive IgG anti-GM3 antibody. Cerebrospinal fluid (CSF) examination showed a normal protein level (25 mg/dL) and cell count ($1/mm^3$) at admission, however, on day 14, a mildly elevated protein level (55.1 mg/dL) and a cell count of up to $9/mm^3$ were observed. SARS-CoV-2 RNA with the N501Y mutation was detected in the nasopharyngeal swab but was negative in the CSF. Nerve conduction studies (NCS) on admission showed prolonged distal latency (DL) in the left median nerve and posterior tibial nerve. Though compound muscle action potential (CMAP) elicited at distal stimulations was within the normal range, proximal CMAP was eliminated in the posterior tibial nerve and decreased in the median nerve. The left median and sural nerves showed decreased sensory conduction velocity (SCV) and normal sensory nerve evoked potentials (SNAPs) (Table 1).

Based on these findings, he was diagnosed with Guillain–Barré syndrome according to the Brighton criteria with level 2 diagnostic certainty. We also considered critical illness polyneuropathy due to COVID-19 as a differential diagnosis. However, we determined that Guillain–Barré syndrome was more appropriate because motor symptoms appeared after COVID-19 symptoms with an improvement of serum inflammatory markers over time. He was administered intravenous immunoglobulin (400 mg/kg/day for 5 days) on the day of admission. His muscle weakness progressed rapidly, and he developed mild difficulty in swallowing on the third day. Additional intravenous methylprednisolone (1000 mg/day for 3 days) was administered, considering the complications of a prolonged proinflammatory state with COVID-19. On day 7, when his symptoms were at their worst, he was almost completely paralyzed with MRC grade 1 (trace muscle activation, such as a twitch, without achieving full range of motion) muscle weakness in his neck and extremities, dysphagia, and respiratory difficulties. His symptom severity was at grade 4 on the Hughes functional grading scale, and the modified Erasmus Guillain–Barré syndrome outcome score was 10. On day 14, he was released from isolation and underwent further rehabilitation. He was able to walk on parallel bars on day 15, walk unaided on day 21, and was transferred to a rehabilitation hospital on day 26. He was discharged on day 40 with minimal muscle fatigue (Figure 1). The NCS on day 14 revealed an improvement in DL and CMAP. However, lower MCV in the left medial nerve and posterior tibial nerve persisted. Prolonged *F*-wave latency in the left ulnar nerve and posterior tibial nerves, as well as the conduction block in the left posterior tibial nerve, were observed. On day 48, CMAP was further improved, and the conduction block disappeared. However, the decreasing SNAP of the left median and sural nerves persisted until day 48 (Table 1).

3. Discussion

We report a case of Guillain–Barré syndrome that developed after COVID-19. The symptoms progressed rapidly, with prolonged distal latency on NCS immediately after symptom onset. However, both clinical and electrophysiological findings improved shortly after immunological treatments.

It is reported that Guillain–Barré syndrome associated with COVID-19 develops on average 12.1 days after COVID-19 and is characterized by demyelination, albuminocytological dissociation, absence of SARS-CoV-2 RNA in CSF, and a good response to immunological treatments [2, 4]. In our case report, Guillain–Barré syndrome developed 10 days after COVID-19 onset. Although the rapid progression and severity of the symptoms implied a poor prognosis, the progression of the disease stopped on day 7 after Guillain–Barré syndrome onset due to immunological treatment. So far, three cases of Guillain–Barré syndrome associated with COVID-19 have been reported in Japan; one case of axonal neuropathy, [5] one of acute inflammatory demyelinating polyneuropathy, [6] and an unidentified case [7]. In these cases, Guillain–Barré syndrome developed 16 to 20 days after the onset of COVID-19. Although clinical manifestations varied widely among patients with Guillain–Barré syndrome associated with COVID-19, all patients showed good improvement with or without immunotherapy (Table 2).

The present case showed prolonged DL and CMAP reduction between distal and proximal stimuli in the left median nerve and posterior tibial nerve. These findings improved on day 14 and recover on day 48 without remyelination processes, indicating an acute motor axonal neuropathy (AMAN) with reversible conduction failure [8] (Figure 2) Many cohort studies were published on Guillain–Barré syndrome after COVID-19, however, these studies included very few cases from the East Asian population. Considering current and previous reports, there seem to be cases of AMAN as well as demyelinating neuropathy in Japan. As with classic Guillain–Barré syndrome,

TABLE 1: Results of the nerve conduction studies during the clinical course.

	Distal latency (ms)	CMAP distal (mV)	CMAP proximal (mV)	MCV (m/s)	*F*-wave minimal latency (ms)	SNAP (uV)	SCV (m/s)
Median L							
Day 2	6.26	6.16	2.25	38.5	NA	21.90	25.6
Day 14	3.8	8.8	8.8	38.0	34.9	13.8	48.2
Day 48	4.1	15.4	14.8	51.4	30.9	15.5	60.0
Ulnar L							
Day 2	4.04	6.15	3.14	42.8	NA	NA	NA
Day 14	2.8	9.2	5.9	55.8	37.3	17.3	53.6
Day 48	2.9	11.8	11.2	54.1	32.0	21.5	55.6
Tibial L							
Day 14	4.4	11.0	4.5	34.1	61.4		
Day 48	3.3	18.6	12.2	45.4	53.7		
Sural L							
Day 2						10.70	31.2
Day 14						7.9	45.8
Day 48						8.4	50.0

Abbreviations: L, left; CMAP, compound motor action potential; MCV, motor conduction velocity; SNAP, sensory nerve action potential; SCV, sensory conduction velocity; NA, not available.

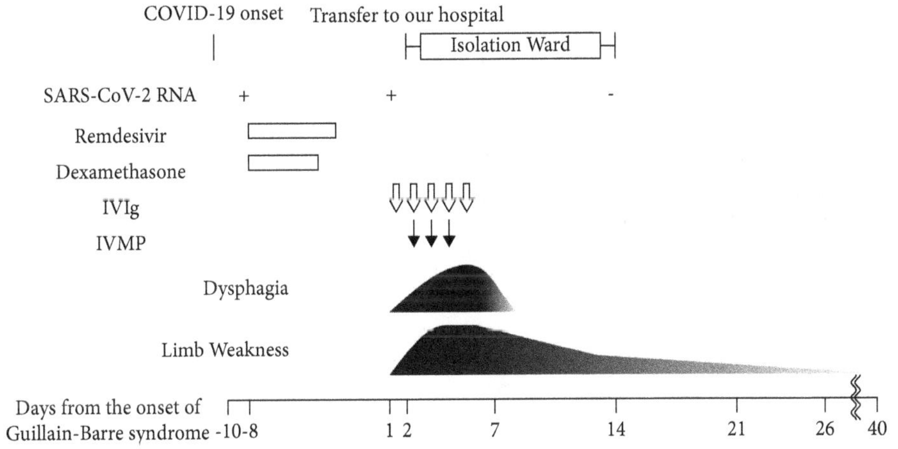

FIGURE 1: Clinical course of the disease. The diagram shows the clinical severity of dysphagia and weakness of the limbs from the onset of Guillain–Barré syndrome on day 1. The arrows indicate Guillain–Barré syndrome treatment with intravenous immunoglobulin (white) and intravenous methylprednisolone (black). On day 7, he showed severe muscle weakness in his neck and extremities, dysphagia, and respiratory difficulties. Thereafter, each symptom improved, and he was discharged on day 40 with minimal muscle fatigue. Abbreviations: IVIg, intravenous immunoglobulin; IVMP, intravenous methylprednisolone; SARS-CoV-2 RNA, severe acute respiratory syndrome coronavirus 2 ribonucleic acid.

AMAN may be more common in the Japanese population. Therefore, further epidemiological investigations are needed in Japanese and Asian populations.

The pathogenesis of Guillain–Barré syndrome associated with COVID-19 is thought to involve immune-mediated mechanisms rather than direct damage due to SARS-CoV-2 [9]. In this case, anti-GM3 antibodies were detected. Antibodies against the common epitopes of GM3, GD1a, and GT1b have been reported to be associated with the pathogenesis of bulbar palsy and respiratory failure [10]. There have been reports of Guillain-Barré syndrome with anti-GM3 antibodies, but these cases were copositive with other antiganglioside antibodies, such as GM1, GD3, and GT3 [11, 12]. Thus, although the pathological significance of pure anti-GM3 antibodies is unclear, it is possible that anti-GM3 or coexisting antiganglioside antibodies were involved in the development of Guillain–Barré syndrome in this case.

In addition, pathological findings in patients with COVID-19 revealed the expression of myxovirus resistance protein A (MxA), which is expressed in the capillaries around the peripheral nerves affected by type I interferon as an antiviral cytokine. This suggests that a COVID-19-induced cytokine storm is involved in peripheral nerve injury [13]. Corticosteroids are sometimes administered to treat central nervous system inflammatory complications associated with COVID-19 [14]. There is a possibility that corticosteroid therapy is effective for peripheral nerve inflammation. In this case, we administered corticosteroid

Table 2: Demographics of previous and present cases of Guillain-Barré syndrome associated with COVID-19 in Japan.

Case	Age	Sex	Clinical feature	GBS onset from the onset of COVID-19	GBS onset from COVID-19 recovery	GBS electrophysiological subtype	Anti-ganglioside antibody	CSF protein (mg/dL)	Immunological treatment
Wada et al. [7]	69	Male	Absence of cough reflex, muscle weakness, areflexia	Not described	Not described	Not described	Anti-Gal-C antibody	202	IVIg
Hirayama et al. [5]	54	Female	Muscle weakness, numbness, and areflexia in the lower limb	20	Approximately 1 week	Axonal type	Negative	Normal level	No treatment
Kakumoto et al. [6]	22	Male	Muscle weakness, hypesthesia, dysarthria, dysphagia, left-sided facial numbness, and dysautonomia	16	6	AIDP	Negative	307	IVIg
Present case	52	Male	Muscle weakness, dysphagia, areflexia, hyperhidrosis	10	1	AIDP	Anti-GM3 antibody	55	IVIg, IVMP

Abbreviations: GBS, Guillain–Barré syndrome; CSF, cerebrospinal fluid; AIDP, acute inflammatory demyelinating polyneuropathy; IVIg, intravenous immunoglobulin; IVMP, intravenous methylprednisolone.

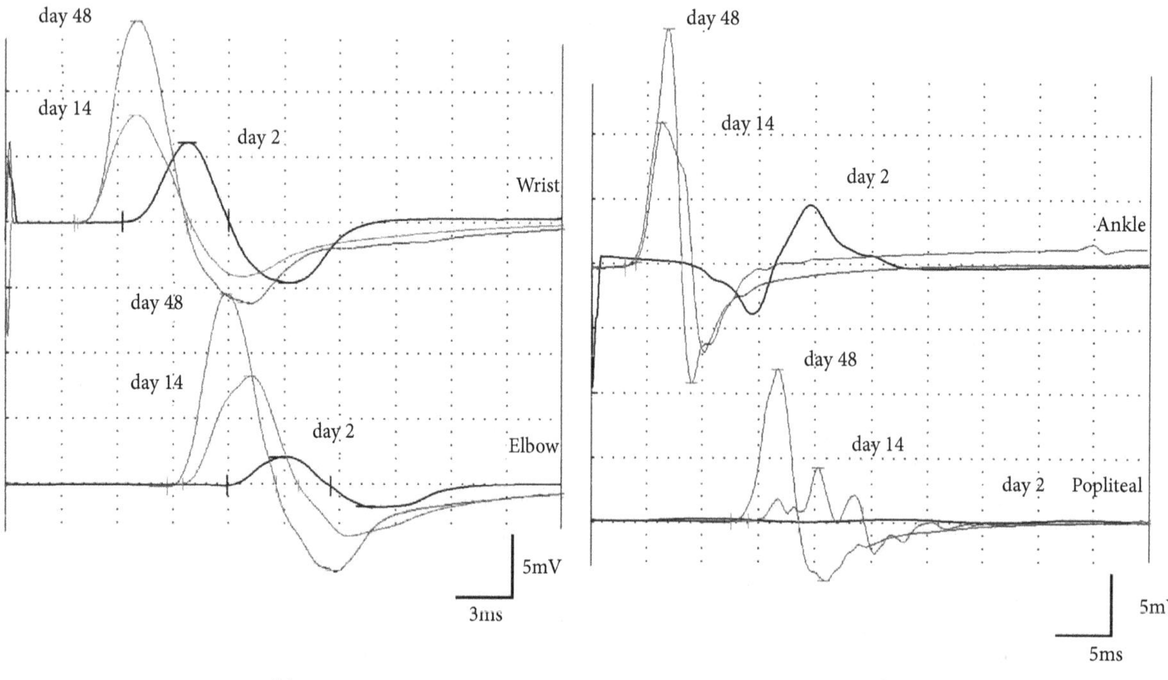

Figure 2: Serial nerve conduction tracings in the case. Serial recordings of compound muscle action potentials (CMAP) of the left median nerve (a) and the left posterior tibial nerve (b) on days 2, 14, and 48. Prolonged distal latencies (DL) were shown in the left median nerve and posterior tibial nerve on day 2. Distal CMAP was within the normal range; however, proximal CMAP was eliminated in the posterior tibial nerve and decreased in the median nerve. DL and CMAP improved over time on day 14 and day 48.

therapy combined with IVIG. Peripheral polyneuropathy following systemic inflammatory reactions is also known as critical illness polyneuropathy. For its treatment, it is suggested that the aggressive management of medical conditions and glycemic control is vital [15]. In such a scenario, the use of glucocorticoids may be refrained. Further studies are needed to assess the effectiveness of this combined therapy.

Although pathological associations between COVID-19 and Guillain–Barré syndrome development have been suggested, epidemiological data did not show an increased incidence of Guillain–Barré syndrome per patient with COVID-19 in 2020 [16]. Therefore, there may be a weak causal relationship between SARS-CoV-2 and Guillain–Barré syndrome, as opposed to the pattern observed with the Zika virus [17].

The incidence of COVID-19 remains high in Japan in 2022. Although Guillain–Barré syndrome associated with COVID-19 is expected to have a good prognosis, early diagnosis and treatment are still important. In conclusion, Guillain–Barré syndrome should be considered as a differential diagnosis when muscle weakness is suspected during or after COVID-19 treatment.

Consent

Written informed consent was obtained from the patient for publication of this report.

Acknowledgments

The authors would like to thank Editage (https://www.editage.com) for their help with English language editing. The authors would also like to thank Dr. Atsuro Chiba and Dr. Ayumi Uchibori, Department of Neurology, Kyorin University, for helping with antiganglioside antibody measurements.

References

[1] R. W. Paterson, R. L. Brown, L. Benjamin et al., "The emerging spectrum of COVID-19 neurology: clinical, radiological and laboratory findings," *Brain*, vol. 143, no. 10, pp. 3104–3120, 2020.

[2] L. Palaiodimou, M. Stefanou, A. H. Katsanos et al., "Prevalence, clinical characteristics and outcomes of Guillain-Barré syndrome spectrum associated with COVID-19: a systematic review and meta-analysis," *European Journal of Neurology*, vol. 28, no. 10, pp. 3517–3529, 2021.

[3] A. Y. Doets, C. Verboon, B. van den Berg et al., "Regional variation of Guillain-Barré syndrome," *Brain*, vol. 141, no. 10, pp. 2866–2877, 2018.

[4] S. Abu-Rumeileh, A. Abdelhak, M. Foschi, H. Tumani, and M. Otto, "Guillain-Barré syndrome spectrum associated with COVID-19: an up-to-date systematic review of 73 cases," *Journal of Neurology*, vol. 268, no. 4, pp. 1133–1170, 2021.

[5] T. Hirayama, Y. Hongo, K. Kaida, and O. Kano, "Guillain-Barré syndrome after COVID-19 in Japan," *BMJ Case Reports*, vol. 13, no. 10, Article ID e239218, 2020.

[6] T. Kakumoto, S. Kobayashi, H. Yuuki et al., "Cranial nerve involvement and dysautonomia in post-COVID-19 Guillain-Barré syndrome," *Internal Medicine (Tokyo, Japan)*, vol. 60, 2021.

[7] S. Wada, Y. Nagasaki, Y. Arimizu et al., "Neurological disorders identified during treatment of a SARS-CoV-2 infection," *Internal Medicine*, vol. 59, no. 17, pp. 2187–2189, 2020.

[8] Y. C. Chan, A. M. Punzalan-Sotelo, T. A. Kannan et al., "Electrodiagnosis of reversible conduction failure in Guillain-Barré syndrome," *Muscle & Nerve*, vol. 56, no. 5, pp. 919–924, 2017.

[9] S. Shoraka, M. L. B. Ferreira, S. R. Mohebbi, and A. Ghaemi, "SARS-CoV-2 infection and Guillain-Barré syndrome: a review on potential pathogenic mechanisms," *Frontiers in Immunology*, vol. 12, Article ID 674922, 2021.

[10] R. Rojas-Garcia, E. Gallardo, N. De Luna et al., "Bulbar involvement in patients with antiganglioside antibodies against NeuNAc (alpha2-3)Gal," *Journal of Neurology Neurosurgery and Psychiatry*, vol. 81, no. 6, pp. 623–628, 2010.

[11] K. Kaida, T. Ariga, and R. K. Yu, "Antiganglioside antibodies and their pathophysiological effects on Guillain-Barré syndrome and related disorders--a review," *Glycobiology*, vol. 19, no. 7, pp. 676–692, 2009.

[12] K. Aoyama, H. Ishikura, S. Mishima et al., "Guillain-Barré syndrome complicated with hemolytic anemia in association with antiganglioside GM3 antibody," *The American Journal of Medicine*, vol. 110, no. 5, pp. 399-400, 2001.

[13] J. Suh, S. S. Mukerji, S. I. Collens et al., "Skeletal muscle and peripheral nerve histopathology in COVID-19," *Neurology*, vol. 97, no. 8, pp. e849–e858, 2021.

[14] A. Pilotto, S. Odolini, S. Masciocchi et al., "Steroid-responsive encephalitis in coronavirus disease 2019," *Annals of Neurology*, vol. 88, no. 2, pp. 423–427, 2020.

[15] N. Latronico and C. F. Bolton, "Critical illness polyneuropathy and myopathy: a major cause of muscle weakness and paralysis," *The Lancet Neurology*, vol. 10, pp. 931–941, 2011.

[16] S. Keddie, J. Pakpoor, C. Mousele et al., "Epidemiological and cohort study finds no association between COVID-19 and Guillain-Barré syndrome," *Brain*, vol. 144, no. 2, pp. 682–693, 2021.

[17] L. R. Petersen, D. J. Jamieson, A. M. Powers, and M. A. Honein, "Zika virus," *New England Journal of Medicine*, vol. 374, no. 16, pp. 1552–1563, 2016.

23

A Case Report of Extensive Cerebral Venous Sinus Thrombosis as a Presenting Sign of Relapsing Nephrotic Syndrome

Janet K. Lee, Kathleen Murray, and Swetha Renati

University of South Florida, Department of Neurology, Tampa, FL, USA

Correspondence should be addressed to Janet K. Lee; janetlee@usf.edu

Academic Editor: Shahid Nimjee

Nephrotic syndrome is defined by three characteristic features including proteinuria of >3 g in 24 hours, hypoalbuminemia of less than 3 g/dL, and peripheral edema. Multiple nephropathies can result in nephrotic syndrome. Most commonly, minimal change disease is seen in children under the age of 10, while adults are more commonly found to have membranous nephropathy. Hypercoagulability and thrombotic sequela can be seen in nephrotic syndrome, regardless of underlying etiology, and thrombosis is most commonly seen in deep veins of the lower extremities and renal veins. Our case identifies an adult with previously diagnosed and treated for minimal change disease who presented with weight gain, peripheral edema, foamy urine, headache but no neurologic deficits. The patient was found to have near to complete occlusion of the entire superior sagittal sinus, near complete occlusion of the left transverse and sigmoid sinuses, and nonocclusive thrombus in the right sigmoid sinus. She was treated with heparin and IV steroids then transitioned to warfarin and PO steroids, respectively, with resolution of symptoms. This case report emphasizes on the importance of recognizing CVST as a potential complication of nephrotic syndrome at both initial presentation and relapse.

1. Introduction

Nephrotic syndrome is characterized by proteinuria, hypoalbuminemia, edema, and hyperlipidemia. It is associated with hypercoagulability with thrombosis occurring most frequently in the deep veins of lower extremities and renal veins [1]. Cerebral venous sinus thrombosis (CVST) is a rare complication of nephrotic syndrome.

2. Case Report

A female in her early 20s with a recent diagnosis of biopsy proven Minimal Change Disease (MCD) presented with headache, neck pain, photophobia, nausea, and vomiting. Patient was diagnosed with MCD approximately 2 months prior and started on prednisone. During follow-up, proteinuria improved from 7 g/day to 0.5 g/day and hypoalbuminemia improved from 0.5 g/dL to 2.2 g/dL. Given improvement she was started on a taper of the steroids. As the prednisone was being tapered off she started having symptoms of foamy urine, edema, and weight gain. Her headache started 8 days prior to presentation. She was seen at an outside hospital 1-week prior for headache and was treated with sumatriptan and acetaminophen/butalbital/caffeine with only minimal improvement. Her headache continued to worsen with associated blurry vision and photophobia. On examination, vitals were within normal range and the neurologic exam was significant only for bilateral Grade 1 papilledema. CT angiogram of the head with venous phase showed near to complete occlusion of the entire superior sagittal sinus, near complete occlusion of the left transverse and sigmoid sinuses, and nonocclusive thrombus in the right sigmoid sinus (Figure 1). The patient was admitted and a continuous unfractionated heparin infusion was started. She was found to have a relapse of her nephrotic syndrome and was started on intravenous corticosteroids. Albumin levels were low at 1.6 g/dL. However, renal function was within normal limits. No prior thrombotic history was reported and hypercoagulable labs were unrevealing. She was transitioned to warfarin and was treated for nephrotic syndrome with prednisone 1 mg/kg/day. Oral contraceptive was discontinued. Patient's headache improved with no residual neurological deficits.

Following discharge, the patient was continued on high dose prednisone and a weaning trial was attempted but

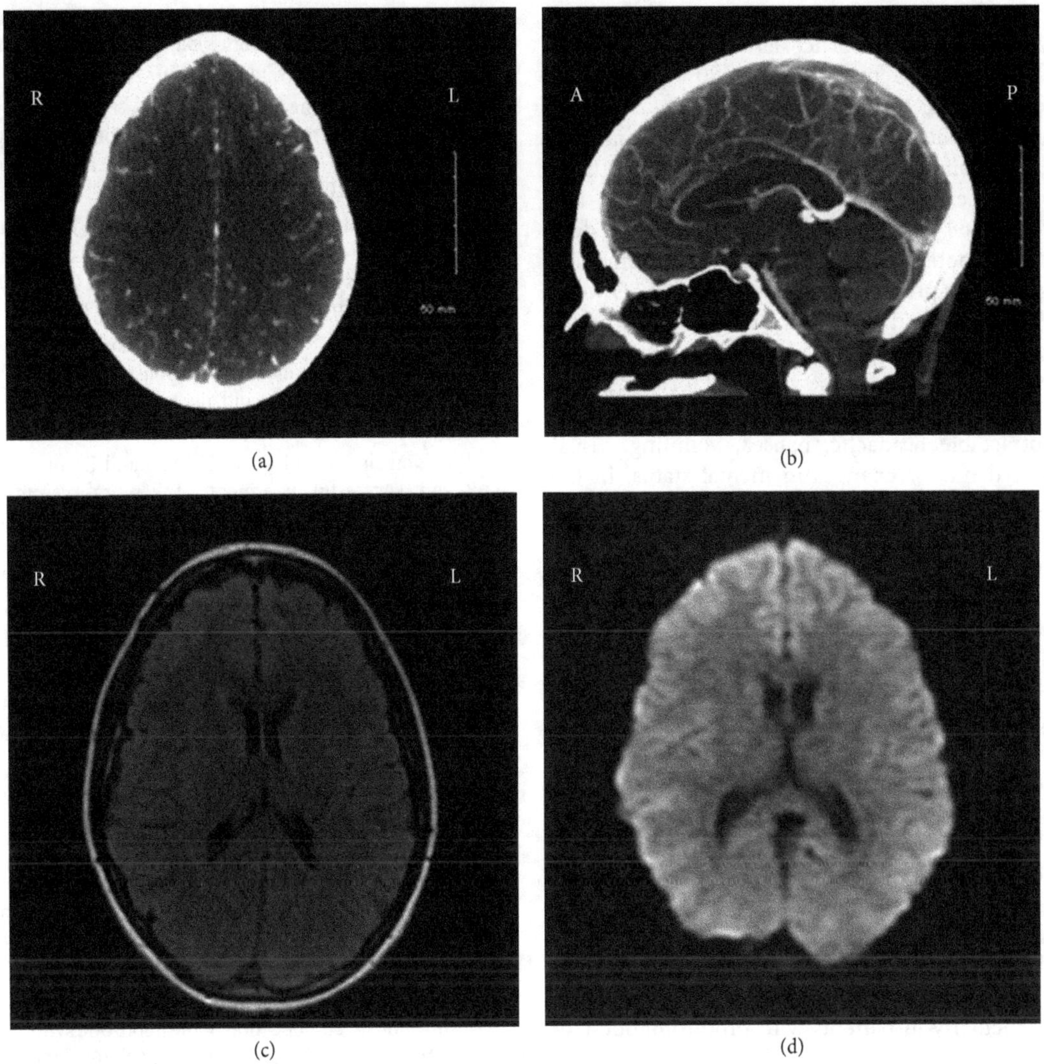

(a) (b) (c) (d)

Figure 1: CTV and MRI showing extensive cerebral sinus thrombosis. (a) CT venogram. Axial view. Showing empty delta sign and thrombus in the superior sagittal sinus. (b) CT venogram. Sagittal view. Showing filling defect in the superior sagittal sinus consistent with thrombotic occlusion of superior sagittal sinus. (c) MRI brain T2 Fluid-attenuated Inversion Recovery (FLAIR). Axial view. Showing no parenchymal involvement. (d) MRI brain Diffusion weighted imaging (DWI). Axial view. Showing no acute ischemia or cytotoxic injury.

resulted in worsening of nephrotic syndrome symptoms. She was eventually started on mycophenolate and successfully weaned off prednisone. Warfarin was continued for 10 months and discontinued following improvement of her nephrotic syndrome. At the time of anticoagulation discontinuation, her albumin improved to 4.8 g/dL. Neurologically, she remained asymptomatic with no recurrence of symptoms.

3. Discussion

Nephrotic syndrome is associated with hypercoagulability. While the mechanism remains poorly understood, it is generally thought to be caused by an imbalance of procoagulant and anticoagulant factors [2]. The risk of thrombotic complications in nephrotic syndrome is highest earlier in the disease course [2] and increases at lower albumin levels with the risk highest in membranous nephropathy. Lionaki et al. found that those with albumin levels <2.8 g/dL have a 2.5-fold increased risk of thromboembolic events [3]. Other risk factors include high proteinuria and age, with adults having a 7-8 fold increase in incidence compared to children [1]. Venous thrombosis is more frequent, and most commonly reported in the deep veins of the lower extremities followed by the renal veins [1]. Patients with nephrotic syndrome also have an increased risk of pulmonary emboli, likely secondary to the increased risk of deep vein thrombosis (DVT). Cerebral venous sinus thrombosis remains a rare or possibly underdiagnosed complication of nephrotic syndrome. In children, only 35 cases were reported from 1980 to 2005 [4]. For adults, the incidence of CVST in the context of nephrotic syndrome and specifically minimal change disease is unknown.

Minimal Change Disease (MCD) causes approximately 90% of cases of nephrotic syndrome in children but is estimated to cause only 10–25% of nephrotic syndrome cases in adults [5]. Compared to children, adults with MCD more commonly present with acute kidney injury and respond less rapidly to steroid therapy [5]. Corticosteroid therapy has been shown to lead to complete remission in over 80% of adults but often requires 12–16 weeks of therapy [5].

In our review of the literature, there are few documented cases of cerebral thrombosis in the context of adult MCD. Only 10 cases involved cerebral venous sinus thrombosis [6–14]. Patients were 20 to 68 years old, with one patient having documented prothrombotic risk factors of OCP use and smoking history. Most patients presented with new onset MCD while at least three documented cases were relapsing. Clinically, patients presented with progressive yet vague neurological complaints. Symptoms included new onset of focal or generalized seizures or signs of increased intracranial pressure including: intractable headache, nausea, vomiting, visual changes, papilledema, or changes in mental status. In the majority of cases with CVST, the superior sagittal sinus was involved followed by transverse sinuses.

Treatment of CVST in the setting of nephrotic syndrome includes the use of corticosteroids and anticoagulation. Anticoagulation with a continuous unfractionated heparin infusion followed by warfarin is preferred. In CVST from a provoked transient risk factor (such as OCP) it is reasonable to continue anticoagulation for 3–6 months based on clinical and imaging improvement [15]. However nephrotic syndrome presents a unique scenario where anticoagulation may need to be continued longer in high risk patients with hypoalbuminemia. Given the increased risk of thrombosis at lower albumin concentrations it has been proposed that prophylactic anticoagulation should be considered in high risk patients with serum albumin <2.0 g/dL [16].

Although rare, our case emphasizes the importance of recognizing CVST as a potential complication of nephrotic syndrome, particularly in patients with prothrombotic risk factors.

References

[1] H. F. Al-Azzawi, O. C. Obi, J. Safi, and M. Song, "Nephrotic syndrome-induced thromboembolism in adults," *International Journal of Critical Illness and Injury Science*, vol. 6, no. 2, pp. 85–88, 2016.

[2] B. A. Kerlin, R. Ayoob, and W. E. Smoyer, "Epidemiology and pathophysiology of nephrotic syndrome-associated thromboembolic disease," *Clinical Journal of the American Society of Nephrology*, vol. 7, no. 3, pp. 513–520, 2012.

[3] S. Lionaki, V. K. Derebail, S. L. Hogan et al., "Venous thromboembolism in patients with membranous nephropathy," *Clinical Journal of the American Society of Nephrology*, vol. 7, no. 1, pp. 43–51, 2012.

[4] L. Ghedira Besbes, S. Haddad, A. Gabsi, M. Hassine, Ch. Ben Meriem, and M. N. Guediche, "Cerebral sinovenous thrombosis in a child with idiopathic nephrotic syndrome," *Case Reports in Nephrology*, vol. 2011, Article ID 724950, 5 pages, 2011.

[5] J. Hogan and J. Radhakrishnan, "The treatment of minimal change disease in adults," *Journal of the American Society of Nephrology*, vol. 24, no. 5, pp. 702–711, 2013.

[6] Y. Wang, R. Meng, J. G. Duan et al., "Nephrotic syndrome may be one of the important etiologies of cerebral venous sinus thrombosis," *Journal of Stroke and Cerebrovascular Diseases*, vol. 25, no. 10, pp. 2415–2422, 2016.

[7] S. P. Nagaraju, M. Bairy, R. P. Attur, and C. J. Sambhaji, "Cerebral venous thrombosis and secondary polycythemia in case of nephrotic syndrome," *Saudi Journal of Kidney Diseases and Transplantation*, vol. 27, no. 2, pp. 391–394, 2016.

[8] Z. Zivanovic, K. Barlinn, C. Balucani, P. Palazzo, and A. V. Alexandrov, "Headache and aphasia in a young woman with protein S deficiency and nephrotic syndrome," *Acta Clinica Croatia*, vol. 50, no. 4, pp. 619–621, 2011.

[9] H. Komaba, H. Kadoguchi, N. Igaki, and T. Goto, "Early detection and successful treatment of cerebral venous thrombosis associated with minimal change nephrotic syndrome," *Clinical Nephrology*, vol. 68, no. 3, pp. 179–181, 2007.

[10] S. P. Friemel, D. W. Mackey, A. Z. Fenves, J. H. Hise, E. H. Cheung, and M. J. Stone, "Nephrotic syndrome presenting as dural sinus thrombosis," *The American Journal of Medicine*, vol. 113, no. 3, pp. 258–260, 2002.

[11] M. Hirata, M. Kuroda, and I. Koni, "Cerebral venous thrombosis in minimal change nephrotic syndrome," *Nihon Junzo Gakkai Shi*, vol. 41, no. 4, pp. 464–468, 1999.

[12] C. Urch and C. D. Pusey, "Sagittal sinus thrombosis in adult minimal change nephrotic syndrome," *Clinical Nephrology*, vol. 45, no. 2, pp. 131–132, 1996.

[13] A. Burns, E. Wilson, M. Harber, C. Brunton, and P. Sweny, "Cerebral venous sinus thrombosis in minimal change nephrotic syndrome," *Nephrology, Dialysis, and Transplantation*, vol. 10, no. 1, pp. 30–34, 1995.

[14] M. Barthelemy, M. G. Bousser, and C. Jacobs, "Cerebral venous thrombosis, complication of the nephrotic syndrome," *Nouvelle Presse Medicale*, vol. 9, no. 6, pp. 367–369, 1980.

[15] G. Saposnik, F. Barinagarrementeria, R. D. Brown et al., "Diagnosis and management of cerebral venous thrombosis," *Stroke*, vol. 42, no. 4, pp. 1158–1192, 2011.

[16] J. Gordon-Cappitelli and M. J. Choi, "Prophylactic anticoagulation in adult patients with nephrotic syndrome," *Clinical Journal of American Society of Nephrology*, 2019.

24

Neurogenic Pulmonary Edema Following a Seizure: A Case Report and Literature Review

Mostafa Suhail Najim, Riyadh Ali Mohammed Hammamy, and Sreethish Sasi

Department of Internal Medicine, Hamad Medical Corporation, Doha, Qatar

Correspondence should be addressed to Mostafa Suhail Najim; drmostafanajim@gmail.com

Academic Editor: Dennis J. Rivet

Acute pulmonary edema is one of the frequent causes of dyspnea encountered in everyday practice. It is broadly attributed to be either cardiogenic or noncardiogenic. It is usually treated with diuretics in addition to other medications depending on the underlying pathology. Here, we report a case of a female patient who presented with shortness of breath after developing a seizure. Further investigations excluded cardiogenic etiology and showed critically low phenytoin level. It improved within 48 h of supportive care without giving diuretics favoring the diagnosis of neurogenic pulmonary edema as the primary pathology. The goal of our case report is to keep neurogenic pulmonary edema in mind, and hence provide the appropriate management, when dealing with similar cases.

1. Introduction

Neurogenic pulmonary edema (NPE) refers to acute pulmonary edema developing within hours after an acute injury to the central nervous system [1]. NPE is usually overlooked due to its low prevalence, and absence of clear diagnostic criteria [2]. It occurs following a wide spectrum of neurological insults with cerebral hemorrhage being the commonest and only 2% are reported following a convulsion [3]. Despite this rarity, almost 80% of epileptic patients who died unexpectedly after a seizure were noted to have NPE [4]. Clinically, NPE is broadly classified into early (within minutes to hours) and delayed (12–24 h) following a neurologic insult. It presents with dyspnea, hypoxia, pink frothy sputum, and bilateral crackles on chest auscultation that correlates with bilateral chest radiograph infiltrates [2]. It is usually diagnosed after the exclusion of clear cardiogenic and intrinsic pulmonary factors contributing to the development of acute pulmonary edema [1].

2. Case Report

A 51-year-old lady presented with cough and shortness of breath. The symptoms started in the morning after waking up from sleeping. The cough was productive of pink-colored sputum and she was using accessory muscles to breathe. The family members noticed that she was also drowsy, confused, and not responding to them for about 30 min. Afterwards, she was fully aware of the surroundings; however, she could not recall what happened. They measured her blood glucose and it was 8.5 mmol/L. The past medical history was significant for a resected right temporal meningioma 3 years back and type 2 diabetes mellitus with well controlled HbA1c. Home medications are phenytoin 200 mg twice daily, lamotrigine 200 mg three times daily, escitalopram 10 mg once daily, and metformin/sitagliptin 1000/50 mg twice daily. The patient is known to experience seizures despite those anti-epileptic medications.

On examination, she was afebrile (37.3°C), hypotensive (89/47 mmHg), and hypoxic (82% oxygen saturation on room air). Respiratory exam showed bilateral crackles up to the mid zones bilaterally. Neurological examination did not reveal any abnormality. The initial laboratory tests ordered upon admission are shown in Table 1.

2.1. Blood Gases

Arterial Blood Gases (ABG) on Room Air. pH 7.41 (7.35–7.45), PaO_2 48.8 mmHg (83–108), $PaCO_2$ 35 mmHg (35–45), HCO_3

Table 1: Laboratory tests*.

Laboratory test	Patient's values	Normal reference range
General hematology		
White blood cells ($10^3/\mu L$)	9.6 *Normal*	4–10
Hemoglobin (g/dL)	10.9	12–15
Platelet ($10^3/\mu L$)	340	150–400
General chemistry		
Urea (mmol/L)	5.7	2.76–8.07
Creatinine (μmol/L)	31	53–97
Sodium (mmol/L)	138	135–145
Potassium (mmol/L)	4.2	3.6–5.1
Chloride (mmol/L)	100	96–110
Magnesium (mmol/L)	0.77	0.66–1.07
Glucose (mmol/L)	11.2	3.3–5.5
Bicarbonate (mmol/L)	22.9	24–30
Albumin (g/L)	40	35–50
Corrected calcium (mmol/L)	2.16	2.1–2.6
Phosphorus (mmol/L)	1.08	0.87–1.45
Bilirubin total (μmol/L)	4.5	3.5–24
ALT (U/L)	12	0–30
AST (U/L)	15	0–31
NT-pro BNP (pg/mL)	717	0–300
Troponin T highly sensitive (ng/L) three sets	24.8 → 20.6 → 16.4	0–14
C-reactive protein (mg/L)	23 *High*	0–5
Procalcitonin (ng/mL)	0.26 *Normal*	0–0.5
Lactic acid (mmol/L)	1.5	0.5–1.6
Microbiology		
Blood culture (2 sets)	*Negative*	—
Sputum culture	*Negative*	—
Drug level		
Phenytoin level (μmol/L)	3.6 *Critical Low*	40–79

*Lamotrigine and escitalopram levels are not available.

22.5 mmol/L (21–28), PaO_2/FiO_2 ratio: 232 (normal ratio is approximately 500).

ABG on Room Air after 2 Days. pH 7.43 (7.35–7.45), PaO_2 90 mmHg (83–108), $PaCO_2$ 36 mmHg (35–45), HCO_3 24.5 mmol/L (21–28), PaO_2/FiO_2 ratio: 429 (normal ratio is approximately 500).

2.2. Diagnostic Work-Up

CXR on Admission. Multiple confluent and patchy air space opacities noticed diffusely involving both lung fields (Figure 1).

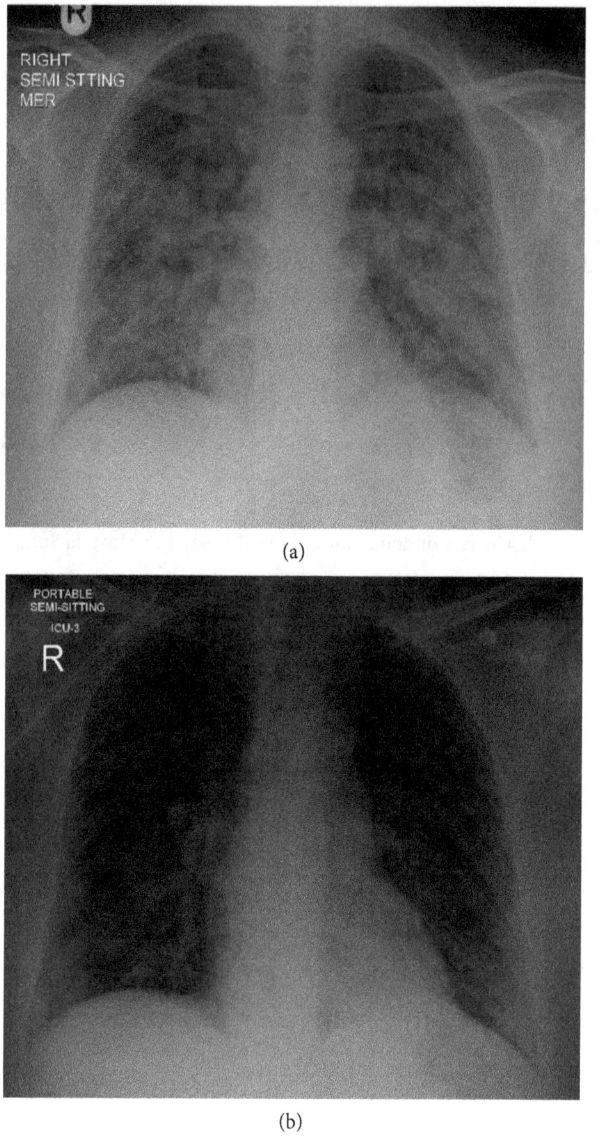

Figure 1: (a) CXR on admission showing multiple confluent and patchy air space opacities noticed diffusely involving both lung fields. (b) CXR after 2 days showing the bilateral lung opacities appear significantly resolved as compared to the previous chest radiograph.

CXR after 2 Days. Bilateral lung opacities appear significantly resolved as compared to the previous chest radiograph (Figure 1).

ECG. Sinus tachycardia with premature ventricular complexes (Figure 2).

Trans-Thoracic Echocardiography. Good global contractility and no resting regional wall motion abnormality. Normal Left ventricle systolic function. Ejection fraction 58%–60%.

2.3. Hospital Course. The patient received 1.5 L of intravenous normal saline boluses, she was connected to noninvasive ventilator—Continuous positive airway pressure (CPAP) machine with empirical IV. antibiotic to cover aspiration pneumonia and admitted to MICU for observation. There, she stayed for 2 days and showed marked improvement

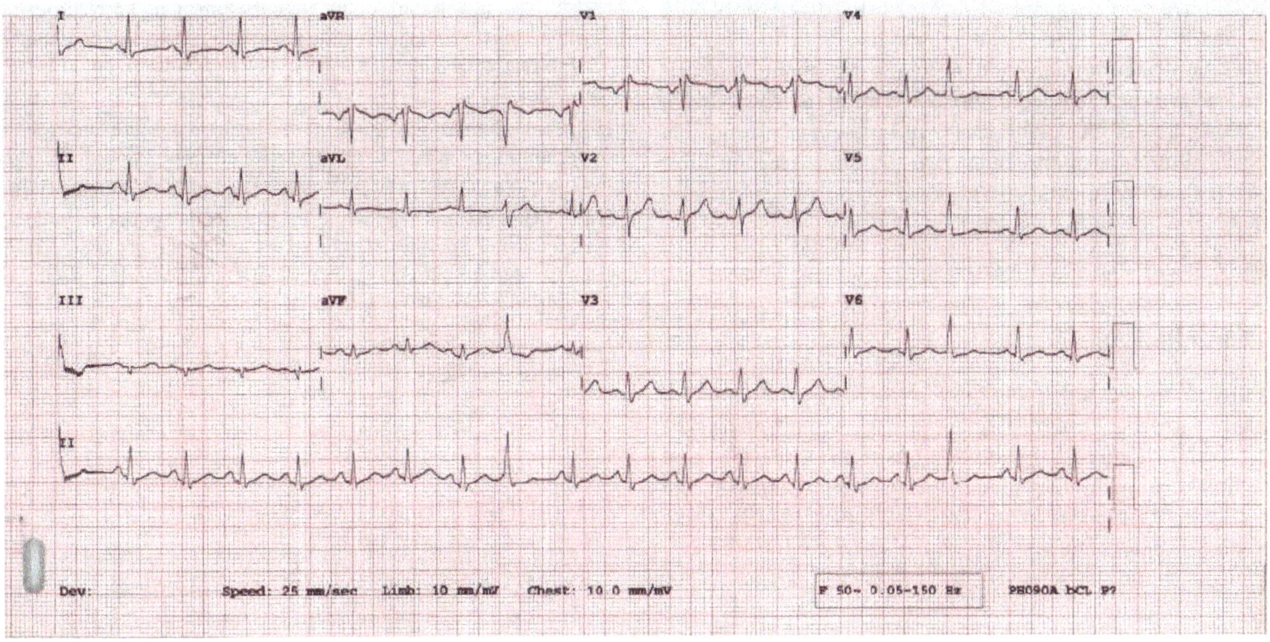

FIGURE 2: ECG showing sinus tachycardia with premature ventricular complexes.

TABLE 2: Neurogenic pulmonary edema (NPE) vs. aspiration pneumonia (AP) [1].

Diagnosis	Onset	Fever	PaO_2/FiO_2 ratio	Chest X-ray findings	WBC	CRP	Procalcitonin	Evolution duration
NPE	Hours	Yes/No	↓	Bilateral	Normal/↑	Normal/↑	Normal	1–3 days
AP	24 h	Yes	Normal/↓	Uni/bilateral	↑	↑	Normal/↑	1–3 weeks

PaO_2: arterial partial pressure of oxygen; FiO_2: inspiratory fraction of oxygen; WBC: white blood cells; CRP: C-reactive protein; PCT: procalcitonin.

clinically and in the requirements of oxygen. Repeated CXR showed dramatic resolution of bilateral lung opacities without giving furosemide (Figure 1). Compliance to anticonvulsant medications was emphasized, and she was maintaining oxygen saturation above 95% on room air upon discharge.

3. Discussion

The pathophysiology behind NPE is not fully understood. Increased intracranial pressure (ICP) is thought to be involved in the pathogenesis of NPE via catecholamine release that causes intense pulmonary and systemic vasoconstriction leading to an increase in capillary hydrostatic pressure and capillary permeability [5–7]. This theory is supported by the demonstration of NPE mitigation when using sympatholytic agents in animal studies [8]. Furthermore, a previous case report had demonstrated a noncardiogenic pulmonary edema as the sole clinical presentation of pheochromocytoma and it was attributed to the catecholamines surge [9]. Another proposed mechanism of NPE involves the central release of the inflammatory mediators secondary to endothelial damage into the systemic circulation. This increases the pulmonary capillary permeability leading to NPE formation [1]. Hypoxemia might be a contributing factor for the development of NPE. Severe ictal hypoxemia has been reported in different types of seizures especially the generalized convulsive ones [10]. Hypoxemia causes peripheral and pulmonary vasoconstriction with shunting of blood to pulmonary vasculature further compromising pulmonary hemodynamics. Hypoxemia also interferes with the alveolar epithelial Na, K-ATPase active transport that is necessary for clearance of NPE fluid [11].

In one retrospective study that involves reviewing chest CT scan for patients presenting with seizures as part of their emergency diagnostics, it was found that NPE was more frequent in cases of generalized convulsive seizures [12]. Recurrent NPE was also reported as the cause of two consecutive intensive care unit admissions following generalized convulsive seizures [13].

NPE is a diagnosis of exclusion. Cardiac etiology should be ruled out first. In addition, it requires the demonstration of hypoxemia and bilateral pulmonary infiltrates, in the presence of a genuine central nervous system insult raising the intracranial pressure [2].

In our case report, there are several clues to diagnose NPE. The witnessed postictal phase, the shortness of breath with oxygen desaturation, the bilateral infiltrates on chest radiograph, the rapid resolution within 48 h without diuretics, the critically subtherapeutic serum level of phenytoin, and the

exclusion of cardiac causes, all have made the diagnosis of NPE on the top of the differential diagnosis list.
Aspiration pneumonia is one of the most relevant diagnosis that needs to be excluded before confirming the diagnosis of NPE [1]. The clinical, laboratory, and imaging findings that help to differentiate between the two are summarized in Table 2. In the setting of extubation, negative pressure pulmonary edema may mimic NPE [14].

4. Conclusion

Acute pulmonary edema is most commonly cardiogenic in origin. However, noncardiogenic causes should always be investigated. Diuretics, in addition to specific disease-related medications, are implemented in the management plan except in selected cases as in neurogenic pulmonary edema where supportive care is the mainstay of treatment.

References

[1] A. Baumann, G. Audibert, J. McDonnell, and P. M. Mertes, "Neurogenic pulmonary edema," *Acta Anaesthesiologica Scandinavica*, vol. 51, no. 4, pp. 447-455, 2007.

[2] D. L. Davison, M. Terek, and L. S. Chawla, "Neurogenic pulmonary edema," *Critical Care*, vol. 16, no. 2, p. 212, 2012.

[3] A. M. Brambrink and W. F. Dick, "Neurogenic pulmonary edema," *Der Anaesthesist*, vol. 46, no. 11, pp. 953-963, 1997.

[4] R. P. Simon, "Neurogenic pulmonary edema," *Neurologic Clinics*, vol. 11, no. 2, pp. 309–323, 1993.

[5] R. Demling and R. Riessen, "Pulmonary dysfunction after cerebral injury," *Critical Care Medicine*, vol. 18, no. 7, pp. 768–774, 1990.

[6] J. D. Kennedy, K. A. Hardin, P. Parikh, C.-S. Li, and M. Seyal, "Pulmonary edema following generalized tonic clonic seizures is directly associated with seizure duration," *Seizure*, vol. 27, pp. 19–24, 2015.

[7] H. Zhao, G. Lin, M. Shi et al., "The mechanism of neurogenic pulmonary edema in epilepsy," *The Journal of Physiological Sciences*, vol. 64, no. 1, pp. 65–72, 2014.

[8] R. E. Brashear and J. C. Ross, "Hemodynamic effects of elevated cerebrospinal fluid pressure: alterations with adrenergic blockade," *Journal of Clinical Investigation*, vol. 49, no. 7, pp. 1324–1333, 1970.

[9] P. W. De Leeuw, F. L. Waltman, and W. H. Birkenhäger, "Noncardiogenic pulmonary edema as the sole manifestation of pheochromocytoma," *Hypertension*, vol. 8, no. 9, pp. 810–812, 1986.

[10] L. M. Bateman, C.-S. Li, and M. Seyal, "Ictal hypoxemia in localization-related epilepsy: analysis of incidence, severity and risk factors," *Brain*, vol. 131, no. 12, pp. 3239–3245, 2008.

[11] I. Vadasz, S. Raviv, and J. I. Sznajder, "Alveolar epithelium and Na, K-ATPase in acute lung injury," *Intensive Care Medicine*, vol. 33, no. 7, pp. 1243–1251, 2007.

[12] Y. Mahdavi, R. Surges, O. Nikoubashman et al., "Neurogenic pulmonary edema following seizures: a retrospective computed tomography study," *Epilepsy & Behavior*, vol. 94, pp. 112–117, 2019.

[13] D. C. Sacher and E. J. Yoo, "Recurrent acute neurogenic pulmonary edema after uncontrolled seizures," *Case Reports in Pulmonology*, vol. 2018, Article ID 3483282, 4 pages, 2018.

[14] D. G. Lorch and S. A. Sahn, "Post-extubation pulmonary edema following anesthesia induced by upper airway obstruction. Are certain patients at increased risk?," *Chest*, vol. 90, no. 6, pp. 802–805, 1986.

25

Composite Anatomical Variations between the Sciatic Nerve and the Piriformis Muscle: A Nepalese Cadaveric Study

Ameet Kumar Jha[1] **and Prakash Baral**[2]

[1]*University of Central Nicaragua, Managua, Nicaragua*
[2]*Department of Anatomy, Gandaki Medical College, Pokhara, Nepal*

Correspondence should be addressed to Ameet Kumar Jha; ameetjha197@gmail.com

Academic Editor: Peter Berlit

Piriformis syndrome is a rare syndrome which is one of the main causes of nondiscogenic sciatica causing severe low back pain due to entrapment of sciatic nerve either by the hypertrophy or by inflammation of the piriformis muscle. We have carried out dissection in 20 Nepalese cadavers. Out of 40 dissected gluteal regions, 37 exhibited typical appearance of sciatic nerve, piriformis muscle, and their relations resembling type-a, whereas 3 gluteal regions showed composite structural variations resembling type-b and type-c based on Beaton and Anson's classification. Knowledge pertaining to such variations will be helpful during a surgical intervention in the gluteal region and in turn reduces the risk of injuring these nerves which are more susceptible to damage. Our study reports such variations in Nepalese population which will be helpful during evaluation of the pain induction in various test positions and also useful for analysis of the range of the neurological deficiency in sciatic nerve neuropathies. The present study also explains the basis of the unsuccessful attempt of the sciatic nerve block during popliteal block anaesthesia.

1. Introduction

Sciatic nerve is the largest nerve carrying ventral rami of L4-S3 spinal nerves, which lies inferior to the piriformis muscle in the gluteal region [1]. It descends along the posterior aspect of the thigh and splits into the tibial and common peroneal components in the popliteal fossa [2, 3]. The provenance of the anatomical variation in pelvic region most likely originates from the existence of such structures as separate entities during the developmental period. Piriformis muscle originates from the pelvic surface of S2–S4 sacral segments, the superior margin of the greater sciatic notch, and the sacrotuberous ligament. Further, it exits through the greater sciatic foramen along with the sciatic nerve and inserts to the greater trochanter of the femur [1].

Sciatic nerve compression throughout its course can results into clinical conditions like sciatica and piriformis syndrome. Piriformis syndrome is a painful condition resembling sciatica, secondary to sciatic nerve entrapment, and is responsible for 6% of low back pain cases [4, 5]. It is one of the nondiscogenic causes of sciatica resulting due to the trauma, inflammation, and degenerative changes to the piriformis muscle. However, rare structural variations can be one of the main causes for this syndrome [6, 7]. It is essential to understand the anatomical variation of the sciatic nerve and piriformis muscle while performing the total hip arthroplasty, sciatic nerve block, and gluteal or pelvic surgery to avoid the iatrogenic injuries which may arise during these procedures [8]. Sciatic neuropathy results due to the compression or damage to the sciatic nerve, leading to the neurological deficits [9]. The structural variation of sciatic nerve, piriformis muscle, and their relations were first classified by Beaton and Anson into six different categories in 1937. Various researchers adopted this classification to categorize their findings. The two common groups of variations are the undivided sciatic nerve passing below unsplit muscle and variation where the sciatic nerve exits into the gluteal region through the greater sciatic foramen as two presplit branches, tibial and common peroneal nerve [8].

Beaton and Anson classified the anatomical relationship between the sciatic nerve and the piriformis muscle as follows:

Type-a: undivided nerve below undivided muscle

Type-b: divisions of nerve between and below undivided muscle

Type-c: divisions above and below undivided muscle

Type-d: undivided nerve between heads

Type-e: divisions between and above heads

Type-f: undivided nerve above undivided muscle [10, 11]

The aim of our study was to provide a compendious and evidence-based evaluation of composite anatomical variations of the sciatic nerve, piriformis muscle, and their relationship during routine dissection of Nepalese cadavers.

2. Methods

The current study was conducted on 40 gluteal regions of 20 formalin fixed human cadavers (18 males and 2 females) during routine dissection in the Anatomy Lab of Gandaki Medical College, Pokhara, Nepal.

The gluteal regions of these cadavers were carefully dissected followed by the retraction of the gluteus maximus muscle to expose the piriformis muscle and sciatic nerve. The sciatic nerve emerges inferior to the piriformis muscle and descends in the inferolateral direction. The variations in division of the sciatic nerve, abnormal origin of piriformis muscle, and their relations in all the specimens were carefully observed, noted, and photographed. Those structural variations were identified and classified based on the Beaton and Anson classification system. The pathological cadavers were excluded. No clinical data on them were available, and therefore, it was not known whether any of them had presented piriformis syndrome when alive. Some of these cadavers were unclaimed bodies, and therefore, the age groups were unknown; however, many of them were between the ages of 45 and 65 years.

We declare that appropriate ethical principles were followed during the procedures according to the regulations outlined in the Helsinki Declaration of the World Medical Association.

3. Case Series

In the current study, 37 (92.5%) out of 40 dissected gluteal regions of the human cadavers showed typical anatomical appearance of sciatic nerve, piriformis muscle, and their relations which resembled type-a based on Beaton and Anson's classification. However, three (7.5%) gluteal regions out of 40 showed composite structural variation of sciatic nerve, piriformis muscle, and their relations.

3.1. Case I. A 54-year-old male cadaver during routine dissection showed composite piriformis muscle with peculiar arrangements of the two heads varying from its usual appearance and early splitting of the left sciatic nerve with tibial and common peroneal components (Figures 1(a) and 1(b)). The common peroneal component passes between the two heads of the piriformis muscle, whereas the tibial component had its usual course.

3.2. Case II. A 47-year-old male cadaver during similar routine dissection showed early splitting of the right sciatic nerve where the common peroneal component descends posterolateral to the piriformis muscle, whereas the tibial component had its usual course (Figure 2). The result corresponded with Beaton and Anson type-c (2.5%).

3.3. Case III. A similar unilateral variation in the formation of sciatic nerve and its unusual relation with the piriformis muscle was encountered in the left gluteal region of a 51-year-old male cadaver. Additionally, an accessory belly of the piriformis muscle at its insertion was observed in the right gluteal region beneath the gluteus maximus of the same cadaver. The relationship of the sciatic nerve and piriformis muscle in this case was classified under type-c (2.5%). There were no any gross anomalic appearance or any surgical intervention in these cadavers near the dissected area.

4. Discussion

Piriformis syndrome is considered to be an atypical, contentious neuromuscular disorder resulted from a compression of the sciatic nerve at the level of the piriformis muscle. The diagnosis has been a major challenge due to difficulties in finding the exact cause of the pain and a paucity of confirmed clinical and definitive diagnostic criteria like radioimaging or electrodiagnostic testing [6, 13].

The anomalic variation of sciatic nerve, piriformis muscle, and their variable relationship can lead to entrapment and compression of the nerve, resulting into piriformis syndrome [14]. Such variations have to be emphasized as it plays a crucial role in the basis of sciatica and the pain etiology [12]. The branching patterns of the two main divisions of the sciatic nerve, the tibial, and the common fibular nerve are responsible for these variations [7].

Piriformis syndrome narrates the presence of pain in the buttock and posterior hip region caused from nondiscogenic and extrapelvic entrapment of the sciatic nerve [15]. The current study aims to explore the Nepalese cadavers to provide awareness and strengthen the findings of the sciatic nerve variations and its relation to the piriformis as a probable cause for the nondiscogenic sciatica as well as other pain etiologies.

In the present study, we have encountered 37 (92.5%) type-a, 1 (2.5%) type-b, and 2 (5%) type-c nerve-muscle relations out of 40 dissected gluteal regions in the Nepalese cadavers (Table 1). Adibatti et al. reported a similar finding with 92% of type-a, 2% of type-b, and 6% of type-c with dissection on 50 gluteal regions of the Indian population [14]. Desalegn et al. found 91.7% of type-a, 2.8% of type-b, and 5.5% of type-c while dissecting 36 gluteal regions of the northern Ethiopian population [16]. A similar study on 30 Polish cadavers revealed 76.7% of type-a, 20% of type-b, and 3.3% of type-c [17]. Berihu et al. with their research on 56

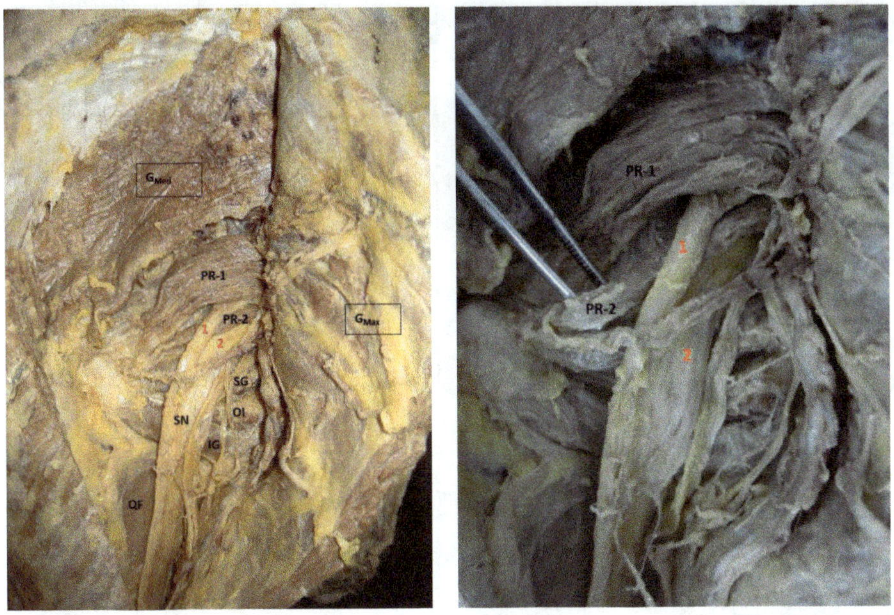

(a) (b)

FIGURE 1: (a) Higher division of sciatic nerve and split piriformis muscle with two heads. 1: common peroneal superior head of piriformis; 2: tibial component; PR-1: inferior component; PR-2: head of piriformis; G_{Max}: gluteus maximus; G_{Med}: gluteus medius; SN: sciatic nerve; SG: superior gemellus. (b) Higher division of the sciatic nerve and split piriformis muscle with two heads. Forceps tip showing the inferior head of piriformis component. 1: common peroneal component; 2: tibial component; PR-1: inferior component; PR-2: head of piriformis.

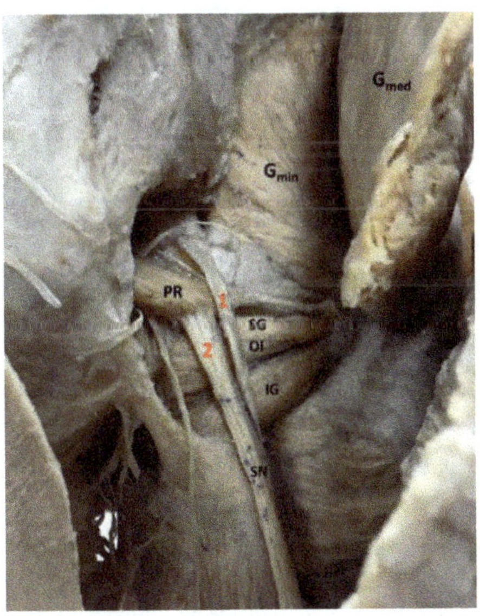

FIGURE 2: Higher division of sciatic nerve and a complete piriformis muscle. 1: common peroneal component; 2: tibial component; PR: piriformis muscle; G_{med} gluteus medius; G_{min}: gluteus minimus; SN: sciatic nerve; SG: superior gemellus.

Ethiopian cadavers marked 89.3% of type-a, 8.9% of type-b and 1.8% of type-c relations [2].

Güvençer et al., Patel et al., Brooks et al., and Ogeng'o et al., with their research on Turkish, Indian, Brazilian, and Kenyan cadavers reported 76%, 91.9%, 90%, and 89.7% type-a relations and 24%, 8.1%, 10%, and 10.3% of type b-f relations, respectively [18–21].

TABLE 1: Summary of sex-wise distribution of dissected gluteal regions and their classification based on Beaton and Anson.

Sex	No. of gluteal regions dissected		Type-a		Type-b		Type-c	
	Right	Left	Right	Left	Right	Left	Right	Left
Male	18	18	17	16	0	1	1	1
Female	2	2	2	2	0	0	0	0

An extensive research on the Czech Republican cadavers revealed 79.1% type-a, 14.3% type-b, 4.4% type-c, and 2.2% type-d relationship between the sciatic nerve and piriformis muscle [22]. Almost a similar type of finding was noted by Sinha et al. who researched on 100 Indian cadavers and showed 85% type-a, 9% type-b, 3% type-c, and 3% type-d relations [23]. Pokorny et al., Brooks et al., Natsis et al., and Sinha et al., also found 2.2%, 10%, 0.35%, and 3% type-d relations, respectively [7, 20, 22, 23]. Natsis et al., with their research on 290 Greek cadavers revealed 0.35% extremely rare type-f relation [7]. However, the current study did not find any type-d and type-f relations probably due to limitation of small sample size (Figure 3).

Studies on 24 Malaysian and 102 American cadavers have reported 83.4% and 88.2% type-a relations and 16.6% and 11.8% type b-f relations, respectively; however, type-d, type-e, and type-f relations were absent, which was also noticed in current study [24, 25]. A research on 120 American cadavers detected 97.5% type-a and 2.5% type-b relations, which was almost similar to our study [12].

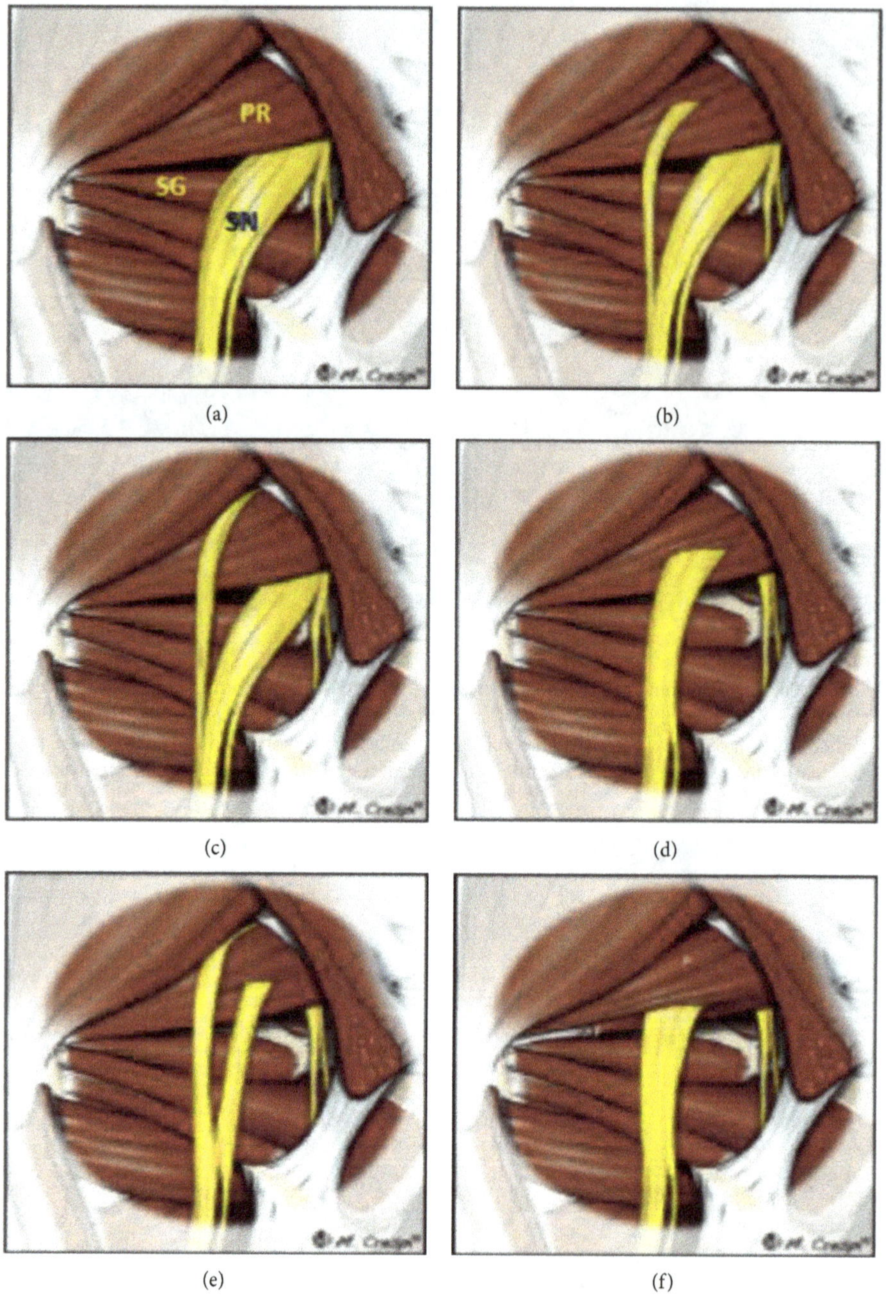

FIGURE 3: Anatomic variations of the relationship between the piriformis muscle and sciatic nerve. Diagrams illustrate the six variants, originally described by Beaton and Anson. (a) An undivided nerve comes out below the piriformis muscle (normal course). (b) A divided sciatic nerve passing through and below the piriformis muscle. (c) A divided nerve passing above and below an undivided muscle. (d) An undivided sciatic nerve passing through the piriformis muscle. (e) A divided nerve passing through and above the muscle heads. (f) Diagram showing an unreported additional variation of d-type consisting of an accessory piriformis (AP) muscle head with its own separate tendon. SN: sciatic nerve; PR: piriformis muscle; SG: superior gemellus [12].

This relationship of sciatic nerve and piriformis muscle was classified as type-b (2.5%). However, in this case, we also observed an altered anatomical variation where a higher division of the sciatic nerve occurs and the common peroneal component passes between the two heads of the piriformis muscle.

A substantial research on 400 fetal cadavers in Turkey revealed 98% type-a 1.2% type b, and 0.8% type c relations [29]. The current study showed similar results; however, the fetal cadavers were not included due to unavailability.

The probability of anatomical variation in cadavers makes it essential among clinicians and surgeons to be aware of the potential complications during medical or surgical interventions [30].

There are several potential etiologies of posterior hip and buttock pain. Jonathan et al. focused on the structural variation that plays a significant role in causing piriformis syndrome; however, the variations unassociated to piriformis syndrome were ruled out due to the difficulty in their identification [12]. In some rare circumstances, anatomic variations may be the source of refractory sciatic pain. Although the variations were recognized in the early 1900s, these findings are uncommon and not readily seen on diagnostic imaging studies. Diagnosis for this syndrome has been historically problematic due to difficulties finding objective evidence as the source of pain. It is usually a diagnosis of exclusion which is made by clinical findings [31]. Neuroimaging techniques are emerging and gaining its popularity, and therefore, researchers and neurophysicians will be able to benefit more precisely in recognizing, diagnosing, treating, and managing the pain associated with nerve entrapment due to composite piriformis-sciatic nerve anomalies. The present study provides awareness of additional sciatic nerve entrapments that are possible within the gluteal regions in the Nepalese population. As a future implication, it is important to emphasize on the study of the embryological basis of these structural variations and their origins.

5. Conclusion

It is important to be aware of anatomical variation in sciatic nerve during a surgical intervention in the gluteal region so as to reduce the risk of injuring these nerves which are more susceptible to be injured. A detailed anatomical study of such variations will be helpful for evaluating the pain in various test positions. The present study provides awareness of additional sciatic nerve entrapments that are possible within the gluteal regions in the Nepalese population. This study is useful for analysis of the range of the neurological deficiency in sciatic nerve neuropathies and explains the basis of the unsuccessful attempt of the sciatic nerve block during popliteal block anaesthesia.

6. Limitations

One of the limitations of this study is small sample size. Therefore, increased sample size has to be considered in future studies. Our research lacks the information on family and medical history of the donors which would have revealed more inference in pain etiology and management.

Acknowledgments

The authors would like to express their sincere thanks to Dr. Pendru Raghunath, Professor of Microbiology, and their colleagues for their precious suggestions and support during preparation of the report. The authors extend their gratitude to all the scholars, authors, editors, and publishers whose articles are reviewed, cited, and included in the references of this report.

References

[1] K. L. Moore, A. F. Dalley, and A. M. R. Agur, *Clinically Oriented Anatomy*, Wolters Kluwer, Philadelphia, PA, USA, 8th edition, 2018.

[2] B. A. Berihu and Y. G. Debeb, "Anatomical variation in bifurcation & trifurcations of sciatic nerve & its clinical implications: in selected university in Ethiopia," *BMC Research Notes*, vol. 8, no. 1, p. 633, 2015.

[3] U.S. Department of Health and Human Services. Health, United States, Centers for Disease Control and Prevention, 2006, https://www.cdc.gov/nchs/data/hus/hus06.pdf.

[4] S. R. Mitra, S. Roy, A. S. Dutta, A. Ghosh, R. Roy, and A. K. Jha, "Piriformis syndrome: a review," *Journal of Evolution of Medical and Dental Sciences*, vol. 3, no. 14, pp. 3804–3814, 2014.

[5] W. Yeoman, "The relation of arthritis of the sacro-iliac joint to sciatica, with an analysis of 100 cases," *The Lancet*, vol. 212, no. 5492, pp. 1119–1123, 1928.

[6] T. H. Ro and L. Edmonds, "Diagnosis and management of piriformis syndrome: a rare anatomic variant analyzed by magnetic resonance imaging," *Journal of Clinical Imaging Science*, vol. 8, no. 6, pp. 1–4, 2018.

[7] K. Natsis, T. Totlis, G. A. Konstantinidis, G. Paraskevas, M. Piagkou, and J. Koebke, "Anatomical variations between the sciatic nerve and the piriformis muscle: a contribution to surgical anatomy in piriformis syndrome," *Surgical and Radiologic Anatomy*, vol. 36, no. 3, pp. 273–280, 2014.

[8] K. A. Tomaszewski, M. J. Graves, B. M. Henry et al., "Surgical anatomy of the sciatic nerve: a meta-analysis," *Journal of Orthopaedic Research*, vol. 34, no. 10, pp. 1820–1827, 2016.

[9] B. A. K. Prakash, M. N. Devi, N. S. Sridevi, P. K. Rao, and G. Singh, "Sciatic nerve division: a cadaver study in the Indian population and review of literature," *Singapore Medical Journal*, vol. 51, pp. 721–723, 2010.

[10] L. E. Beaton and B. J. Anson, "The relation of the sciatic nerve and of its subdivisions to the piriformis muscle," *The Anatomical Record*, vol. 70, no. 1, pp. 1–5, 1937.

[11] L. E. Beaton, "The sciatic nerve and piriform muscle: their interrelations possible cause of coccygodynia," *J Bone Joint Surg Am*, vol. 20, pp. 686–688, 1938.

[12] Van Erdewyk and I. Jonathan, "Anatomical variations of the sciatic nerve divisions in relation to the piriformis muscle and clinical implications," Theses & Dissertations, vol. 194, University of Nebraska Medical Center, Omaha, Nebraska, 2017, http://digitalcommons.unmc.edu/etd/194.

[13] T. A. Miller, K. P. White, and D. C. Ross, "The diagnosis and management of piriformis syndrome: myths and facts," *Canadian Journal of Neurological Sciences/Journal Canadien des Sciences Neurologiques*, vol. 39, no. 5, pp. 577–583, 2012.

[14] M. Adibatti, "Study on variant anatomy of sciatic nerve," *Journal of Clinical and Diagnostic Research: JCDR*, vol. 8, no. 8, pp. AC07–9, 2014.

[15] D. G. Kulcu and S. Naderi, "Differential diagnosis of intraspinal and extraspinal non-discogenic sciatica," *Journal of Clinical Neuroscience*, vol. 15, no. 11, pp. 1246–1252, 2008.

[16] M. Desalegn and A. Tesfay, "Variations of sciatic nerve its exit in relation to piriformis muscle in the northern Ethiopia," *International Journal of Pharmaceutical Sciences and Research*, vol. 5, no. 12, pp. 953–956, 2014.

[17] R. Haladaj, M. Pingot, M. Polguj, G. Wysiadecki, and M. Topol, "Anthropometric study of the piriformis muscle and sciatic nerve: a morphological analysis in a polish population," *Medical Science Monitor: International Medical*

Journal of Experimental and Clinical Research, vol. 21, pp. 3760–3768, 2015.

[18] M. Güvençer, C. Iyem, P. Akyer, S. Tetik, and S. Naderi, "Variations in the high division of the sciatic nerve and relationship between the sciatic nerve and the piriformis," *Turkish Neurosurgery*, vol. 19, no. 19, pp. 139–144, 2009.

[19] S. Patel, M. Shah, R. Vora, A. Zalawadia, and S. P. Rathod, "A variation in the high division of the sciatic nerve and its relation with piriformis muscle," *National Journal of Medical Research*, vol. 1, no. 2, pp. 27–30, 2011.

[20] J. B. B. Brooks, C. A. C. Silva, S. A. Soares, M. R. Kai, R. H. Cabral, and Y. D. Fragoso, "Variações anatômicas do nervo ciático em um grupo de cadáveres brasileiros," *Revista Dor*, vol. 12, no. 4, pp. 332–336, 2011.

[21] J. A. Ogeng'o, H. El-Busaidy, P. M. Mwika, M. M. Khanbhai, and J. Munguti, "Variant anatomy of sciatic nerve in a black Kenyan population," *Folia Morphol*, vol. 70, no. 3, pp. 175–179, 2016.

[22] D. Pokorný, D. Jahoda, D. Veigl, V. Pinskerová, and A. Sosna, "Topographic variations of the relationship of the sciatic nerve and the piriformis muscle and its relevance to palsy after total hip arthroplasty," *Surgical and Radiologic Anatomy*, vol. 28, no. 1, pp. 88–91, 2006.

[23] M. B. Sinha, A. Aggarwal, D. Sahni, K. Harjeet, R. Gupta, and H. P. Sinha, "Morphological variations of sciatic nerve and piriformis muscle in gluteal region during fetal period," *European Journal of Anatomy*, vol. 18, no. 4, pp. 261–266, 2014.

[24] A. A. Khan, M. A. Asari, and M. A. Pasha, "The sciatic nerve in human cadavers-high division or low formation?" *Folia Morphologica*, vol. 75, no. 3, pp. 306–310, 2016.

[25] S. Lewis, J. Jurak, C. Lee, R. Lewis, and T. Gest, "Anatomical variations of the sciatic nerve, in relation to the piriformis muscle," *Translational Research in Anatomy*, vol. 5, pp. 15–19, 2016.

[26] A. K. Singh and R. C. Sharma, "Relationship between the sciatic nerve and piriformis muscle," *Neuroscience Research Letters*, vol. 2, no. 1, pp. 26–28, 2011.

[27] A. D. Shewale, R. R. Karambelkar, and B. N. Umarji, "Study of variations in the divisions, course and termination of the sciatic nerve," *Journal of Krishna Institute of Medical Sciences University*, vol. 2, no. 1, pp. 62–68, 2013.

[28] T. Muthu Kumar, Srimathi, A. Rani, and S. Latha, "A cadaveric study of sciatic nerve and it's level of bifurcation," *Journal of Clinical and Diagnostic Research*, vol. 5, no. 8, pp. 1502–1504, 2011.

[29] O. Sulak, B. Sakalli, G. Ozguner, and Y. Kastamoni, "Anatomical relation between sciatic nerve and piriformis muscle and its bifurcation level during fetal period in human," *Surgical and Radiologic Anatomy*, vol. 36, no. 3, pp. 265–272, 2014.

[30] N. R. Smoll, "Variations of the piriformis and sciatic nerve with clinical consequence: a review," *Clinical Anatomy*, vol. 23, no. 1, pp. 8–17, 2010.

[31] L. Cassidy, A. Walters, K. Bubb et al., "Piriformis syndrome: implications of anatomical variations, diagnostic techniques, and treatment options," *Surgical and Radiologic Anatomy*, vol. 34, no. 6, pp. 479–486, 2012.

26

Cervical Spine Ischemic Stroke Complicated by Spastic Quadriparesis and Ogilvie Syndrome: A Case Report and Literature Review

Salman Assad, Justin Nolte, Dharampreet Singh, Samrina Hanif, and Paul Ferguson

Department of Neurology, Marshall University School of Medicine, Huntington, WV, USA

Correspondence should be addressed to Salman Assad; salmanassad91@gmail.com

Academic Editor: Peter Berlit

Infarction or ischemia of the spinal cord is a rare entity and is often misdiagnosed as inflammatory myelopathy in acute settings. Atherosclerotic disease can affect spinal arteries, leading to cord ischemia with clinical presentation mixed with myelopathy. We present a case of a 66-year-old male who came to the hospital with unsteady gait and numbness of all extremities without associated pain for the past 48 hours. The neurological examination on admission directed the diagnosis towards myelopathy of the cervical spine. However, the initial magnetic resonance imaging (MRI) of the cervical spine demonstrated gliosis and restricted diffusion of the cord with multilevel neuroforaminal stenosis but without central canal stenosis or cord compression. The MRI brain, cerebrospinal fluid analysis, and rheumatologic evaluation were unremarkable. Four days into the clinical course, the patient developed weakness and spasticity of all extremities prompting further evaluation. Computed tomography angiography (CTA) scan of the head and neck revealed right vertebral artery occlusion and intracranial atherosclerotic disease. He was started on aspirin and clopidogrel for secondary risk reduction. The hospital course was further complicated by Ogilvie syndrome (OS), and the patient underwent uncomplicated cecostomy.

1. Introduction

Spinal cord ischemia is caused by a vascular interruption that can lead to cord dysfunction, ischemia, and infarction [1]. The blood supply of the spinal cord consists of anterior and posterior spinal arteries. The cervical cord lesions can typically present with either acute quadriparesis or paraparesis. Three vessels arising from vertebral arteries supply the spinal cord in the neck consisting of anterior and two posterior spinal arteries [2]. The manifestation of cord infarction is spontaneous with unknown etiology. Vascular aneurysm, dissection, and post-surgical complications should be ruled out when suspecting a cord ischemic stroke [3]. We present a unique and first-ever report of cryptogenic cervical cord acute ischemic infarction with late-onset development of Ogilvie syndrome.

2. Case Presentation

A 66-year-old male with a past medical history of hypertension, hyperlipidemia, coronary artery disease, prostate cancer, and gastroesophageal reflux disease presented to the emergency department with intermittent symptoms of disequilibrium, gait instability, and progressive numbness of all extremities. The patient also developed hypotension and required vasopressors and intravenous fluid support after his neurologic symptomatology further evolved into weakness and spasticity. Laboratory investigation revealed hypercholesterolemia with normal thyroid-stimulating hormone, vitamin B12, and folate levels. Transthoracic echocardiography showed ejection fraction >55%, no wall abnormalities, and no patent foramen ovale. The MRI of the brain was unremarkable. The computed tomography angiography (CTA) of the head and neck showed right vertebral artery occlusion with moderate diffuse intracranial atherosclerosis (Figure 1). On day 2 of admission, the patient's weakness of all four extremities worsened and became acutely myelopathic with Babinski and Hoffman's sign in the setting of diffuse hyperreflexia and quadriparesis. An MRI of the cervical spine with and without gadolinium demonstrated a restriction on diffusion-weighted imaging (DWI)

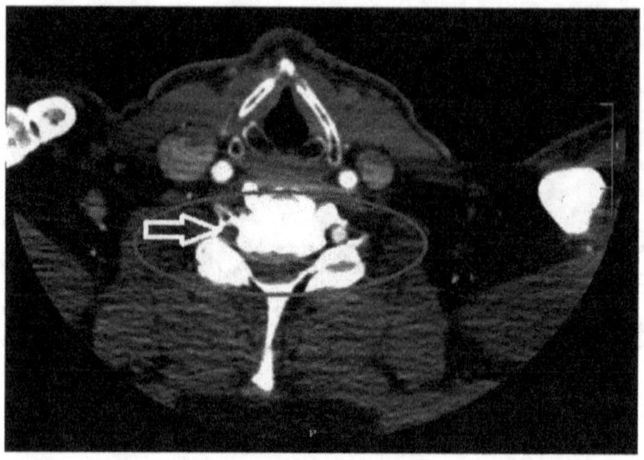

Figure 1: The computed tomography angiography (CTA) of the the head and neck showed right vertebral artery occlusion with moderate diffuse intracranial atherosclerosis.

corresponding to the signal abnormality foci seen on short-TI inversion recovery (STIR) images (Figure 2).

He further developed urinary retention and Ogilvie's (acute colonic pseudo-obstruction) syndrome. The MRI of the thoracolumbar region did not reveal any abnormality. For spasticity, the patient was given baclofen 20 mg three times per day and tizanidine 2 mg every 8 hours. For Ogilvie's syndrome, cecostomy was performed by the surgery team. The lumbar puncture and cerebrospinal fluid analysis showed normal IgG index 0.6 (normal range 0.0–0.7), high myelin basic protein 12 (normal range 0–1.2 nanograms/milliliter (ng/ml)), no oligo clonal bands, negative neuromyelitis optica spectrum disorders (NMOSD) antibody, and negative myelin oligodendrocyte glycoprotein (MOG) antibody. The blood cultures, urine cultures, and CSF diagnostic workup for viral, bacterial, or fungal infections were noncontributory. The patient was started on subcutaneous heparin for deep venous thrombosis prophylaxis, aspirin 81 mg daily, clopidogrel 75 mg daily, and atorvastatin 40 mg daily for secondary risk reduction. The patient was discharged to a rehabilitation facility.

3. Discussion

The onset of spinal cord ischemia or infarction symptomatology is usually abrupt like that noted in cerebral ischemia. A diffuse atherosclerotic process can affect spinal arteries and can lead to focal or nonfocal neurological deficits [3]. Cigarette smoking, uncontrolled hypertension, diabetes, positive family history of vascular insults, and hyperlipidemia are the major risk factors for spinal cord infarction [4]. The vertebrobasilar insufficiency can present with a multitude of symptoms such as bilateral body weakness, headaches, vomiting, diplopia, blindness, dizziness, and gait instability [5]. The symptoms of bladder dysfunction, quadriparesis, bilateral loss of pain, temperature sensation with intact proprioception, and vibration sensation are indicative of anterior spinal artery (ASA) syndrome [5]. The patient in our case has occluded right nondominant vertebral artery indicative of vertebrobasilar insufficiency. The functional outcome with spinal cord infarction is promising due to the noninvolvement of cognitive deficits [6]. Elzamly et al. reported a case of posterior cervical cord infarction after the neuro-endovascular intervention for vertebrobasilar insufficiency [7]. It is imperative to mention that we did not consider thrombolysis in our case as cord infarction might have happened due to hypotensive episode. The patient in our report also developed neurogenic bladder and Ogilvie syndrome (colonic pseudo-obstruction), which is usually common with lesions below thoracic spine vertebra level 10 (T10) as reported by Korsten et al. [8].

Davda and Osman also mentioned a similar anterior spinal cord infarct with an affected spinothalamic tract involving the pain and temperature sensation [9]. This finding is in contrast to our report where both vibration and fine touch with pain and temperature sensations were affected, highlighting the involvement of both anterior and posterior spinal arteries. Ota et al. mentioned a patient who initially presented with sudden onset quadriplegia with an MRI cervical spine indicative of myelopathy [10]. After almost one week of the worsening of neurological symptoms, DWI and ADC images of the MRI cervical spine were obtained that showed acute cord infarction [10]. On the other hand, our patient developed spastic quadriplegia almost after 10 days of onset with intermittent episodes of unsteady gait. Müller et al. and Restrepo et al. mentioned the prompt recovery within few days of ASA syndrome in patients presented within 3 hours of symptoms and treated with intravenous recombinant tissue plasminogen activator (tPA) [4, 11]. It is also necessary to look for vascular dissection, aneurysm, or malformations before giving tPA [11]. The fluid resuscitation and use of dual antiplatelet therapy (DAPT) with statins were found to be associated with good outcomes in ASA syndrome patients [4]. The role of a mechanical thrombectomy or neuroendovascular procedures in such cases is still debatable and will require future studies.

The first limitation of our case presentation was not taking into consideration the magnetic resonance angiography (MRA) or conventional angiogram of the cervical spine in the beginning. The second limitation was not ordering a repeat MRI or MRA of the thoracolumbar spine on day 14 of hospitalization after the patient developed Ogilvie syndrome to rule out thoracolumbar infarction. However,

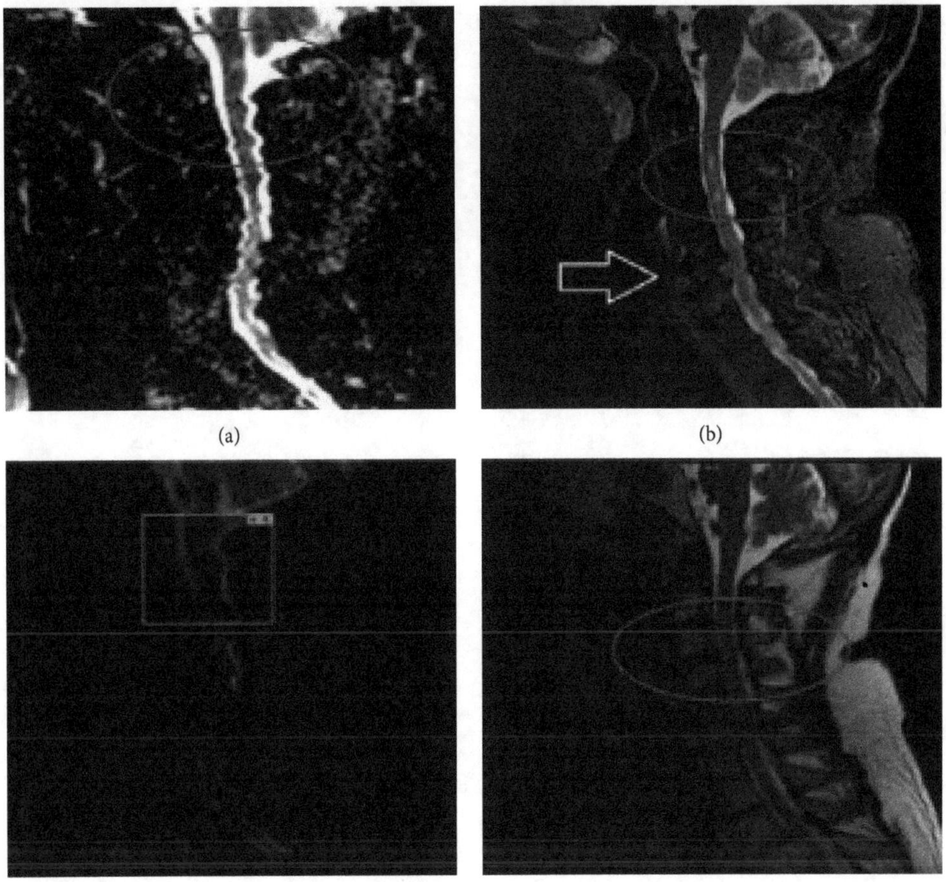

(a) (b) (c) (d)

FIGURE 2: (a–d) MRI of the cervical spine with and without gadolinium demonstrated a restriction on diffusion-weighted imaging (DWI) (a) corresponding to the signal abnormality foci seen on short-TI inversion recovery (STIR) images (red circles in (b) and (d) and white marker image in (c)) and anterior compression from displaced cervical discs (white arrow in (b)).

the CTA of the head and neck was done and vascular dissection or aneurysm was not reported which in the past has been associated with spinal cord vascular syndromes. We conclude that the timely diagnosis of cord ischemia is important and MRI with DWI/ADC, MRA, or conventional angiogram should be considered in such cases. If within the window, tPA can be considered followed by DAPT for 3–6 months based on clinical discretion until clinical trials are available in the literature.

References

[1] M.-Y. Cheng, R.-K. Lyu, Y.-J. Chang et al., "Spinal cord infarction in Chinese patients. Clinical features, risk factors, imaging and prognosis," *Cerebrovascular Diseases*, vol. 26, no. 5, pp. 502–508, 2008.

[2] S. Prasad, R. S. Price, S. M. Kranick, J. H. Woo, R. W. Hurst, and S. Galetta, "Clinical reasoning: a 59-year-old woman with acute paraplegia," *Neurology*, vol. 69, no. 24, pp. E41–E47, 2007.

[3] T. A. Bley, C. C. Duffek, C. J. François et al., "Presurgical localization of the artery of adamkiewicz with time-resolved 3.0-T MR angiography," *Radiology*, vol. 255, no. 3, pp. 873–881, 2010.

[4] K. I. Müller, L. H. Steffensen, and S. H. Johnsen, "Thrombolysis in anterior spinal artery syndrome," *BMJ Case Reports*, vol. 2012, no. 2, 2012.

[5] A. Lima Neto, R. Bittar, G. Gattas et al., "Pathophysiology and diagnosis of vertebrobasilar insufficiency: a review of the literature," *International Archives of Otorhinolaryngology*, vol. 21, no. 3, pp. 302–307, 2017.

[6] K. Nedeltchev, T. J. Loher, F. Stepper et al., "Long-term outcome of acute spinal cord ischemia syndrome," *Stroke*, vol. 35, no. 2, pp. 560–565, 2004.

[7] K. Elzamly, C. Nobleza, E. Parker, and R. Sugg, "Unilateral upper cervical posterior spinal cord infarction after a neuroendovascular intervention: a case report," *Case Reports in Neurological Medicine*, vol. 2018, Article ID 5070712, 3 pages, 2018.

[8] M. A. Korsten, A. S. Rosman, A. Ng et al., "Infusion of neostigmine-glycopyrrolate for bowel evacuation in persons with spinal cord injury," *The American Journal of Gastroenterology*, vol. 100, no. 7, pp. 1560–1565, 2005.

[9] N. Davda and C. Osman, "Anterior spinal cord infarct: a rare yet disabling stroke," *BMJ Case Reports*, vol. 7, pp. 22017–221655, 2018.

[10] K. Ota, R. Iida, K. Ota et al., "Atypical spinal cord infarction: a case report," *Medicine (Baltimore)*, vol. 97, no. 23, Article ID e11058, 2018.
[11] L. Restrepo and J. F. Guttin, "Acute spinal cord ischemia during aortography treated with intravenous thrombolytic therapy," *Texas Heart Institute Journal*, vol. 33, no. 1, pp. 74–77, 2006.

27

A Novel SPAST/SPG4 Splice-Site Variant in a Family with Dominant Hereditary Spastic Paraplegia

Nathaniel M. Robbins,[1] Jillian R. Ozmore,[2] Thomas L. Winder,[3] Pedro Gonzalez-Alegre,[4] and Tanya M. Bardakjian[4]

[1]*Department of Neurology, Geisel Dartmouth School of Medicine, Hanover, USA*
[2]*Department of Medical Genetics, Dartmouth-Hitchcock Medical Center, Lebanon, USA*
[3]*Invitae Corporation, San Francisco, USA*
[4]*Department of Neurology, The University of Pennsylvania, Philadelphia, USA*

Correspondence should be addressed to Nathaniel M. Robbins; nathaniel.m.robbins@dartmouth.edu

Academic Editor: Mathias Toft

Some causes of spastic paraplegia are treatable and many are not. Diagnostic work-up to determine the etiology can be costly and invasive. Here we report the case of a man with slowly progressive spastic paraparesis. Using a multigene next-generation sequencing (NGS) panel, we identified a novel variant in the consensus splice site of the SPAST gene (exon 13, c.1536G>A, heterozygous), affecting codon 512 of the SPAST mRNA. The observed variant segregated with the disease in four tested family members. In this case, genetic confirmation obviated the need for additional testing such as MRI and lumbar puncture and helped the patient and his family understand his condition and prognosis. We conclude with a brief discussion of the SPG4/SPAST gene and the role of multigene panels in the diagnosis and management of hereditary spastic paraplegia.

1. Case Presentation

A 46-year-old man presented with insidiously progressive gait and balance difficulties over fifteen years. His legs felt stiff. Gait was slow. He could trip from catching his toes on the ground. The lateral part of his shoes wore away asymmetrically. He endorsed urinary frequency but normal bowel function. He had occasional cramps but no significant pain. He had mild memory complaints but continued to work, drive, and do all other independent activities of daily living. He took no medications; reported no trauma; and denied substance use.

The proband's father developed symptoms around age 45 and cognitive problems (no additional details available) before he died at 75. A paternal cousin developed gait problems in her 30 s. She later developed urinary and bowel dysfunction as well as anosmia, ageusia, and sensorineural hearing loss. Cognition remained normal. Figure 1 details the family history.

Neurologic examination revealed a spastic paraparesis, with symmetrically brisk (3 out of 4) patellar and ankles reflexes, and bilateral extensor responses with plantar stimulation. Ankle eversion was slightly weak (Medical Research Council 5-/5) but other distal (i.e., toe and ankle extension, foot inversion) and proximal muscles were strong. He could stand on his toes but not his heels. Vibration sensation was slightly reduced distally, but pinprick and light touch were normal. Gait was scissoring. He scored 25 of 30 on a Montreal Cognitive Assessment, losing three points for delayed recall, and one point each for clock draw and tapping "A's." Mental status, cranial nerve, and arm examination were otherwise normal. He was clinically diagnosed with a thoracic myelopathy, presumed to be hereditary. Vitamin B12 was normal.

A twelve-gene panel looking for autosomal dominant hereditary spastic paraparesis (HSP) was sent to Invitae (San Francisco, CA—see below and Appendix for genetic testing methods). NGS identified a variant of uncertain significance

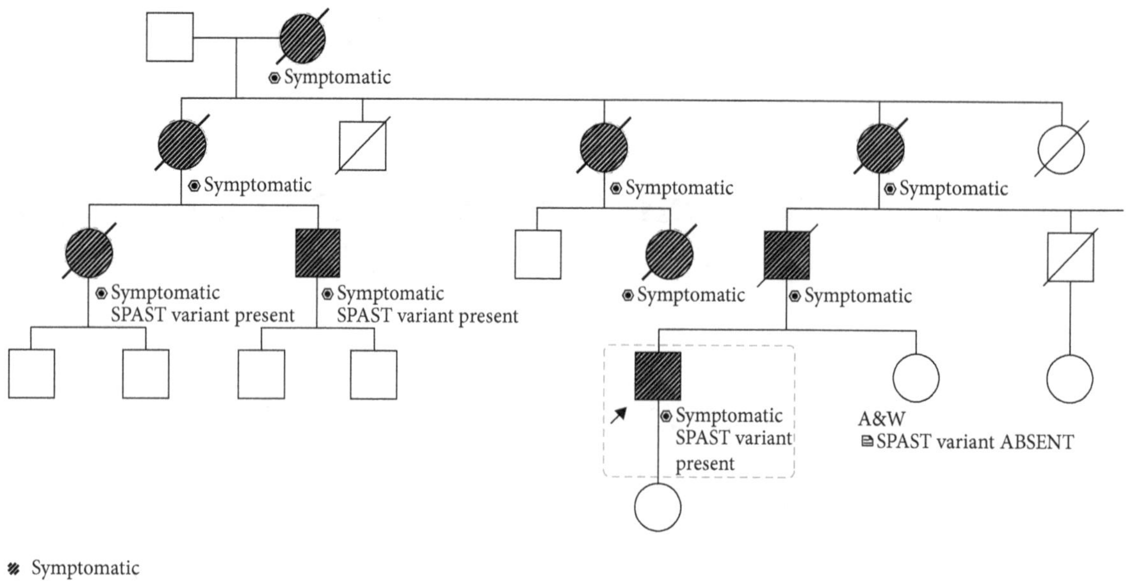

Figure 1: Pedigree of the family.

(VUS) in the SPAST gene (exon 13, c.1536G>A, heterozygous), affecting codon 512 of the SPAST mRNA (NM_014946.3). This variant was not present in any standard population or clinical databases (see Appendix for databases queried, or the following web page: https://www.invitae.com/static/data/WhitePaper_Variant-Classification-Method.pdf). This variant fell at the last nucleotide of exon 13, which is part of the consensus splice site. A novel pathogenic variant was suspected since nucleotide substitutions within the consensus splice site are a relatively common cause of aberrant splicing [1] and since a different variant affecting this nucleotide (c.1536G>C) was previously reported as probably pathogenic using RT-PCR for mRNA analysis and familial segregation analysis [2]. In silico splice models were used to analyze the c.1536G>A variant (see Appendix for methods), and all models suggest this variant interferes with normal splicing, though this has not been confirmed by published transcriptional studies. Saliva from the patient's sister and father's affected cousin was then tested. Testing demonstrated the identical variant in the affected cousin, but not the unaffected sister (see pedigree—Figure 1), supporting the hypothesis that this novel variant is pathogenic, though functional expression studies were not done.

2. Genetic Testing Methods

The following 13 genes were analyzed for sequence changes and exonic deletions/duplications using NGS: *ALDH18A1, ATL1, BSCL2, HSPD1, KIF1A, KIF5A, NIPA1, REEP1, REEP2, RTN2, SPAST, VAMP1*, and *WASHC5*. As previously described [3–5], genomic DNA obtained from the proband's blood and family members' saliva was subjected to target enrichment using hybridization capture with a custom bait pool and sequenced using Illumina sequencing chemistry. A validated bioinformatics pipeline incorporating community standard and custom algorithms was used to identify sequence changes and exonic deletions/duplications simultaneously. Clinically significant observations were confirmed by orthogonal technologies, except individually validated variants and variants previously confirmed in a first-degree relative. Depending on the variant type, confirmation technologies may include any of the following: Sanger sequencing, Pacific Biosciences SMRT sequencing, MLPA, MLPA-seq, and Array CGH. Variants were evaluated and classified using a refinement of the five-tier system for grading evidence for pathogenicity by American College of Medical Genetics and Genomics (ACMG) [6, 7]. Appendix illustrates more detailed methods.

3. Discussion

A mutated SPAST gene, which encodes the microtubule-severing protein spastin, is the most common cause of HSP, accounting for 15–40% of all HSP cases [8, 9]. Autosomal dominant HSP-SPG4 is usually "uncomplicated," causing lower limb spasticity only without shortening lifespan. However, cognitive impairment has been described, and up to 50% of patients can have autonomic symptoms [8–11]. The mechanisms by which a mutated SPAST causes dysfunction are complex and remain incompletely understood [8].

Known pathogenic variants in SPAST/SPG4 include missense, nonsense, deletions, insertions, and splice-site variants [2, 8, 9]. Age of onset ranges from infancy through senescence, and functional impairment is highly variable [2, 8, 9, 11]. Penetrance is incomplete though typically symptomatic and age-dependent, with 50% and 80% showing symptoms at age 27 and 50, respectively [8].

Insidious spastic paraparesis with few sensory symptoms and a positive family history strongly suggests HSP. However, in the absence of genetic confirmation, HSP is a diagnosis of exclusion, which can lead to expensive and superfluous MRIs, lumbar punctures, and blood tests looking for metabolic, infectious, and inflammatory causes of myelopathy. Genetic confirmation can curtail this misdirected testing and help patients to obtain psychological closure, better understand prognosis, and gain entry into clinical trials and support groups that require a diagnosis. Since more than 80 genes and many more variants have thus far been associated with HSP, NGS panels have become essential for diagnosis and should be considered first-line in the right clinical scenario [12]. Cost of NGS varies widely based on insurance coverage, but can be as little as 250 USD: far less than MRI.

Here NGS and family comparison testing identified a novel variant in SPAST associated with classic HSP-SPG4, thereby expanding the known genetic spectrum of this heterogeneous disease. A genetically confirmed diagnosis obviated the need for additional testing.

Appendix

Genetic testing methods used by Invitae

Clinical genetic testing for autosomal dominant hereditary spastic paraparesis was performed at Invitae (San Francisco, California). The following 13 genes were analyzed for sequence changes and exonic deletions/duplications using next-generation sequencing: ALDH18A1, ATL1, BSCL2, HSPD1, KIF1A, KIF5A, NIPA1, REEP1, REEP2, RTN2, SPAST, VAMP1, and WASHC5. As previously described [3-5], genomic DNA obtained from the proband's blood and family members' saliva was subjected to target enrichment using hybridization capture with a custom bait pool and sequenced using Illumina sequencing chemistry. A validated bioinformatics pipeline incorporating community standard and custom algorithms was used to identify sequence changes and exonic deletions/duplications simultaneously. Clinically significant observations were confirmed by orthogonal technologies, except individually validated variants and variants previously confirmed in a first-degree relative. Depending on the variant type, confirmation technologies may include any of the following: Sanger sequencing, Pacific Biosciences SMRT sequencing, MLPA, MLPA-seq, and Array CGH. Variants were evaluated and classified using a refinement of the five-tier system for grading evidence for pathogenicity by American College of Medical Genetics and Genomics (ACMG) [6, 7]. In silico splicing programs used are as follows: GeneSplicer, NNSPLICE, MaxEntScan, and SpliceSiteFinder-like.

Disclosure

This manuscript was presented in abbreviated form at the 2020 American Academy of Neurology Annual meeting.

Acknowledgments

The authors would like to thank Drs. Sean Zadeh and Nicky Wu for their assistance with that abstract and presentation.

References

[1] M. Zhang, "Statistical features of human exons and their flanking regions," *Human Molecular Genetics*, vol. 7, no. 5, pp. 919–932, 1998.

[2] C. Patrono, C. Casali, A. Tessa et al., "Missense and splice site mutations in SPG4 suggest loss-of-function in dominant spastic paraplegia," *Journal of Neurology*, vol. 249, no. 2, pp. 200–205, 2002.

[3] R. Truty, J. Paul, M. Kennemer et al., "Prevalence and properties of intragenic copy-number variation in Mendelian disease genes," *Genetics in Medicine*, vol. 21, no. 1, pp. 114–123, 2018.

[4] S. E. Lincoln, Y. Kobayashi, M. J. Anderson et al., "A systematic comparison of traditional and multigene panel testing for hereditary breast and ovarian cancer genes in more than 1000 patients," *The Journal of Molecular Diagnostics*, vol. 17, no. 5, pp. 533–544, 2015.

[5] A. W. Kurian, E. E. Hare, M. A. Mills et al., "Clinical evaluation of a multiple-gene sequencing panel for hereditary cancer risk assessment," *Journal of Clinical Oncology*, vol. 32, no. 19, pp. 2001–2009, 2014.

[6] M. M. Li, M. Datto, E. J. Duncavage et al., "Standards and guidelines for the interpretation and reporting of sequence variants in cancer: a joint consensus recommendation of the association for molecular pathology, American Society of Clinical Oncology, and College of American Pathologists," *The Journal of Molecular Diagnostics*, vol. 19, no. 1, pp. 4–23, 2017.

[7] K. Nykamp, M. Anderson, M. Anderson et al., "Sherloc: a comprehensive refinement of the ACMG-AMP variant classification criteria," *Genetics in Medicine*, vol. 19, no. 10, pp. 1105–1117, 2017.

[8] J. M. Solowska and P. W. Baas, "Hereditary spastic paraplegia SPG4: what is known and not known about the disease," *Brain*, vol. 138, no. 9, pp. 2471–2484, 2015.

[9] L. Parodi, S. L. Rydning, C. Tallaksen, and A. Durr, "Spastic paraplegia 4," in *GeneReviews®*, M. P. Adam, R. A. Pagon, H. H. Ardinger et al., Eds., University of Washington, Seattle, WA, USA, 2003.

[10] S. Salinas, C. Proukakis, A. Crosby, and T. T. Warner, "Hereditary spastic paraplegia: clinical features and pathogenetic mechanisms," *The Lancet Neurology*, vol. 7, no. 12, pp. 1127–1138, 2008.

[11] A. Orlacchio, T. Kawarai, A. Totaro et al., "Hereditary spastic paraplegia: clinical genetic study of 15 families," *Archives of Neurology*, vol. 61, no. 6, pp. 849–855, 2004.

[12] L. Travaglini, C. Aiello, F. Stregapede et al., "The impact of next-generation sequencing on the diagnosis of pediatric-onset hereditary spastic paraplegias: new genotype-phenotype correlations for rare HSP-related genes," *Neurogenetics*, vol. 19, no. 2, pp. 111–121, 2018.

28

Unusual Phenotype and Disease Trajectory in Kearns–Sayre Syndrome

Josef Finsterer,[1] **Michael Winklehner**,[2] **Claudia Stöllberger**,[3] **and Thomas Hummel**[4]

[1]*Krankenanstalt Rudolfstiftung, Messerli Institute, Vienna, Austria*
[2]*Institute of Neurology, Medical University of Vienna, Vienna, Austria*
[3]*2nd Medical Department, Krankenanstalt Rudolfstiftung, Vienna, Austria*
[4]*Krankenhaus Stockerau, Stockerau, Austria*

Correspondence should be addressed to Josef Finsterer; fipaps@yahoo.de

Academic Editor: Samuel T. Gontkovsky

Objective. To describe unusual course and unusual phenotypic features in an adult patient with Kearns–Sayre syndrome (KSS). *Case Report.* The patient is a 49-year-old male with KSS, diagnosed clinically upon the core features, namely, onset before the age 20 of years, pigmentary retinopathy, and ophthalmoparesis, and the complementary features, namely, elevated CSF protein, cardiac conduction defects, and cerebellar ataxia. The patient presented also with other previously described features, such as diabetes, short stature, white matter lesions, hypoacusis, migraine, hepatopathy, steatosis hepatis, hypocorticism (hyponatremia), and cataract. Unusual features the patient presented with were congenital anisocoria, severe caries, liver cysts, pituitary enlargement, desquamation of hands and feet, bone chondroma, aortic ectasia, dermoidal cyst, and sinusoidal polyposis. The course was untypical since most of the core phenotypic features developed not earlier than in adulthood. *Conclusions.* KSS is a multisystem disease, but the number of tissues affected is higher than so far anticipated. KSS should be considered even if core features develop not earlier than in adulthood and if unusual features accompany the presentation.

1. Introduction

Kearns–Sayre syndrome (KSS) is a mitochondrial disorder (MID) most frequently due to a single mtDNA deletion and rarely due to mtDNA point mutations [1, 2]. The diagnosis is established clinically if the three core features onset, <20 years of age, chronic progressive external ophthalmoplegia (CPEO), and pigmentary retinopathy, and at least one of the following features are present: cerebrospinal fluid (CSF) protein >100 mg/dl, cardiac conduction defects, or cerebellar dysfunction [1]. Here, we present an adult male with KSS with unusual phenotypic features and disease trajectory.

2. Case Report

The patient is a 49-year-old male, with height 161 cm, weight 85 kg, and a history of preterm birth at gestational week 34 from nonconsanguineous parents, congenital anisocoria, developmental delay, hypoacusis, and tetra-ataxia (Table 1). During childhood general downslowing, chronic fatigue, and sicca syndrome of the eyes occurred. He repeatedly experienced respiratory infections and oral herpetic infections and once painless desquamation of the hands and foot soles (Table 1). He was successfully trained and worked as a hairdresser until the age of 38 years in his parent's hair saloon and retired at the age of 40 years.

At age of 30 years, left anterior hemiblock and right bundle-branch-block were recorded. Since age 35, recurrent mild elevation of creatine-kinase (CK) was noted. Aldolase and myoglobin were also elevated. Since age 35, recurrent electrolyte disturbances (hypokalemia and hyponatremia) and hyperuricemia developed. At age 36, he experienced a first episode of disorientation, impaired cognition, bradyphrenia, and secessus urinae. Clinical exam revealed bilateral ophthalmoparesis and dysarthria. Magnetic resonance imaging (MRI) showed subcortical hyperintensities in a

Table 1: Disease trajectory of the presented patient over 49 years of age.

Onset (age)	Manifestation	Therapy
Intrauterine	Premature birth (7 weeks earlier)	None
Birth	Congenital anisocoria	None
Infancy	Developmental delay	None
Infancy	Hypoacusis	Hearing devices since age 39
Childhood	Downslowing, chronic fatigue	None
Childhood	Sicca syndrome + recurrent conjunctivitis	Eye drops
Childhood	Recurrent respiratory infections	Antibiotics
Childhood	Recurrent herpetic infections, stomatitis	Virostatics
5 y	Painless desquamation of hands and feet	None
6 y	Ophthalmoparesis (first recognised)	None
7 y	Tetra-ataxia	None
18 y	Severe caries	Full prosthesis
27 y	Right-sided inguinal hernia	Bassini surgery
29 y	Sacral dermoidal cyst	Surgery
30 y	Bifascicular block*	None
30 y	Erythema nodosa of feet	Steroids
35 y	Hyper-CKemia	None
35 y	Hyperuricemia	Diet
35 y	Hyponatremia, hypokalemia	NaCl, KCl
36 y	Somnolence, infection, suspected BE, SLE	Antibiotics, virostatics, endobolin, steroids
36 y	Suspected SLE	None
36 y	Elevated CSF protein	None
36 y	Dysarthria	None
36 y	Polyposis of nasal sinuses	None
36 y	Gait disturbance, falls	None
36 y	Neuropsychological deficits	Training
37 y	Arterial hypertension	Antihypertensives
37 y	Hepatopathy	None
37 y	Liver cysts	None
37 y	Rhabdomyolysis (CK: 2673 U/L)	None
38 y	Chondroma/fibroma of the right femur	None
38 y	Steatosis hepatis	None
44 y	Suspected SLE, Na↓, K↓, migraine	Analgesics
45 y	Fall, rib fracture, pneumothorax	Drainage
45 y	Diabetes	Antidiabetics
47 y	Cataract bilaterally	Surgery
49 y	Aortic ectasia	None

*Left anterior hemiblock plus right bundle branch block, SLE: stroke-like episode, nr: not relevant, CSF: cerebrospinal fluid, BE: Bickerstaff encephalitis.

nonvascular distribution, which were hyperintens on diffusion-weighted imaging (DWI) and apparent diffusion coefficient (ADC) (Figure 1). Neuropsychological testing revealed attention deficits, disability of encoding visual contents, adjustment disorder, and depression. The patient was diagnosed with suspected Bickerstaff encephalitis and questionable seizures. Following these episodes, his gait became disturbed with occasional falls due to increased ataxia. At age 37, he experienced an untriggered rhabdomyolysis. Muscle biopsy from the deltoid muscle suggested muscular dystrophy as only fat but no muscle tissue was detected (Table 2). At age 38, he underwent a second muscle biopsy from the left lateral vastus muscle which showed cytochrome-C-oxidase (COX)-negative fibers (Figure 2(a)), glycogen depositions (Figure 2(b)), fiber splitting, and ragged-red fibers (Figure 2(c)). Electron microscopy showed abnormally shaped and structured mitochondria, megaconia, abnormal glycogen and lipid depositions, and dark bodies (Figures 2(d) and 2(e)). At age 44, migraine developed. At age 47, he underwent cataract surgery bilaterally (Table 1). At age 49, diabetes was diagnosed. Transthoracic echocardiography was normal except for mild enlargement of the ascending aorta (Figure 3).

The family history was positive for hypotonia (mother), diabetes (father, brother of father, grandmother from the father's side, grand-grandfather from the father's side), carcinoma (father), and stroke (father). Neurological exam at age 49, revealed short stature, microcephaly, facial dysmorphism, myopathic face, ophthalmoparesis, pupils nonreactive to light, anisocoria (left: 5 mm, right: 3 mm, unrounded), divergence of bulbs, ophthalmoparesis (abduction right bulb 60° abduction left bulb: 15° vertical movements impossible), bilateral ptosis (right > left), reduced corneal reflexes, hypoacusis requiring bilateral hearing devices, dysarthria, dropped head, weakness for right elbow extension and flexion, reduced tendon reflexes on the upper limbs, ataxia and brady-dysdiadochokinesia on the upper limbs, marked wasting of the thighs, ataxia on the lower limbs, truncal ataxia, and ataxic stance, and gait. Gnome calves bilaterally, which were described at age 38

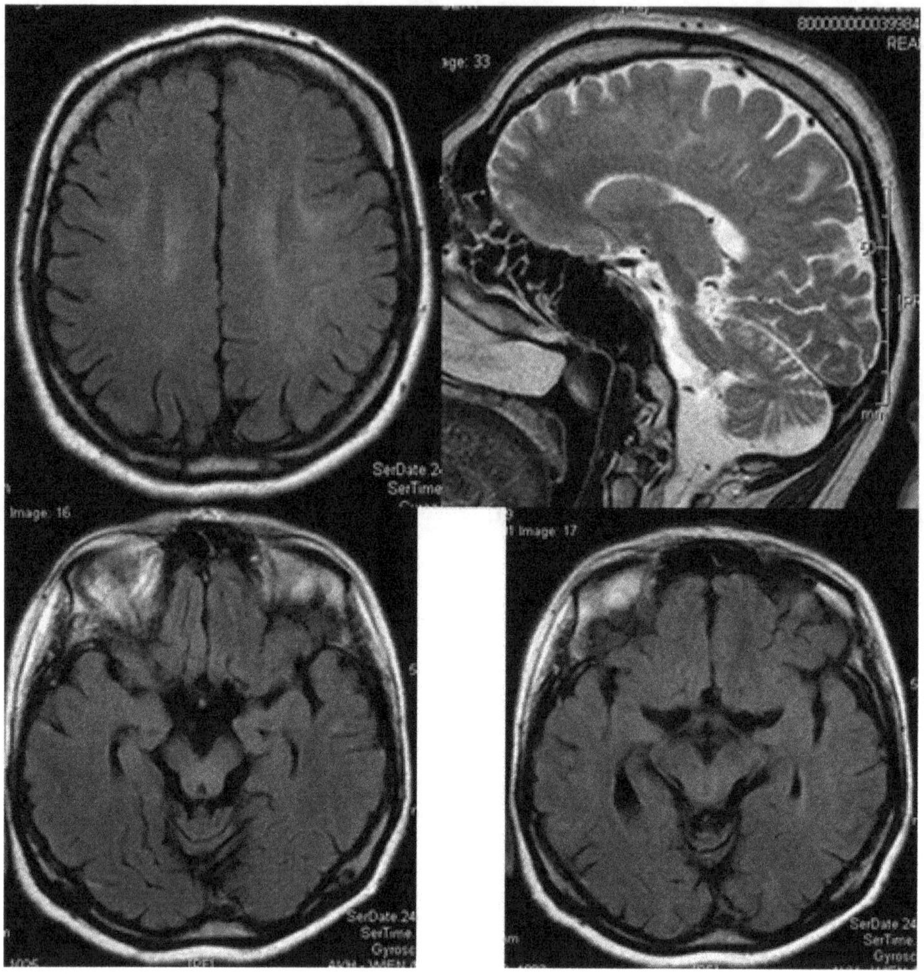

Figure 1: Cerebral MRI at age 36 showing mild, band-like T2-hyperintensities in the white matter bilaterally (upper left) and the midbrain (lower panels) and mild cerebellar atrophy (upper right).

were no longer present. The last medication included indapamide, furosemide/spironolactone, simvastatin, NaCl, KCl, coenzyme-Q (60 mg/d), and vitamin-D.

3. Discussion

The presented patient is interesting in several aspects. Though clinical manifestations of KSS developed already in early infancy and childhood, the majority of the typical phenotypic features (CPEO, pigmentary retinopathy, elevated CSF protein, and cardiac conduction defects) and hepatopathy were recognised not earlier than in adulthood. Possibly, the typical features of KSS required for establishing the diagnosis [1, 2] were present already earlier; however, they were not recognied before age 30. KSS was suspected for the first time at age 39. An argument in favor of the diagnosis of KSS is that the mother was not affected suggesting that there was no transmission of a pathogenic mtDNA variant but rather spontaneous occurrence of a single mtDNA deletion, which is the cause in 96% of cases [3].

Another interesting point is the phenotype. Though the patient fulfilled the diagnostic criteria for KSS, he additionally presented with a plethora of manifestations, of which some have been reported earlier in KSS. In addition to the features required for diagnosing KSS, the patient presented with the known features of diabetes [4], hypocorticism (hyponatremia) [5], short stature [6], white matter lesions [7], hypoacusis [1], migraine [8], hepatopathy [9], steatosis [10], and cataract [11]. Features so far unreported in KSS include congenital anisocoria, severe caries, liver cysts, pituitary enlargement, desquamation of hands and feet, bone chondroma, aortic ectasia, dermoidal cyst, and polyposis of nasal sinuses. Whether all these features are truly attributable to the underlying metabolic defect remains speculative and requires further investigations, but from other MIDs it is well known that such features can be part of the phenotype [12]. The reason for the high number of novel phenotypic features could be that previous cases were not thoroughly investigated or that the genetic cause of the present patient was different from that of the previous cases.

Concerning the recurrent deteriorations of the phenotype during infections or spontaneously, it cannot be excluded that these conditions were in fact seizures or stroke-like episodes (SLEs), which remained unrecognized and recovered spontaneously. At least 4 of these episodes were

Table 2: Crucial investigations carried out during the disease trajectory.

Date/age	Investigation	Result
2000, 30 years	Echocardiography	"Pulmonary insufficiency"
1.1.06	Lumbar puncture	Protein 167 mg/dl, otherwise normal
3.1.06	EEG	Normal
3.1.06	Lumbar puncture	Protein 107 mg/dl, otherwise normal
5.1.06, 35 years	Nerve conduction studies	Normal
4.1.06, 36 years	Cerebral MRI	T2-hyperintensities, subcortical, mesencephalon, DWI, ADC hyperintense enlarged pituitary gland, sinusoidal polyposis
12.1.06	Neuropsychological testing	Attention deficit, disability of encoding visual contents, adjustment disorder, and depression
13.1.06	Cerebral MRI	Unchanged to previously
17.1.06	Lumbar puncture	Protein 152 mg/dl, otherwise normal
1/2006	Ophthalmologic investigation	Strabism, fundus tabulates, AM atrophy, papillary excavation
24.2.06	Cerebral MRI	Band-like T2-, DWI-, ADC-hyperintensities in the ML and mesencephalon bilaterally
2.1.06	Abdominal ultrasound	Normal
1/06	Lumbar puncture	Protein 167 mg/dl
16.12.06	Ophthalmologic investigation	Pigmentary epithelium shifts, retinal dystrophy, rod/cone degeneration (RP suspected)
8/07	Muscle biopsy (deltoid)	Fat, no muscle
12.9.07	CK	2673 U/L (rhabdomyolysis)
10.8.07	Myoglobin	152 ng/ml (n, 19–92 ng/ml)
2.8.07	X-ray of the lungs	Normal width of aorta
6.8.07	Echocardiography	Normal
8.8.07	Liver enzymes	Elevated
9.8.07	Abdominal CT	Multiple liver cysts
13.8.07	Muscle biopsy	No muscle tissue, only fat
13.2.08	Muscle MRI	Chondroma right femur
19.2.08, 38 years	Muscle biopsy (left lateral vastus)	Indicates mitochondrial myopathy
15.12.08	Cerebral MRI	Cerebellar atrophy
19.12.08	Needle electromyography	Increased polyphasia exclusively

WMLs: white matter lesions, RP: retinitis pigmentosa.

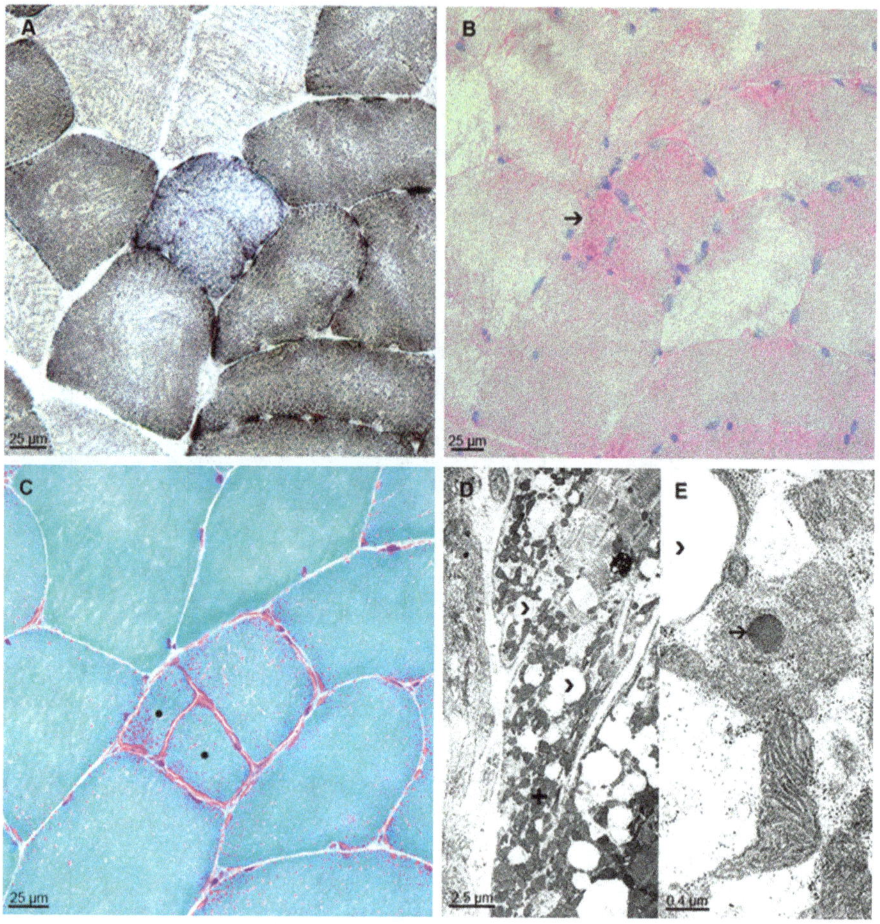

FIGURE 2: (a–c) Neuropathology of muscle biopsy (left vastus lateralis muscle) presents myopathic changes with single COX-negative fibers (a) COX/SDH double-labeling, mildly increased PAS-positivity in few fibers (b) arrow, muscle fiber splitting, and ragged-red fibers (c) Gomori-trichrome stain, asterisk. (d and e) Electron microscopy images illustrate increased numbers of fat vacuoles (d and e, arrow heads) between densly packed subsarcolemmal mitochondria (d) plus. Some mitochondria show single dark bodies in higher magnification (e) arrow.

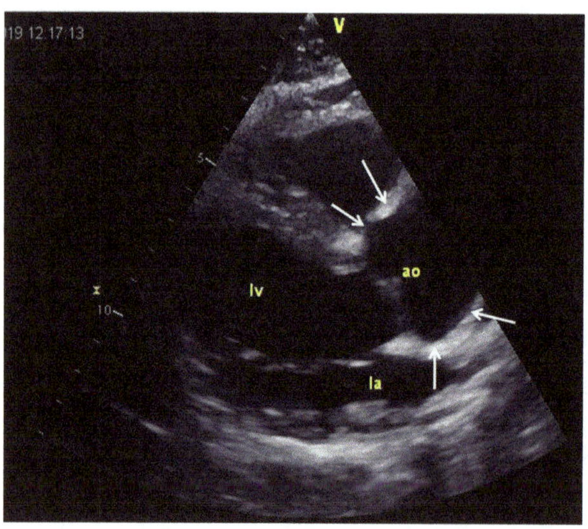

FIGURE 3: Echocardiographic parasternal long axis view showing the ectatic ascending aorta, measuring 37 mm in diameter.

documented. An argument for SLEs is that MRI at the first episode at age 36 showed subcortical T2-hyperintensities, which were also hyperintense on DWI and ADC and not confined to a vascular territory, suggesting a vasogenic edema. Whether arterial hypertension should be regarded as a manifestation of the MID is questionable but there are indications from Chinese studies that arterial hypertension can be in fact a phenotypic feature of an MID [4].

Limitations of the study were that the diagnosis was not confirmed by genetic investigations, that the mother was not investigated for the presence of a MID, and that no biochemical investigations of the muscle homogenate were carried out.

In conclusion, this case shows that KSS is indeed a multisystem disease affecting all types of tissues and that the phenotypic presentation may be broader than so far anticipated.

Authors' Contributions

Josef Finsterer, Michael Winklehner, Claudia Stöllberger, and Thomas Hummel contributed equally.

References

[1] J. Finsterer, "Kearns-Sayre syndrome," *Handbook of Mitochondrial Dysfunction*, Taylor and Francis Group, Boca Raton, FL, USA, 2019.

[2] L. Welzing, J. C. von Kleist-Retzow, A. Kribs, F. Eifinger, C. Huenseler, and N. Sreeram, "Rapid development of life-threatening complete atrioventricular block in Kearns-Sayre syndrome," *European Journal of Pediatrics*, vol. 168, no. 6, pp. 757–759, 2009.

[3] J. Poulton, J. Finsterer, and P. Yu-Wai-Man, "Genetic counselling for maternally inherited mitochondrial disorders," *Molecular Diagnosis & Therapy*, vol. 21, no. 4, pp. 419–429, 2017.

[4] L. Lin, P. Cui, Z. Qiu et al., "The mitochondrial tRNA(Ala) 5587T>C and tRNA(Leu(CUN)) 12280A>G mutations may be associated with hypertension in a Chinese family," *Experimental and Therapeutic Medicine*, vol. 17, pp. 1855–1862, 2019.

[5] H. J. Southgate and M. D. Penney, "Severe recurrent renal salt wasting in a boy with a mitochondrial oxidative phosphorylation defect," *Annals of Clinical Biochemistry*, vol. 37, no. 6, pp. 805–808, 2000.

[6] A. Berio and A. Piazzi, "Multiple endocrinopathies (growth hormone deficiency, autoimmune hypothyroidism and diabetes mellitus) in Kearns-Sayre syndrome," *La Pediatria Medica e Chirurgica*, vol. 35, no. 3, pp. 137–140, 2013.

[7] M. Sacher, G. M. Fatterpekar, S. Edelstein, C. Sansaricq, and T. P. Naidich, "MRI findings in an atypical case of Kearns-Sayre syndrome: a case report," *Neuroradiology*, vol. 47, no. 4, pp. 241–244, 2005.

[8] M. Magner, H. Kolářová, T. Honzik, I. Švandová, and J. Zeman, "Clinical manifestation of mitochondrial diseases," *Developmental Period Medicine*, vol. 19, pp. 441–449, 2015.

[9] C. Ponzetto, N. Bresolin, A. Bordoni et al., "Kearns-Sayre syndrome: different amounts of deleted mitochondrial DNA are present in several autoptic tissues," *Journal of the Neurological Sciences*, vol. 96, no. 2-3, pp. 207–210, 1990.

[10] N. Bresolin, M. Moggio, L. Bet et al., "Progressive cytochromec oxidase deficiency in a case of earns-sayre syndrome: morphological, immunological, and biochemical studies in muscle biopsies and autopsy tissues," *Annals of Neurology*, vol. 21, no. 6, pp. 564–572, 1987.

[11] T. Fritz, K. Wessel, E. Weidle, G. Lenz, and J. Peiffer, "Anästhesie für augenoperationen bei mitochondrialer enzephalomyopathie," *Klinische Monatsblätter für Augenheilkunde*, vol. 193, no. 8, pp. 174–178, 1988.

[12] C. Nesti, A. Rubegni, D. Tolomeo et al., "Complex multisystem phenotype associated with the mitochondrial DNA m.5522G>A mutation," *Neurological Sciences*, vol. 40, no. 8, pp. 1705–1708, 2019.

29

Anti-NMDAR Encephalitis: Higher Suspicious Needed for Earlier Diagnosis (Case Report, Literature Review and Diagnostic Criteria)

Chanaka Amugoda,[1] Noushin Chini Foroush,[2] and Hamed Akhlaghi[3]

[1]*Emergency Department, Werribee Mercy Hospital, Melbourne, Australia*
[2]*Medical Registrar, Austin Health, Melbourne, Australia*
[3]*Emergency Physician, St. Vincent's Hospital, University of Melbourne, Melbourne, Australia*

Correspondence should be addressed to Hamed Akhlaghi; hamed.akhlaghi@svha.org.au

Academic Editor: Dennis J. Rivet

Background. Auto-immune mediated anti-NMDA receptor encephalitis is a very common delayed diagnosed encephalitis which predominately affecting young population. *Objectives.* This encephalitis is relatively unknown amongst emergency physicians and a majority of patients are admitted to psychiatric wards before their diagnosis is confirmed and appropriate treatments are commenced. We reported a case of a 22-year-old female presented to our emergency department with acute psychiatric symptoms. She was initially diagnosed with first presentation of acute psychosis and was hospitalised under mental health act. further assessment in the emergency department identified possible an organic cause for her acute psychosis and she was later admitted under medical team after her mental health assessment order was revoke. Several days later, her CSF result was positive with anti-NMDA receptor antibodies. Appropriate treatments were instituted leading to her full recovery. *Conclusion.* This case was the first confirmed anti-NMDA receptor encephalitis in our emergency department. It highlights the importance of thorough assessment of psychiatric presentations to emergency departments and consideration of auto-immune medicated encephalitis as one of the differential diagnosis in young patients presenting with first acute psychotic episode.

1. Introduction

Encephalitis causes significant morbidity and mortality worldwide. Encephalitis is defined by the Consensus Statement of the *International Encephalitis Consortium* as severe Inflammation of the brain parenchyma associated with debilitating neurologic dysfunction [1]. Traditionally, viral encephalitis was the most recognisable type of encephalitis. However, in the last 15 years with advancements in medical imaging and the development of new neurologic biomarkers, other noninfectious, mainly autoimmune-mediated encephalitis have been identified and reported [2]. Anti-N-methyl-D-aspartate receptor (NMDAR) encephalitis was first described by Dalmau et al. in 2005 [3]. NMDAR encephalitis is a common cause of autoimmune encephalitis [4] frequently misdiagnosed by the treating physician as a psychiatric illness [5]. In this article, we review the clinical presentation, investigation and diagnosis of NMDAR encephalitis in conjunction with a case report. The article concludes with proposed diagnostic criteria for NMDAR encephalitis, developed to assist primary care and emergency physicians should they suspect a possible diagnosis of NMDAR encephalitis.

2. Clinical Presentation

The clinical presentation typically progresses in four stages: the prodromal phase, the psychotic phase, the unresponsive phase and the hyperkinetic phase [6]. During the prodromal phase, patients experience unspecific viral-like symptoms such as low-grade fever, headache, upper respiratory tract symptoms, fatigue, nausea, vomiting and diarrhoea. However, fever and headache more commonly occur after the onset of neuropsychiatric symptoms. The initial phase manifests in 70 to

86 per cent of patients and can last up to 21 days [6, 7]. The psychotic features typically manifest within two weeks following the prodromal phase. Majority of patients seek medical attention during this phase with symptoms of agitation, paranoid delusions, auditory and visual hallucinations, bizarre behaviour, mood liability, insomnia, depression, anxiety, disorganised thoughts, epileptic seizures, cognitive impairment, and memory deficit [7, 8]. Frequently half of NMDAR encephalitis patients is misdiagnosed predominantly due to psychotic features [6]. A seizure is commonly observed in up to 82 per cent of patients. The main manifestations of the unresponsive phase are mutism and akinesia followed by hyperkinetic phase. Patients experience autonomic instability, hypo- or hypertension, hypo- or hyperthermia, cardiac arrhythmia and hypoventilation [6]. In cases with severe hypoventilation, ventilatory support may be required.

Younger patients mainly present with behavioural disturbances instead of frank psychosis hindering the diagnosis of anti-NMDAR encephalitis in children. Frequently they present with nonpsychiatric manifestations such as seizures, dystonia or mutism [9]. In contrast, psychiatric symptoms and memory deficit are the main manifestation of the disease amongst patients over 44 years old [10].

2.1. Disease Pathogenesis. Anti-N-methyl-D-aspartate receptor, mainly found in the forebrain, hippocampus and limbic system, is a tetrameric complex composed of two GluN1 subunits and combination of two GluN2 or GluN3 subunits. The function of this receptor has been linked to learning, memory, cognition, and behaviour [6]. Current evidence suggests that IgG antibodies in the serum and CSF bind specifically to the GluN1 subunit are the cause of disease pathogenesis [8].

Higher incidence of teratoma and post-HSE (herpes-simplex-encephalitis) NMDAR encephalitis suggests malignancies and infections as triggers for this disease. A recent study shows ovarian teratoma contains abnormal CNS neuron leading to extra-axial expression of NMDA receptor, however in 80% of anti-NMDAR encephalitis cases, no tumour is found [11]. Due to correlation between HSE and NMDAR encephalitis, it is suggested that to test Anti-NMDAR antibodies in CSF of patients with relapse post-HSE [2]. Almost 90% of patients with anti-NMDAR encephalitis manifest the prodromal phase, support the idea of infective aetiologies. Nevertheless, extensive CSF sampling and brain biopsies fail to identify direct viral pathogenesis. The underlying pathophysiology of the prodrome phase is unclear, it is uncertain whether it is solely an early manifestation of immune-mediated response or an infection interrupting the normal blood-brain barrier function letting antibodies to cross [12].

2.2. Epidemiology. Anti-NMDAR encephalitis is a female predominant disease, as women represent up to 80 per cent of reported cases [9]. It is also considered a middle-aged person disease, although anti-NMDAR encephalitis has been reported in cases of people aged between two months and 90 years [9, 10, 13]. The male : female ratio is as high as 40 per cent amongst patients over 44 years old [13].

Teratoma is the most common tumour associated with this disease and around 40–50 per cent of female patients with anti-NMDAR encephalitis have been reported to have teratoma. A large series study revealed that 98 per cent of tumours are ovarian teratomas [9]. Detection of other malignancies such as neuroblastoma or Hodgkin's lymphoma is rare [9]. Underlying malignancies are less common in younger or male patients.

Paediatric patients (younger than 18 years old) have a higher incidence of seizures as the first presentation for medical attention compared to adult patients. They have more favourable outcome and less likely to have CSF pleocytosis [14]. The presence of underlying tumour is less common in the paediatric population and in females more likely to be an ovarian teratoma if there is a tumour (90%) [14].

2.3. Diagnosis. Diagnosis of anti-NMDAR encephalitis is based on the presentation of NMDAR antibodies in CSF or serum. The NMDAR antibodies in CSF have higher specificity and sensitivity in comparison to the serum antibodies. Antibodies in CSF are always present at the time of diagnosis nevertheless, to avoid false-negative or false-positive results, it is recommended to test NMDAR antibodies in both CSF and serum [15].

The titre of NMDAR antibodies increases with disease progression and there is a direct correlation between the severity of the disease, clinical presentation, and underlying malignancies with antibody titration [12]. Other abnormal nonspecific findings in CSF are pleocytosis (60–76%), high protein (19%), oligoclonal band (17%) and increased opening pressure in nearly 40% [3, 16, 17]. Glucose and chloride concentrating of CSF is almost always normal [17]. A recent study proposed CSF cell-free mitochondrial DNA as a potential biomarker in anti-NMDAR encephalitis [18], however it takes several years to get into general practice.

Imaging of the brain, although not a widely accepted approach, is mainly requested as part of the initial clinical evaluation of the first episode of acute psychiatric illness or to exclude other causes of acute confusion [19]. Only one-third of patients with anti-NMDAR encephalitis have positive brain imaging results, with changes reported in hippocampi, cerebellar and cerebral cortex, fronto-basal and insular regions, basal ganglia, brainstem or spinal cord [3, 6, 12]. These imaging findings are nonspecific and have poor correlation with disease severity and symptoms and fully resolved after treatment [6]. Recent MRI study showed only half of anti-NMDAR encephalitis showed abnormalities in their brain regions including medial temporal lobe, frontal lobe subcortical white matter and periventricular region [20]. Therefore, the imaging modalities are not a useful and recommended clinical tool in diagnosis of anti-NMDAR encephalitis.

PET scans (FDG-PET) have been suggested as a potential biomarker in diagnosis of autoimmune encephalitis and showed hypometabolism of the occipital lobe in anti-NMDAR encephalitis [6, 21].

EEG findings are abnormal in 90% of patients with anti-NMDAR encephalitis [12, 16]. The most frequent abnormal EEG finding in a series of 100 patients was delta-theta wave which is described as slow-wave with or without epileptic features. In up to the third of anti-NMDAR encephalitis patients, the EEG pattern shows distinct EDB (extreme delta brush) pattern independent of body Circadian rhythm which can lead to diagnosis of the disease in the early stages [22]. Due to higher incidence of malignancies in anti-NMDAR encephalitis, screening with CT, MRI, abdominal and transvaginal ultrasound is recommended.

2.4. Treatment and Outcome. The mainstay of current treatment is conservative management, high-dose corticosteroid, intravenous immunoglobulins (IVIg), plasma exchange (PE), immunotherapy, and tumour removal if present. The first line therapy compromises of corticosteroid, IVIg, and PE with or without tumour removal. Recovery in four weeks has been observed in approximately 50 per cent of patients. The second line therapy consists of immunotherapy with rituximab or cyclophosphamide and is used if patient relapses or the first-line therapy fails.

Currently, there is no high-quality controlled trial evidence on the standard and optimal therapeutic guideline for anti-NMDAR encephalitis. The class IV expert opinion is to start a combination of IVIg and methylprednisolone for five days as the first line, and if there is no clinical improvement after 15 days then the second-line therapy should commence which consists of rituximab with monthly cycle of cyclophosphamide [23].

Patients with no underlying malignancy have shown a higher rate of relapse and resistance to usual treatment, less favourable outcome and prolonged recovery time [16]. The early immunosuppressive therapy and early resection of the tumour are associated with improved outcome and recovery [12, 24, 25]. The intra-thecal treatment has been reported in a case series resistant to first-line and second-line therapies [26]. Symptomatic treatment with lorazepam and ECT for management of catatonia has been reported with efficacy between 80 and 90 per cent [6, 27].

Anti-NMDAR encephalitis tends to have a better outcome in comparison with other autoimmune medicated encephalitis with a full or substantial recovery rate of 80–90 per cent after 24 months [14, 16]. Mortality is around six per cent, and higher mortality rates have been observed amongst older patients or patients with significant CSF pleocytosis at the time of diagnosis [14]. In a case series of 501 patients, early treatment, low severity of symptoms in the early phase and no need for ICU admission, were associated with better outcomes and fewer relapses [16]. Improvement of symptoms is observed after a few weeks post commencement of treatment. However full recovery may take up to three years to return to baseline functioning [6]. Structural hippocampal damage and cognitive deficits such as impairment in attention, working memory, episodic memory and executive function comprise the major burden and long-term morbidity of anti-NMDAR encephalitis [28].

3. Case Report

A 28-years-old female was brought into the hospital by her husband concerned by his wife's recent bizarre and abnormal behaviour in the setting of recent university exam and work-related stress. Her main symptoms were acute behavioural changes for five days including lack of sleep, paranoia, talkative, labile mood, and auditory hallucination. The woman is a PhD student who is bilingual in English and Chinese. Her husband reported that she was hearing voices and has become paranoid. Although his wife was fluent in English, she had begun to communicate in her native language. The patient complained of a headache for one week for which she was taking therapeutic dose of paracetamol. She did not have any recent febrile illness, trauma, or head injury. The patient has no history of psychiatric illness or illicit drugs use. She was not on any regular medication, a nonsmoker, and social alcohol drinker.

TABLE 1: CSF result of the patient.

	Tube 1	Tube 2	Tube 3
Erythrocyte ($* 10^6$/L)	660	1940	7020
White cell ($* 10^6$/L)	200	380	290
Polymorph ($* 10^6$/L)	13	30	35
Mononuclear ($* 10^6$/L)	187	350	255

In the emergency department, the patient presented as paranoid and confused. Vital signs showed intermittent tachycardic with HR between 80 and 150/min and hypertensive with BP 140/80 mmHg. The patient was initially afebrile, and her initial investigations showed only slight elevation of white cell count up to $15 * 10^6$ mmol/L with significant neutrophilia. The rest of the clinical investigations including electrolytes, renal function, liver function, C-reactive protein, urine test, thyroid function test and CT Brain was normal. A neurological examination was completely normal with no signs of meningitis. Patients GCS was fluctuating from 14 to 15. During her emergency stay, she became agitated requiring both oral diazepam 5 mg and intravenous Droperidole 5 mg for sedation. The patient was referred to the psychiatric team and accepted for further management and treatment for the first episode of psychosis.

While the patient was in the emergency department, she became more confused and agitated, and her temperature spiked to 38.5°C. A lumbar puncture was conducted. Her CSF results indicated elevated protein 0.59 gr/L and white cell count of 200 with 13 of polymorphs and 187 mononuclear cells. There were no bacteria seen in the CSF sample (Table 1). The patient was diagnosed with possible infective encephalitis and commenced treatment with intravenous ceftriaxone 1gr/daily and acyclovir to cover for possible HSE was commenced. The previous admission to the psychiatric unit was changed to medical admission.

During her admission under the medical team, she underwent Brain MRI study which was reported normal. Her varicella-zoster and herpes PCR of CSF came back negative alongside with autoimmune panel tests. Her GCS continued to drop to as low as five, and she became verbally unresponsive and more catatonic despite being on intravenous antibiotics.

After one week in conjunction with a neurology input, the diagnosis of autoimmune encephalitis and possible anti-NMDAR encephalitis was suspected, and pelvic ultrasound was requested which showed a $25 * 100 * 90$ mm large multiocular cyst with no vascularity with no solid material suggestive of teratoma. At this point, the patient commenced on intravenous immunoglobulin, methylprednisone and rituximab. During this time the patient underwent laparotomy and a subsequent right-side oophorectomy and was admitted to ICU due to low GCS. Her length of stay in ICU was twenty days. Her admission was complicated with one episode of self-remitting generalised tonic-clonic seizure, autonomic dysfunction and orofacial dyskinesia requiring Botox treatment. The patient's EEG result was consistent with a moderate diffuse encephalopathy, and 24H EEG showed diffuse delta brush wave highly suggestive of anti-NMDAR encephalitis. A subsequent CSF test was positive with NMDAR antibody confirming diagnosis as anti-NMDAR encephalitis.

Upon discharge, the patient needed ongoing cognitive rehabilitation. She was subsequently transferred to rehabilitation centre where she was able to progress positively in terms of behaviour and cognition, returning to pre-morbid functional level and activities and since has not experienced any relapse in symptoms.

4. Discussion

This case report presented a delayed diagnosis of anti-NMDAR encephalitis with most of the typical features and ovarian teratoma. Lack of clinical suspicion and the absence of diagnostic criteria were two important factors that circumvent earlier diagnosis.

This case showed the complexity of patient symptoms and nonspecific nature of anti-NMDAR encephalitis. Our case was referred to the psychiatric unit for treatment of first psychosis because the initial investigations failed to reveal an organic cause for the patient's presentations. Even after abnormal CSF, the patient was diagnosed with possible viral or bacterial encephalitis. The alternative diagnosis of auto-immune encephalitis and anti-NMDAR encephalitis was considered when the patient failed to respond to initial treatment and her level of consciousness continued to decline.

Diagnostic criteria for autoimmune encephalitis depend on detection of autoantibodies and response to immunotherapy which are not available at the time of presentation to emergency department or early clinical evaluation. Besides, the capability for detection of the antibody may not be readily available, and in most cases, it takes several weeks for the result to become available which potentially delays the diagnosis while early treatment of anti-NMDAR encephalitis is associated with more favourable outcome. The following clinical diagnostic approach was proposed by a group of neurologists to assist with early diagnosis and treatment of anti-NMDAR encephalitis [2].

4.1. Diagnostic Criteria for Probable Anti-NMDAR Encephalitis [2]

(A) Rapid onset (less than three months) of at least four of the six following major groups of symptoms (or three at the presence of underlying tumour such as teratoma):

(1) Abnormal (psychiatric) behaviour or cognitive dysfunction.
(2) Speech dysfunction (pressured speech, verbal reduction, mutism).
(3) Seizure.
(4) Movement disorder, dyskinesias or rigidity/abnormal postures.
(5) Decreased level of consciousness.
(6) Autonomic dysfunction or central hypoventilation.

(B) At least one of the following laboratory study results:

(1) Abnormal EEG (focal or diffuse slow or disorganised activity, epileptic activity, or extreme delta brush).
(2) CSF with pleocytosis or oligoclonal bands.

(C) Reasonable exclusion of other disorders such as CNS infection, herpes simplex virus encephalitis, epileptic disorders, or known psychiatric disease.

Memory testing is not part of the criteria due to poor accuracy for memory assessment during acute psychosis, abnormal behaviours or agitation. It is recommended to start immunotherapy once the criteria are met whilst checking for underlying malignancies or tumour [2].

The proposed diagnostic criteria have high sensitivity of 90 per cent and specificity of 96 per cent. However, duration between onset of symptoms until symptoms could fulfil the proposed diagnostic criteria could take up to two weeks [29].

The patient exhibited acute behavioural changes accompanied by autonomic dysfunction, decreased level of consciousness, speech difficulty and cognitive disturbances. Using the criteria, our patient could have been diagnosed as possible anti-NMDAR encephalitis, and definitive treatment could have commenced sooner.

It is important to increase awareness of primary care physicians and emergency doctors of possible organic and auto-immune aetiology for psychiatric presentations and share the understanding that normal initial investigations do not completely exclude organic causes. A high level of suspicious and detailed history taking is required to consider an alternative diagnosis such as anti-NMDAR encephalitis.

Therefore, once a patient (particularly those aged in their twenties and thirties), presents to the emergency department or primary care physician with acute onset psychiatric symptoms or seizure while manifesting four of the six criteria, CSF testing for pleocytosis or oligoclonal bands should be urgently performed. In most hospitals, the results can be available within a couple of hours. If in-house an EEG service is available, the abnormal EEG findings can confirm the diagnosis and prevent significant delays in commencement of the immunotherapy.

Acknowledgments

We would like to thank the patient who provided consent to share this case report. The patient's identity remains anonymous for patient privacy and confidentiality.

References

[1] A. Venkatesan, A. R Tunkel, K. C. Bloch et al., "Case definitions, diagnostic algorithms, and priorities in encephalitis: consensus statement of the international encephalitis consortium," *Clinical Infectious Diseases*, vol. 57, no. 8, pp. 1114–1128, 2013.

[2] F. Graus, M. J. Titulaer, R. Balu et al., "A clinical approach to diagnosis of autoimmune encephalitis," *The Lancet Neurology*, vol. 15, no. 4, pp. 391–404, 2016.

[3] R. Vitaliani, W. Mason, B. Ances, T. Zwerdling, Z. Jiang, and J. Dalmau, "Paraneoplastic encephalitis, psychiatric symptoms, and hypoventilation in ovarian teratoma," *Annals of Neurology*, vol. 58, no. 4, pp. 594–604, 2005.

[4] H. Barry, S. Byrne, E. Barrett, K. C. Murphy, and D. R. Cotter, "Anti-*N*-methyl-D-aspartate receptor encephalitis: review of clinical presentation, diagnosis, and treatment," *BJPsych Bulletin*, vol. 39, no. 1, pp. 19–23, 2015.

[5] Y. Shimoyama, O. Umegaki, T. Agui, N. Kadono, and T. Minami, "Anti-NMDA receptor encephalitis presenting as an acute psychotic episode misdiagnosed as dissociative disorder: a case report," *JA Clinical Reports*, vol. 2, no. 1, p. 22, 2016.

[6] A. Venkatesan and K. Adatia, "Anti-NMDA-receptor encephalitis: from bench to clinic," *ACS Chemical Neuroscience*, vol. 8, no. 12, pp. 2586–2595, 2017.

[7] T. Hermans, P. Santens, C. Matton et al., "Anti-NMDA receptor encephalitis: still unknown and underdiagnosed by physicians and especially by psychiatrists?" *Acta Clinica Belgica*, vol. 73, no. 5, pp. 364–367, 2018.

[8] K. P. Wandinger, S. Saschenbrecker, W. Stoecker, and J. Dalmau, "Anti-NMDA-receptor encephalitis: a severe, multistage, treatable disorder presenting with psychosis," *Journal of Neuroimmunology*, vol. 231, no. 1-2, pp. 86–91, 2011.

[9] J. Dalmau, E. Lancaster, E. Martinez-Hernandez, M. R. Rosenfeld, and R. Balice-Gordon, "Clinical experience and laboratory investigations in patients with anti-NMDAR encephalitis," *The Lancet Neurology*, vol. 10, no. 1, pp. 63–74, 2011.

[10] L. Zhang, X. Liu, X. Y. Jiang, Y. H. Wang, J. M. Li, and D. Zhou, "Late-onset anti-N-methyl-D-aspartate receptor encephalitis in China," *Epilepsy & Behavior*, vol. 84, pp. 22–28, 2018.

[11] G. S. Day, S. Laiq, D. F. Tang-Wai, and D. G. Munoz, "Abnormal neurons in teratomas in NMDAR encephalitis," *JAMA Neurology*, vol. 71, no. 6, pp. 717–724, 2014.

[12] J. Dalmau, A. J. Gleichman, E. G. Hughes et al., "Anti-NMDA-receptor encephalitis: case series and analysis of the effects of antibodies," *The Lancet Neurology*, vol. 7, no. 12, pp. 1091–1098, 2008.

[13] M. J. Titulaer, L. McCracken, I. Gabilondo et al., "Late-onset anti-NMDA receptor encephalitis," *Neurology*, vol. 81, no. 12, pp. 1058–1063, 2013.

[14] L. Zhang, M. Q. Wu, Z. L. Hao et al., "Clinical characteristics, treatments, and outcomes of patients with anti-N-methyl-D-aspartate receptor encephalitis: a systematic review of reported cases," *Epilepsy & Behavior*, vol. 68, pp. 57–65, 2017.

[15] N. Gresa-Arribas, M. J. Titulaer, A. Torrents et al., "Antibody titres at diagnosis and during follow-up of anti-NMDA receptor encephalitis: a retrospective study," *The Lancet Neurology*, vol. 13, no. 2, pp. 167–177, 2014.

[16] M. J. Titulaer, L. McCracken, I. Gabilondo et al., "Treatment and prognostic factors for long-term outcome in patients with anti-NMDA receptor encephalitis: an observational cohort study," *The Lancet Neurology*, vol. 12, no. 2, pp. 157–165, 2013.

[17] R. Wang, H. Z. Guan, H. T. Ren, W. Wang, Z. Hong, and D. Zhou, "CSF findings in patients with anti-N-methyl-D-aspartate receptor-encephalitis," *Seizure*, vol. 29, pp. 137–142, 2015.

[18] Y. Peng, D. Zheng, X. Zhang et al., "Cell-free mitochondrial DNA in the CSF: a potential prognostic biomarker of anti-NMDAR encephalitis," *Frontiers in Immunology*, vol. 10, p. 103, 2019.

[19] K. Goulet, B. Deschamps, F. Evoy, and J. F. Trudel, "Use of brain imaging (computed tomography and magnetic resonance imaging) in first-episode psychosis: review and retrospective study," *The Canadian Journal of Psychiatry*, vol. 54, no. 7, pp. 493–501, 2009.

[20] S. Bacchi, K. Franke, D. Wewegama, E. Needham, S. Patel, and D. Menon, "Magnetic resonance imaging and positron emission tomography in anti-NMDA receptor encephalitis: a systematic review," *Journal of Clinical Neuroscience*, vol. 52, pp. 54–59, 2018.

[21] J. C. Probasco, L. Solnes, A. Nalluri et al., "Abnormal brain metabolism on FDG-PET/CT is a common early finding in autoimmune encephalitis," *Neurology—Neuroimmunology Neuroinflammation*, vol. 4, no. 4, p. 352, 2017.

[22] S. E. Schmitt, K. Pargeon, E. S. Frechette, L. J. Hirsch, J. Dalmau, and D. Friedman, "Extreme delta brush: a unique EEG pattern in adults with anti-NMDA receptor encephalitis," *Neurology*, vol. 79, no. 11, pp. 1094–1100, 2012.

[23] L. Bartolini, "Practice current: how do you treat anti-NMDA receptor encephalitis?" *Neurology: Clinical Practice*, vol. 6, no. 1, pp. 69–72, 2016.

[24] S. Byrne, B. McCoy, B. Lynch, D. Webb, and M. D. King, "Does early treatment improve outcomes in N-methyl-D-aspartate receptor encephalitis?" *Developmental Medicine & Child Neurology*, vol. 56, no. 8, pp. 794–796, 2014.

[25] J. N. Brenton, J. Kim, and R. H. Schwartz, "Approach to the management of pediatric-onset anti-N-Methyl-D-aspartate (Anti-NMDA) receptor encephalitis: a case series," *Journal of Child Neurology*, vol. 31, no. 9, pp. 1150–1155, 2016.

[26] S. Tatencloux, P. Chretien, V. Rogemond, J. Honnorat, M. Tardieu, and K. Deiva, "Intrathecal treatment of anti-N-Methyl-D-aspartate receptor encephalitis in children," *Developmental Medicine & Child Neurology*, vol. 57, no. 1, pp. 95–99, 2015.

[27] M. R. Chapman and H. E. Vause, "Anti-NMDA receptor encephalitis: diagnosis, psychiatric presentation, and treatment," *American Journal of Psychiatry*, vol. 168, no. 3, pp. 245–251, 2011.

[28] C. Finke, U. A. Kopp, A. Pajkert et al., "Structural hippocampal damage following anti-N-Methyl-D-aspartate receptor encephalitis," *Biological Psychiatry*, vol. 79, no. 9, pp. 727–734, 2016.

[29] A. C. C. Ho, S. S. Mohammad, S. C. Pillai et al., "High sensitivity and specificity in proposed clinical diagnostic criteria for anti-N-methyl-D-aspartate receptor encephalitis," *Developmental Medicine & Child Neurology*, vol. 59, no. 12, pp. 1256–1260, 2017.

30

CAPN1 Variants as Cause of Hereditary Spastic Paraplegia Type 76

Jesus Eduardo Garcia-Berlanga,[1] Mariana Moscovich,[2] Isaac Jair Palacios,[1] 4 Alejandro Banegas-Lagos,[1] Augusto Rojas-Martinez,[1] and Daniel Martinez-Ramirez[1]

[1]*Tecnologico de Monterrey, Escuela de Medicina y Ciencias de la Salud, Monterrey, Nuevo Leon, Mexico*
[2]*Department of Neurology, Christian-Albrechts University, Kiel, Germany*

Correspondence should be addressed to Daniel Martinez-Ramirez; daniel.martinez@medicos.tecsalud.mx

Academic Editor: Federico Micheli

Background. Autosomal recessive hereditary spastic paraplegias (HSP) are a rare group of hereditary neurodegenerative disorders characterized by spasticity with or without other symptoms. *SPG11* gene is the most common cause of autosomal recessive HSP. We report a case of autosomal recessive spastic paraplegia type 76 due to heterozygous variants of *CAPN1* in an Argentinean subject. *Case Presentation.* A 38-year-old Argentinean female presented with progressive gait problems and instability of 15-year duration. Oculomotor abnormalities, ataxia, bradykinesia, cervical dystonia, and lower limb pyramidal signs were observed. Brain MRI was unremarkable. Whole-exome sequencing analysis identified two heterozygous variants in *CAPN1*. *Conclusions.* Clinicians should screen for *CAPN1* mutation in a young female patient without significant family history with a spastic paraplegia syndrome associated with other symptoms.

1. Background

Hereditary spastic paraplegias (HSP) are a group of heterogeneous degenerative disorders characterized by lower limb spasticity and weakness due to progressive degeneration of corticospinal tracts [1]. HSP can present as a pure form only with pyramidal symptoms, or as a complex form associated with other symptoms. HSP are transmitted in all modes of inheritance [2]. The autosomal dominant mode of inheritance is the most prevalent representing 70% of cases. Mutation in *SPAST* gene accounts for 40% of the autosomal dominant HSP. In the recessive HSP, the most frequent mutation is in *SPG11*. We report a case of autosomal recessive spastic paraplegia type 76 (SPG76, OMIM #616907) due to heterozygous variants of *CAPN1* in an Argentinean subject.

2. Case Presentation

A 38-year-old Argentinean female presented with slowly progressive unsteadiness noticed first at age 23. She reported pronounced instability and gait problems as disease progressed. Her gait problems were described as short steps, with starting hesitation, fear of falling, and needing to hold from walls to avoid falling. She also reported several falls, dizziness, neck pain, and constipation. Symptoms progressed over the years affecting her mobility and functionality. She currently needs assistance for moving around. No relevant medical, family, or psychosocial history was reported. No past interventions were reported.

On neurological examination (Video 1), she presented dysarthria, interrupted slow horizontal and vertical eye movements, and slow horizontal saccades. She manifested spasticity and hyperreflexia more pronounced in her lower extremities. Mild cervical dystonia with bradykinesia was also observed. She showed ataxic symptoms more pronounced on her left upper extremity. Gait was spastic and no cognitive abnormalities were observed.

Brain MRI with and without contrast was unremarkable. Due to the presence of a slowly progressive adult onset spastic-ataxia syndrome, associated with other neurological abnormalities, and facing the challenge of poor financial

Table 1: Clinical and genetical characteristics of SPG76 cases reported in the literature.

	Ethnicity	Age at onset	Age at diagnosis	Gender	Lower limbs spasticity	Upper limbs spasticity	Ataxia	Dysarthria	Oculomotor Impairment	Exon or Intron affected	Mutation	Type	Heterozygous /Homozygous	Consanguinity	Brain MRI	NCS and SSEP
1	Latin American	NA	NA	NA	+	+	-	-	-	-	c.1176G>A p.Trp392*	Stop gain mutation	Homozygous	+	NA	NA
2	Latin American	NA	NA	NA	+	+	-	-	-	-	c.1176G>A p.Trp392*	NA	Homozygous	+	NA	NA
3	Latin American	NA	NA	NA	+	+	-	-	-	-	c.1176G>A p.Trp392*	NA	Homozygous	+	NA	NA
4	Latin American	22	37	F	+	+	-	-	-	-	c.1176G>A p.Trp392*	NA	Homozygous	-	NA	NA
5	Caucasian	20	46	F	+	+	+	-	-	-	c.675C>A p.Tyr225*	Novel LoF Mutation	Homozygous	-	NA	NA
6	Caucasian	35	51	M	+	+	+	-	-	-	c.675C>A p.Tyr225*	Novel LoF Mutation	Homozygous	-	NA	NA
7	Latin American	30	42	F	+	+	+	-	-	-	c.1176G>A p.Trp392* c.618_619delAG p.Gly208Glnfs*7	LoF Mutation	Heterozygous	+	NA	NA
8	Latin American	38	-	M	+	+	+	-	-	-	c.1176G>A p.Trp392*	LoF Mutation	Homozygous	+	NA	NA
9	Arab	20	31	F	+	+	-	+	-	Ex:8	c.884G>C p.Arg295Pro	LoF Mutation	Homozygous	+	NA	Normal
10	Arab	NA	NA	NA	NA	NA	NA	NA	NA	Ex:8	c.884G>C p.Arg295Pro	LoF Mutation	Homozygous	+	NA	NA
11	Arab	NA	NA	NA	NA	NA	NA	NA	NA	Ex:8	c.884G>C p.Arg295Pro	LoF Mutation	Homozygous	+	NA	NA
12	Arab	35	47	M	+	+	-	+	-	Ex:14	c.1579C>T p.Gln527	Stop variant	Homozygous	+	NA	Moderate Sensory Axonal Neuropathy
13	Arab	36	44	F	+	+	+	+	-	Ex:14	c.1579C>T p.Gln527	Stop variant	Homozygous	+	NA	Moderate Sensory Axonal Neuropathy
14	Arab	22	42	M	+	+	-	+	-	Ex:14	c.1579C>T p.Gln527	Stop variant	Homozygous	+	Normal	NA
15	Arab	39	40	M	+	+	+	+	-	Ex:14	c.1579C>T p.Gln527	Stop variant	Homozygous	+	NA	NA
16	Arab	NA	NA	NA	NA	NA	NA	NA	NA	Ex:14	c.1579C>T p.Gln527	Stop variant	Homozygous	+	NA	NA
17	Arab	NA	NA	NA	NA	NA	NA	NA	NA	Ex:14	c.1579C>T p.Gln527	Stop variant	Homozygous	+	NA	NA
18	Arab	NA	NA	NA	NA	NA	NA	NA	NA	Ex:14	c.1579C>T p.Gln527	Stop variant	Homozygous	+	NA	NA
19	Caucasian	24	30	F	+	-	-	-	-	Ex:4	c.406delC p.Pro136Argfs*40	Deletion	Heterozygous	-	NA	Normal

Table 1: Continued.

	Ethnicity	Age at onset	Age at diagnosis	Gender	Lower limbs spasticity	Upper limbs spasticity	Ataxia	Dysarthria	Oculomotor Impairment	Exon or Intron affected	Mutation	Type	Heterozygous /Homozygous	Consanguinity	Brain MRI	NCS and SSEP
20	Caucasian	33	35	M	+	-	-	-	-	Ex:4	c.406delC p.Pro136Argfs*40	Deletion	Heterozygous	-	Atrophy of spinal cord	NA
21	Caucasian	19	22	F	+	+	+	-	-	Ex:4	c.1605+5G>A	Mutation Splicing	Heterozygous	-	Normal	NA
22	Indian	33	43	F	+	+	+	+	-	Ex:3	c.337+1G>A	Splice Mutation	Homozygous	+	Mild cerebellar atrophy	Normal
23	Indian	NA	NA	F	NA	NA	NA	NA	NA	Ex:3	c.337+1G>A	Splice Mutation	Homozygous	+	NA	NA
24	Caucasian	29	39	F	+	+	+	+	+	Ex:6	c.759+1G>A	Donor splice site	Homozygous	+	Mild cerebellar vermal atrophy	NA
25	Caucasian	33	37	F	+	+	+	+	-	Ex:6	c.759+1G>A	Donor splice site	Homozygous	+	NA	NA
26	Caucasian	5	16	M	+	-	-	-	-	-	c.221GNA/ p.(G74D) c.911CNT/ p.(T304M) c.1418GNT/ p.(R473L)	missense	Heterozygous	-	Normal	Normal
27	Arab	21	37	F	+	+	+	+	-	-	c.994G>A P.Gly.332Arg	NA	Homozygous	+	Normal	Normal
28	Arab	30	54	F	+	+	+	+	-	Ex10	c. 1176G>A p. Trp392	Nucleotide substitution	Heterozygous	+	Normal	Normal
29	Arab	15	30	F	+	+	+	+	-	Ex:10	c. 1176G>A p. Trp392	Nucleotide substitution	Heterozygous	+	Normal	Normal
30	Asian	37	42	F	+	+	+	-	-	-	c.2118+1G>T	Donor Splice site	Homozygous	NA	NA	NA
31	Caucasian	23	23	M	+	-	-	-	-	-	c.397C>T	NA	Homozygous	+	NA	NA
32	Caucasian	20	20	F	+	-	-	-	-	-	c.397C>T	Mutation in DYSF	Homozygous	+	NA	NA
33	Asian	37	37	M	+	+	+	-	-	-	c.843+1G>C	Donor Splice Site	Homozygous	+	NA	NA
34	Caucasian	13	14	F	+	+	+	-	-	Ex: 13	c.1534C>T p.Arg512Cys	NA	Homozygous	-	Small midbrain and ponds, cerebellar atrophy	Delayed cortical wave defective conduction of large sensory fibers
35 (our case)	Latin American	23	38	F	+	+	+	+	+	In: 12 and 16	c.1729+1G>A c.1353+2T>C	Donor Splice Mutation	Heterozygous	NA	Normal	NA

Abbreviations. F: female, M: male, +: present, -: absent, LoF: loss of function, DYSF: dysferlin, MRI: magnetic resonance image, C: cerebral, S: spinal, NCS: nerve conduction studies, SSEP: somatosensory evoked potentials, NA: not available.

access, we decided to optimize our resources studying the patient using whole-exome sequencing (CentoDX™, Centogene AG, Germany). The analysis identified two variants in *CAPN1* (MIM:114220) considered as probably pathogenic Class 2, according to the American College of Medical Genetics and Genomics criteria. She was heterozygous for a splicing mutation in intron 16 (c.1729+1G>A) and a second splicing mutation in intron 12 (c.1353+2T>C). Carrier testing in the parents was not performed. Due to the strong phenotypic overlap between the symptoms and previously reported cases, we consider the detected variants as pathogenic of SPG76.

3. Discussion

We report two pathogenic variants of *CAPN1* gene and the first case affecting two noncoding regions (introns) in a Latin-American patient. Table 1 describes all SPG76 reported cases in the literature [3, 4]. We observed that female patients are more commonly (67%) affected, with a mean age of onset of 19.8 years (Min. = 5, Max. = 39), most had family history of consanguinity (71%), and most were homozygous (77%). All initiated with lower limb spasticity, 85% reported upper limb spasticity, 58% showed ataxia, and 41% reported dysarthria. Our case also presented with oculomotor abnormalities. Three cases showed cerebellar atrophy and 1 spinal atrophy on MRI.

In comparison with other published cases, we found similarities in that all of them presented lower limb spasticity and ataxia. The difference from our case was the oculomotor abnormalities, which was also reported in only one other case [5]. We suggest that the combined phenotype of spasticity and ataxia with oculomotor abnormalities, in a young female patient of Arab origin, could be a diagnostic clue for SPG76. The age of onset of our case was similar to that previously reported. All of the subjects experienced pronounced instability and gait problems as disease progresses [6].

CAPN1 mutations account for 2.2% of autosomal recessive HSP. *CAPN1* is located in chromosome 11q13 and encodes calpain 1, a calcium-activated cysteine protease that is widely present in the central nervous system. The exact role of calpain 1 in humans is unclear; however, studies in animal models suggest that calpain 1 is involved in synaptic plasticity, neuronal migration, neuronal necrosis, and maintenance [7].

4. Conclusions

Our report adds to the clinical and genetical spectrum of *CAPN1*-related SPG76 disorders. We recommend clinicians to consider screening for *CAPN1* in a young female patient with spastic paraplegia with additional neurological symptoms without significant family history.

Abbreviations

HSP: Hereditary spastic paraplegia
SPAST: Spastin gene
SPG: Spastic paraplegia gene
CAPN1: Calpain 1 gene
MRI: Magnetic resonance imaging.

Consent

Written informed consent was obtained from the patient for publication of this case report and any accompanying images or videos.

Authors' Contributions

Daniel Martinez-Ramirez and Jesus Eduardo Garcia-Berlanga were responsible for conception, organization, and execution. All the authors were responsible for the preparation of the manuscript: writing of the first draft, review and critique, and reading and approving the final version of the manuscript.

Acknowledgments

We would like to thank the patient for authorizing us to use her clinical data to make it available for the medical community.

References

[1] C. Blackstone, "Hereditary spastic paraplegia," *Handbook of Clinical Neurology*, vol. 148, pp. 633–652, 2018.

[2] J. Finsterer, W. Löscher, S. Quasthoff, J. Wanschitz, M. Auer-Grumbach, and G. Stevanin, "Hereditary spastic paraplegias with autosomal dominant, recessive, X-linked, or maternal trait of inheritance," *Journal of the Neurological Sciences*, vol. 318, no. 1-2, pp. 1–18, 2012.

[3] J. Lambe, B. Monaghan, T. Munteanu, and J. Redmond, "*CAPN1* mutations broadening the hereditary spastic paraplegia/spinocerebellar ataxia phenotype," *Practical Neurology*, vol. 18, no. 5, pp. 369–372, 2018.

[4] C. Kocoglu, A. Gundogdu, G. Kocaman et al., "Homozygous CAPN1 mutations causing a spastic-ataxia phenotype in 2 families," *Neurology: Genetics*, vol. 4, no. 1, p. e218, 2018.

[5] Z. Gan-Or, N. Bouslam, N. Birouk et al., "Mutations in CAPN1 cause autosomal-recessive hereditary spastic paraplegia," *American Journal of Human Genetics*, vol. 98, no. 6, p. 1271, 2016.

[6] F. Peng, Y. Sun, C. Quan, J. Wang, and J. Wu, "Two novel homozygous mutations of CAPN1 in Chinese patients with hereditary spastic paraplegia and literatures review," *Orphanet Journal of Rare Diseases*, vol. 14, no. 1, p. 83, 2019.

[7] M. Baudry and X. Bi, "Calpain-1 and calpain-2: the yin and yang of synaptic plasticity and neurodegeneration," *Trends in Neurosciences*, vol. 39, no. 4, pp. 235–245, 2016.

31

Postpartum-Onset Moyamoya Disease: A Rare Cause of Stroke in Unexpected

Muhammet Ozer,[1] **Khadija Merchant,**[1] **Zulfiya Manning,**[1] **Suleyman Yasin Goksu,**[2] **Kirti Juneja,**[3] **and Vernard S. Fennell**[4]

[1]*Department of Internal Medicine, Capital Health Regional Medical Center, Trenton, NJ, USA*
[2]*Department of Internal Medicine, University of Texas Southwestern Medical School, Dallas, TX, USA*
[3]*Bharati Vidyapeeth Deemed University Medical College, Pune, Maharashtra, India*
[4]*Division of Endovascular Neurosurgery, Capital Health Regional Medical Center, Trenton, NJ, USA*

Correspondence should be addressed to Muhammet Ozer; muh.ozer@gmail.com

Academic Editor: Majaz Moonis

Moyamoya disease (MMD) is a chronic cerebrovascular occlusive disease that is characterized by progressive bilateral stenosis of the terminal portion of the internal carotid artery and its main branches. Cerebrovascular events are the primary presenting symptoms and are related both to stenosis and occlusion of the ICAs and their main branches. Detection of bilateral stenosis by cerebral angiography is considered the gold standard, but computed tomography angiography (CTA) is also an acceptable method of diagnosis. In the current literature, there are no precise data on the incidence of moyamoya disease in Europe and the United States. Also, the pathogenesis of MMD remains obscure, and genetic factors and inflammation are the two most representative mechanisms. Here, we report the case of MMD in a 29-year-old African American female who presented with an ischemic stroke for the second time that manifested after pregnancy. This case is important to increase awareness of the probability of this rare disease in Western countries as well as to call attention to pregnancy's accelerating effects of MMD. Careful, long-term neurologic and radiologic follow-up is essential in adult patients with MMD to prevent additional stroke events and improve outcomes.

1. Introduction

Moyamoya disease (MMD) is a chronic progressive cerebrovascular occlusive disease characterized by bilateral stenosis of the terminal portion of the internal carotid artery and its main branches accompanied by an abnormal vascular formation of collateral vessels at the base of the brain. Significant presenting symptoms of MMD are transient ischemic attacks or strokes. Takeuchi, for the first time, described MMD in 1957 in Japan [1]. Moyamoya means "a puff of smoke" in Japanese. The reason why the name was given is due to the typical appearance of collateral blood vessels that develop at the base of the brain and resemble a puff of smoke.

Besides being a rare condition, epidemiological studies showed that MMD is most prevalent in East Asian countries with an estimated prevalence of 3.2–10.5 per 1,000,000 and estimated annual incidence of 0.43–0.94 per 100,000 [2]. The incidence and prevalence of MMD are increasing with recent advances in neuroradiological diagnostic modalities. In the current literature, there are no precise data on the incidence of MMD in Europe and the United States. Most recent US study estimated overall incidence as 0.086 per 100,000 [3]. Between Western countries, MMD is exceptionally rare in African Americans; it presumably remains a misdiagnosed cause of ischemic and/or hemorrhagic stroke. MMD has two age peaks: in childhood and in young adults. Worldwide studies showed women are more frequently affected than men [4].

Although several hypotheses have been investigated, the pathogenesis of this enigmatic disease remains obscure. Here, we report the case of MMD in a 29-year-old African American female who presented with an ischemic stroke for the second time that manifested after pregnancy. This case is important to increase awareness of the probability of this rare disease in Western countries as well as to call attention to pregnancy's accelerating effects of MMD. Pregnancy and puerperium have some potential deleterious effect on MMD, but mechanisms remain unclear [5].

2. Case Description

The patient is a 29-year-old African American female, G1P1A0, with a history of stroke in multiple areas in the brain approximately two months ago; she was eight months postpartum following an uneventful pregnancy and normal vaginal delivery. At this time, the patient presented with confusion, unusual behavior pattern, headache, involuntary movements, and forgetfulness for the last three days. Patient reported that she had difficulty in performing easy tasks such as putting a bottle together, getting out of the car, and changing her baby. She also reported that, at times, she got lost in her home. She denied having weakness, numbness, seizures, chest pain, shortness of breath, fever, or chills. The patient had a previous ischemic stroke affecting her left side but no residual weakness at this time; however, she did report urinary incontinence since then. Multiple members in her family had a stroke when they were young. The patient was awake, alert, and oriented with no focal neurologic deficits. National Institutes of Health Stroke Scale (NIHSS) score was zero. The first stroke was two months ago, and at that time, she presented with left-sided weakness and cognitive deficits. She was found to have acute cerebral ischemic infarcts primarily noted in the right cerebral hemisphere (Figures 1(a)–1(d)). Subsequently, she underwent a CT angiogram (CTA), which showed questionable stenosis of the bilateral middle cerebral artery (MCA) and distal right vertebral artery. On this admission, she had further progression of intracranial stenosis and ischemic infarcts noted bilaterally (Figures 1(e)–1(h)). CTA of the head revealed moderate to severe narrowing of the supraclinoid segment of both internal carotid arteries (ICA) and extensive narrowing of both M1 segments of the MCAs and both A1 segments of anterior cerebral arteries (ACA). Cerebral perfusion imaging revealed diminished cerebral blood flow in the ACA, MCA, and watershed territories, compatible with ischemia. A diagnostic digital subtraction cerebral angiography showed progressive arteriopathy in both ICA terminals, M1, and A1 with prominent lateral lenticulostriate branches, indicating early collateralization of flow (Figures 2(a) and 2(b)). Based on these clinical and radiological findings, our diagnostic considerations were MMD, primary CNS vasculitis, hypertensive disorder preceding multiple strokes, or hypercoagulability disorders. During this admission, her blood pressure was well controlled. There were no skipped lesions found to support vasculitidies. She denied the previous history of photosensitivity and rash on the face or limbs. There was no history of oral or nasal ulcers, hemoptysis, hematemesis, and recurrent urine infections. She denied a history of Raynaud phenomenon, and there was no history of blood clots that she is aware of. Detailed history and review of systems did not elicit any suspicion of rheumatologic disease. Basic blood work was within normal limits. Specific tests for hypercoagulability, antiphospholipid syndrome, and rheumatologic disorders were negative. CSF analysis was also unremarkable. In following with diagnostic criteria, we diagnosed our patient with MMD. We discharged patients with antihypertensive medications, high-dose statin, and dual antiplatelet therapy.

3. Discussion

MMD is an important diagnosis to consider when evaluating cerebrovascular events in children, young adults, and Asian ethnicity. Cerebrovascular events are the primary presenting symptoms and are related both to the occlusion of the ICAs and their main branches. The incidence of MMD in Europe and the United States is not well studied, but literature analysis suggests that the incidence in Western countries is lower than in Asian countries [3, 6]. Clinical and demographic presentation of MMD cases is quite different between ethnicities. The results of the US-based studies suggest that Caucasian patients are characterized by an older average age of presentation and without bimodal age distribution [7]. Comparing to Asian cases, Caucasian patients mostly present with ischemic strokes with more benign symptoms and less common familial occurrence [4, 8, 9]. MMD is especially rare in African American ethnicity. Uchino et al. [3] detected only 27 MMD cases in African American race, 13 of whom were diagnosed with moyamoya syndrome with having concurrent sickle cell disease.

The diagnosis of MMD requires detection of steno-occlusive changes in the ICA either by CTA, MRA, or cerebral angiography. In patients with unilateral stenosis, cerebral angiography is needed for definitive diagnosis, while bilateral cases can be promptly diagnosed with either CTA or MRA. Cerebral angiography is more sensitive than CTA to show small saccular aneurysms and collateral moyamoya vessels that is why cerebral angiography is considered the gold standard in diagnosis of MMD [10]. Angiographic staging of the MMD was described by Suzuki and Takaku [11] to represent the natural course of the angioarchitecture in affected patients. Although Suzuki's angiographic staging explains compensatory mechanisms of ischemic changes, it is not able to reflect the severity of the MMD. Recently, Czabanka et al. [12] described more specific grading criteria which allow to stratify angiographic severity and clinical symptomatology in MMD patients. There are no remarkable specific CSF changes in patients with MMD. Electroencephalography (EEG) appearances can be abnormal but are usually nonspecific. Infectious processes and primary central nervous system vasculitis should be in the main differential diagnosis. All rheumatologic workups were negative including CSF analysis.

Currently, the pathophysiological mechanisms of MMD are mainly unknown. Investigators described genetic factors and inflammatory changes as the two most representative mechanisms. Recent genetic studies pointed RNF213 as an important susceptibility gene of MMD. A big study on zebrafish vasculature showed that RNF213 is involved in a novel signaling pathway in intracranial angiogenesis [13]. Further studies are needed to explain how the mechanisms of RNF213 mutations are leading to clinical features of MMD. In addition to underlying genetic factors,

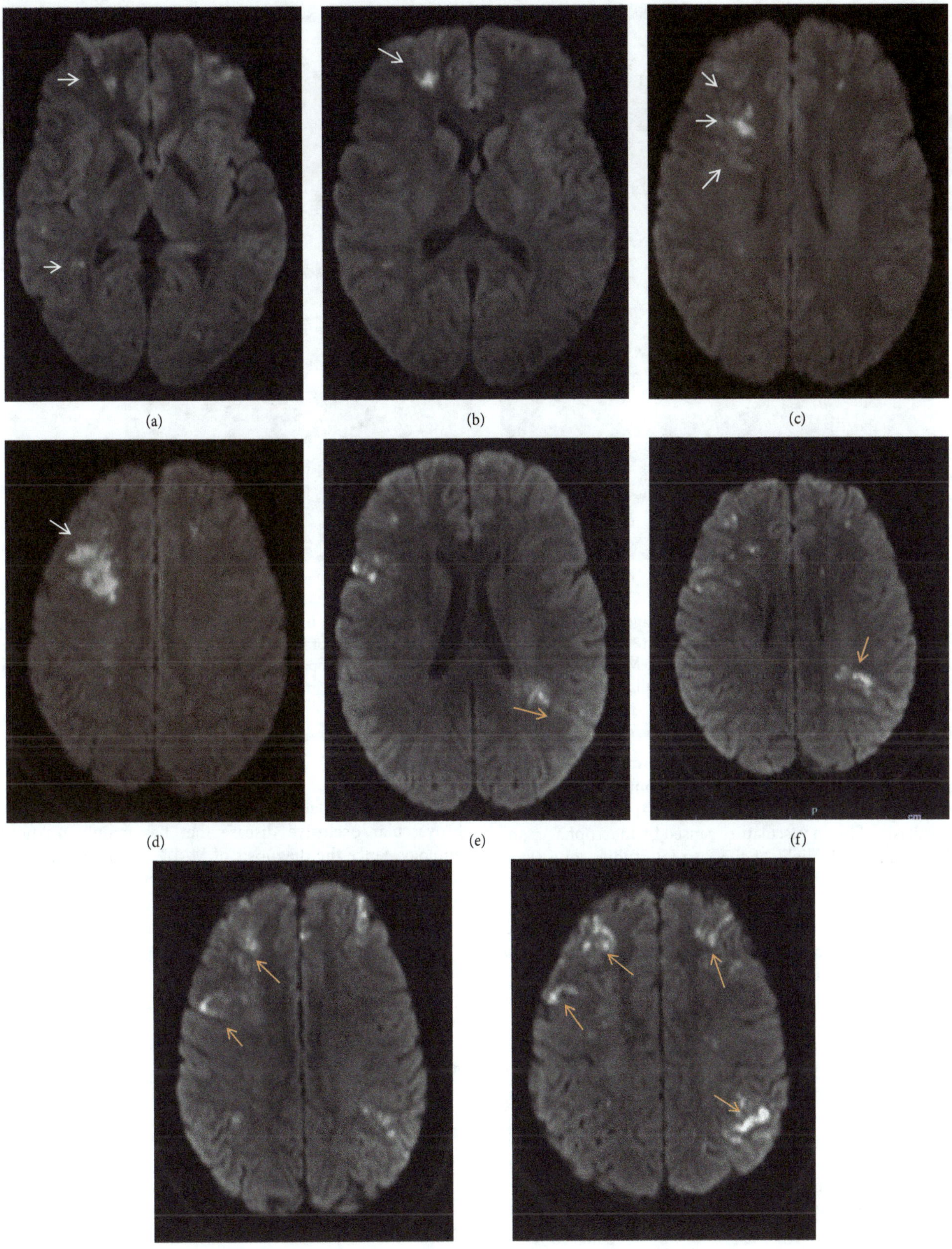

FIGURE 1: Axial MRI brain imaging: (a)—(d) images from the first episode of stroke, with regions of restricted diffusion indicative of acute ischemia (arrows), primarily noted in the right cerebral hemisphere; (e)—(h) images from the second episode, with progressive bilateral ischemic changes (arrows).

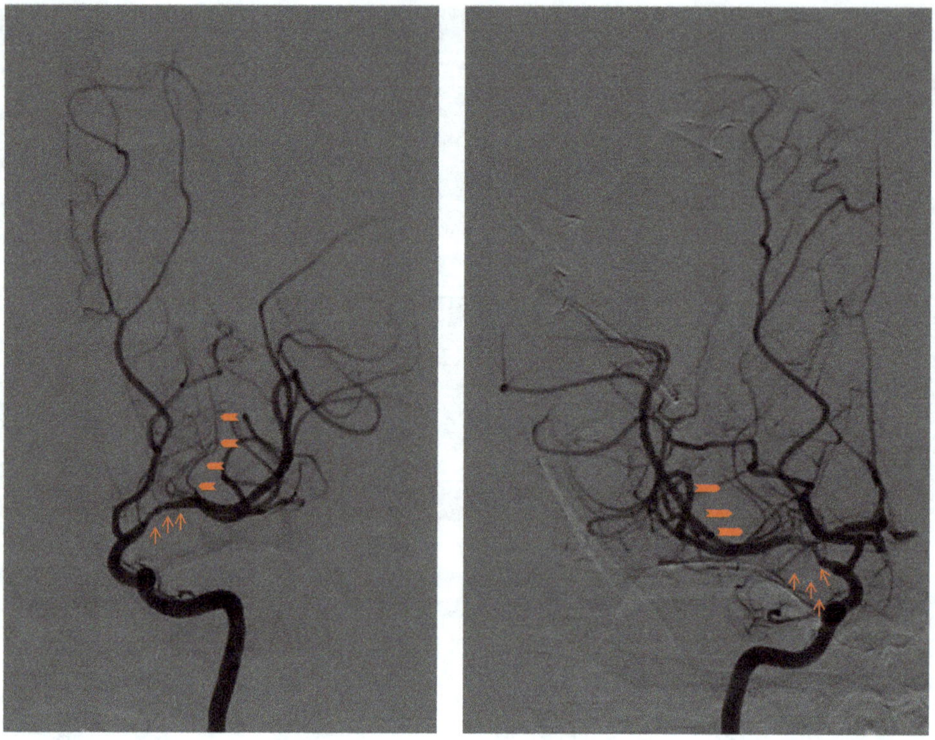

(a) (b)

FIGURE 2: Digital subtraction angiography images: (a) left internal cerebral artery (ICA) with focal distal ICA and proximal M1 arteriopathy (arrows) with prominent lateral lenticulostriate branches, indicating early collateralization of flow (arrowheads); (b) right internal cerebral artery (ICA) with focal distal ICA, proximal MCA (M1), and proximal ACA (A1) arteriopathy (arrows) with prominent lateral lenticulostriate branches, indicating early collateralization of flow (arrowheads).

angiogenesis and vasculogenesis-related inflammatory and autoimmune factors seem to be contributing to the pathophysiology of MMD. Masuda et al. [14] detected intimal hyperplasia of brain vasculature caused by macrophages and T lymphocytes. In light of the current studies, one single mechanism is unable to explain MMD pathogenesis, and further studies are needed.

Unfortunately, there is no definitive treatment described in the literature shown to reverse the intracranial vasculopathy of MMD. Due to the progressive nature of MMD, the prognosis is poor. Current studies show that, within the first year of diagnosis of MMD, the risk of recurrent stroke was approximately 18% but decreased to 5% per year henceforth [7, 15]. Currently, treatment strategies are focused on treating symptoms and halting progression of arteriopathy. The guidelines recommend the use of antiplatelet agents in acute and symptomatic chronic phase patients except in those who present with hemorrhage [16]. The surgical indications and timing of revascularization for MMD have not been established well. Revascularization surgery aims toward improving brain perfusion to prevent recurrent strokes. Due to a wide variety of disease presentation, the decision of revascularization surgery should be specific to each individual's condition. In our case, due to satisfactory response to initial medical management, we did not consider surgical intervention.

4. Conclusion

MMD is a multifactorial, complex, and progressive cerebrovascular occlusive disease that has mainly unknown etiology. Since the diagnosis of MMD is rapidly increasing worldwide, we highly suggest considering MMD as a differential diagnosis in Western countries, especially in young patients who present with progressive cerebrovascular events. Long-term close follow-up is crucial to minimize the risk of future cerebrovascular events and improve outcomes.

Authors' Contributions

S.Y.G. involved in diagnostic steps and interpreting results. K.J. participated in writing up of the manuscript and editing.

References

[1] K. Takeuchi, "Hypoplasia of bilateral internal carotid arteries," *Brain Nerve*, vol. 9, pp. 37–43, 1957.

[2] W. Miao, P.-L. Zhao, Y.-S. Zhang et al., "Epidemiological and clinical features of moyamoya disease in Nanjing, China," *Clinical Neurology and Neurosurgery*, vol. 112, no. 3, pp. 199–203, 2010.

[3] K. Uchino, S. C. Johnston, K. J. Becker, and D. L. Tirschwell, "Moyamoya disease in Washington state and California," *Neurology*, vol. 65, no. 6, pp. 956–958, 2005.

[4] R. Kleinloog, L. Regli, G. J. E. Rinkel, and C. J. M. Klijn, "Regional differences in incidence and patient characteristics of moyamoya disease: a systematic review," *Journal of Neurology, Neurosurgery & Psychiatry*, vol. 83, no. 5, pp. 531–536, 2012.

[5] J. C. Ma and J. M. Burlingame, "Moyamoya disease in pregnancy: a case series and review of management options," *Hawaii Medical Journal*, vol. 70, no. 8, pp. 161–163, 2011.

[6] Y. Goto and Y. Yonekawa, "Worldwide distribution of moyamoya disease," *Neurologia Medico-Chirurgica*, vol. 32, no. 12, pp. 883–886, 1992.

[7] E. Y. Yilmaz, M. B. Pritz, A. Bruno, A. Lopez-Yunez, and J. Biller, "Moyamoya," *Archives of Neurology*, vol. 58, no. 8, pp. 1274–1278, 2001.

[8] G. Acker, S. Goerdes, U. C. Schneider, P. Schmiedek, M. Czabanka, and P. Vajkoczy, "Distinct clinical and radiographic characteristics of moyamoya disease amongst European caucasians," *European Journal of Neurology*, vol. 22, no. 6, pp. 1012–1017, 2015.

[9] D. Kainth, S. A. Chaudhry, H. Kainth, F. K. Suri, and A. I. Qureshi, "Epidemiological and clinical features of moyamoya disease in the USA," *Neuroepidemiology*, vol. 40, no. 4, pp. 282–287, 2013.

[10] I. Yamada, S. Suzuki, and Y. Matsushima, "Moyamoya disease: comparison of assessment with MR angiography and MR imaging versus conventional angiography," *Radiology*, vol. 196, no. 1, pp. 211–218, 1995.

[11] J. Suzuki and A. Takaku, "Cerebrovascular "moyamoya" disease," *Archives of Neurology*, vol. 20, no. 3, pp. 288–299, 1969.

[12] M. Czabanka, P. Peña-Tapia, G. A. Schubert et al., "Proposal for a new grading of moyamoya disease in adult patients," *Cerebrovascular Diseases*, vol. 32, no. 1, pp. 41–50, 2011.

[13] W. Liu, D. Morito, S. Takashima et al., "Identification of RNF213 as a susceptibility gene for moyamoya disease and its possible role in vascular development," *PLoS One*, vol. 6, no. 7, Article ID e22542, 2011.

[14] J. Masuda, J. Ogata, and C. Yutani, "Smooth muscle cell proliferation and localization of macrophages and T cells in the occlusive intracranial major arteries in moyamoya disease," *Stroke*, vol. 24, no. 12, pp. 1960–1967, 1993.

[15] D. Chiu, P. Shedden, P. Bratina, and J. C. Grotta, "Clinical features of moyamoya disease in the United States," *Stroke*, vol. 29, no. 7, pp. 1347–1351, 1998.

[16] "Guidelines for diagnosis and treatment of moyamoya disease (spontaneous occlusion of the circle of willis)," *Neurologia medico-chirurgica (Tokyo)*, vol. 52, no. 5, pp. 245–266, 2012.

32

Fatigue and Exercise Intolerance as Initial Manifestations of a Nonsyndromic Mitochondrial Disorder Due to the Variant m.3243A>G

Josef Finsterer[1] **and Sinda Zarrouk**[2]

[1]*Neurology and Neurophysiology Center, Vienna, Austria*
[2]*University of Tunis El Manar, Tunis, Tunisia*

Correspondence should be addressed to Josef Finsterer; fipaps@yahoo.de

Academic Editor: Peter Berlit

Objectives. Fatigue and exercise intolerance have been only rarely reported as initial- and sole-onset manifestations of a mitochondrial disorder (MID). We present a patient with nonsyndromic MID with fatigue and exercise intolerance as its initial manifestations of the disease. *Case Report.* A 39 yo female experienced fatigue since age 18 and exercise intolerance since age 21. Later on, she developed Hashimoto thyroiditis, recurrent diffuse headache, and double vision upon exercise. Clinical exam revealed short stature, bilateral ptosis, partially reduced tendon reflexes, and hypertrophic calves. Serum lactate was elevated, and the lactate stress test was abnormal. Workup for suspected MID revealed ragged-red fibers and NADH-deficient muscle fibers, and biochemical investigations revealed a mild complex-I defect. mtDNA sequencing revealed the variant m.3243A>G with a heteroplasmy rate of 70% in the muscle. *Conclusions.* This case shows that the initial manifestation of a MID can be fatigue and exercise intolerance. MIDs due to the m.3243A>G variant may have a slowly progressive course and only delayed multisystem involvement. The variant m.3243A>G may not only manifest as syndromic MID, particularly MELAS but also as nonsyndromic phenotype. MIDs should be considered as differentials of chronic fatigue even if no other phenotypic manifestation of a MID is present.

1. Introduction

Mitochondrial disorders (MIDs) can be due to mutations on the mtDNA or in nDNA located genes [1]. They manifest with a broad range of phenotypic features and have an onset between birth and senescence. Though fatigue is a common phenotypic feature of MIDs [1], it has been only rarely reported as the initial and sole manifestation of a MID. Usually, fatigue is one feature among others at onset or develops later in the course. Here, we present the data of a MID patient with fatigue and exercise intolerance as the initial manifestations of the disease. Informed consent was obtained from the patient.

2. Case Report

The patient is a 39 yo female, height 160 cm, with an uneventful previous history until age 18 y when she started to recognise increased tiredness and fatigability. At age 21 y, she developed exercise intolerance initially only during sport activities but later also in association with simple activities of daily living. Overexertion was complicated by nausea and tiredness. Later in the course, Hashimoto thyroiditis was diagnosed and hypothyroidism substituted with L-thyroxin, without a beneficial effect on fatigue. During the further course, she developed episodic nonmigrainous, diffuse headache. Since several months, she noted double vision during episodes of tiredness. She also realised a depressive mood.

Her family history was positive for hypothyroidism, aortic valve replacement therapy at age 52 y because of a bicuspid aortic valve, headache, hypothyroidism, and mental instability in her mother, psychosis, and exercise intolerance in her brother, breast cancer, anxiety disorder, and fatigability in her grandmother from the mother's side (Figure 1).

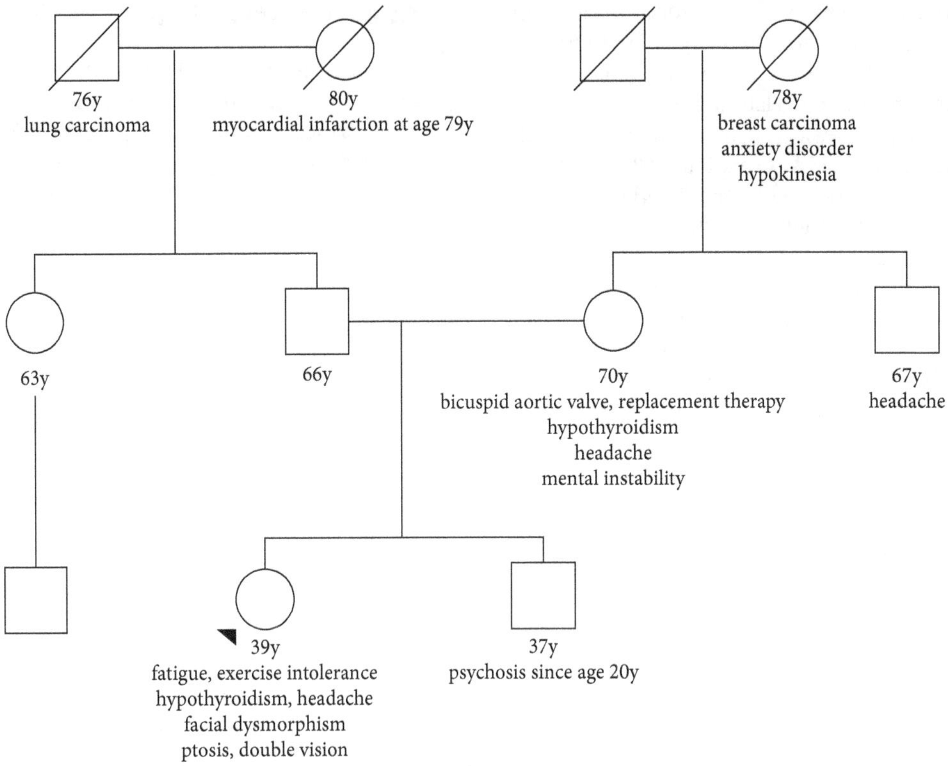

FIGURE 1: Pedigree of the index patient's family revealing that a maternal trait of inheritance is quite likely despite absence of the culprit variant in the mother.

Clinical neurologic exam at age 28 y revealed short stature, bilateral ptosis, hypertelorism, reduced tendon reflexes on the upper limbs, reduced patella tendon reflexes on the lower limbs, and gnome calves.

Workup for a suspected MID revealed lactic acidosis, ragged-red fibers on muscle biopsy, mild complex-I deficiency (complex-1 activity: 27 mU/mU CS (*n*, 28–76 mU/mU CS), and the variant m.3243A>G with a heteroplasmy rate of 70% in muscle. The mutation was not detected in blood or urinary epithelial cells. The mutation could not be detected in blood or urine of her mother either. Cerebral magnetic resonance imaging (MRI), electrocardiography (ECG), and echocardiography were noninformative. She was recommended to regularly take riboflavin (300 mg/d) and coenzyme-Q (300 mg/d) in addition to L-thyroxin with limited benefit.

3. Discussion

The case shows that fatigue and exercise intolerance can be the initial phenotypic manifestation of a MID besides short stature. The case also demonstrates that the disease course of a MID can be slowly progressive over years with only delayed affection of organs other than the muscle. Extramuscular manifestations in the index patient were headache, hypothyroidism, and short stature. Lactic acidosis most likely derived from affection of the skeletal muscles.

Fatigue is a nonspecific term with many different meanings. Fatigue may have an organic or a psychological cause. Among the organic causes, fatigue may derive from a genetic or an acquired defect. Fatigue may be present already without any physical activity or only in association with physical exercise. The latter is also known as exercise intolerance or exhaustibility. Acquired causes of fatigue include disorders of the central nervous system, the peripheral nervous system, the muscles, endocrinologic disorders, cardiac disease, pulmonary dysfunction, renal insufficiency, infectious diseases, immunological diseases, malignancy, malnutrition, or drugs. Among the psychological causes, fatigue may derive from depression, chronic pain, chronic overstimulation, or chronic overload (e.g., seafarer fatigue).

Since the brain, heart, and kidneys were not affected in the index patient, since substitution of hypothyroidism did not resolve fatigue, and since there was no systemic disease, fatigue and exercise intolerance were most likely due to affection of the skeletal muscles. Whether lactic acidosis contributed to fatigue or was the sole cause of fatigue remains speculative. Since lactic acidosis was only mild, it was most likely not responsible for fatigue and exercise intolerance. More likely, the initial manifestations were caused by the mismatch between energy requirements and energy production. A contributing factor to fatigue in the index patient could be the depression. Nocturnal hypoventilation was excluded as a cause of fatigue as polysomnography including oximetry did not reveal desaturations overnight.

Fatigue is a common phenotypic feature of MIDs and has been reported in various types of syndromic and nonsyndromic MIDs, irrespective of an mtDNA or nDNA mutation as the underlying cause, and irrespective if the respiratory chain or other metabolic pathways (e.g. urea cycle, ketone body metabolism, and heme synthesis), receptors, transport proteins, pore proteins, or signalling mitochondrial proteins were involved [2]. In a study of 48 adults with a MID, 71–100% reported fatigue depending on the measure used, and the correlation between severity of fatigue and severity of disease [2]. In a study of 72 MID patients carrying the m.3243A>G variant, 60% showed a high degree of fatigue as assessed by the RAND-SF36 score [3]. In a case series of four patients carrying the m.3243A>G variant, one patient manifested exclusively with exercise intolerance, muscle aching since childhood, and mental and physical fatigue [4]. Unfortunately, heteroplasmy rates were not provided and it was not mentioned which of the manifestations occurred first [4]. Usually, fatigue is one among other features of the m.3243A>G phenotype at onset or develops later in the course [5].

Exercise intolerance is also a frequent manifestation of MIDs or m.3243A>G carriers but usually occurs in association with other phenotypic features [6]. In a study of 47 Chinese families carrying the m.3243A>G variant, the most frequent manifestations in the index patients' mothers were lactic acidosis, exercise intolerance, short stature, and weight loss [7]. In a study of 82 Dutch m.3243A>G carriers, exercise intolerance was reported in 54% of them, being thus the most frequent manifestation after hearing loss and gastrointestinal compromise [8]. In a study of 11 MID patients of whom 5 carried the m.3243A>G variant, a single patient manifested exclusively with exercise intolerance [9]. In a patient with only mild exercise intolerance, normal muscle histochemistry, and normal respiratory chain activity in vitro, the heteroplasmy rate of the variant m.3243A>G was 6% [10]. Despite this low heteroplasmy rate, the maximum rate of ATP production was reduced to 35% in his calf muscles [10].

Despite the absence of the causative mtDNA variant in the index patient's mother in the blood and urine, the variant was regarded as inherited given the clinical presentation of her mother and grandmother from the mother's side and the putative maternal trait of inheritance.

4. Conclusions

This case shows that the initial manifestation of a MID can be fatigue and exercise intolerance, that MIDs due to the m.3243A>G variant may have a slowly progressive course and only delayed multisystem involvement, that the variant m.3243A>G may not only manifest as syndromic MID, particularly MELAS, but also as nonsyndromic phenotype, and that MIDs should be considered as differentials of chronic fatigue even if no other phenotypic manifestation of the MID is present.

Consent

Informed consent was obtained.

Authors' Contributions

JF designed the study and wrote the first draft. JF and SZ performed the literature search, conducted discussion, and provided critical comments. SZ gave the final approval to the manuscript.

References

[1] S. Kanungo, J. Morton, M. Neelakantan, K. Ching, J. Saeedian, and A. Goldstein, "Mitochondrial disorders," *Annals of Translational Medicine*, vol. 6, no. 24, p. 475, 2018.

[2] S. Parikh, R. Galioto, B. Lapin et al., "Fatigue in primary genetic mitochondrial disease: no rest for the weary," *Neuromuscular Disorders*, vol. 29, no. 11, pp. 895–902, 2019.

[3] C. Verhaak, P. de Laat, S. Koene et al., "Quality of life, fatigue and mental health in patients with the m.3243A>G mutation and its correlates with genetic characteristics and disease manifestation," *Orphanet Journal of Rare Diseases*, vol. 11, no. 1, p. 25, 2016.

[4] S. Blum, T. Robertson, S. Klingberg, R. D. Henderson, and P. McCombe, "Atypical clinical presentations of the A3243G mutation, usually associated with MELAS," *Internal Medicine Journal*, vol. 41, no. 2, pp. 199–202, 2011.

[5] K. Komlósi, R. Kellermayer, A. Maász et al., "Maternally inherited deafness and unusual phenotypic manifestations associated with A3243G mitochondrial DNA mutation," *Pathology and Oncology Research*, vol. 11, no. 2, pp. 82–86, 2005.

[6] A. Gál, A. Szabó, K. Pentelényi, and Z. Pál, "Maternally inherited diabetes mellitus, deafness, chronic progressive external ophthalmoplegia and myopathy as the result of A3243G mutation of mtDNA," *Orvosi Hetilap*, vol. 149, no. 34, pp. 1593–1598, 2008.

[7] Y. Ma, F. Fang, Y. Cao et al., "Clinical features of mitochondrial DNA m.3243A>G mutation in 47 Chinese families," *Journal of the Neurological Sciences*, vol. 291, no. 1-2, pp. 17–21, 2010.

[8] P. de Laat, S. Koene, L. P. W. J. van den Heuvel, R. J. T. Rodenburg, M. C. H. Janssen, and J. A. M. Smeitink, "Clinical features and heteroplasmy in blood, urine and saliva in 34 dutch families carrying the m.3243A>G mutation," *Journal of Inherited Metabolic Disease*, vol. 35, no. 6, pp. 1059–1069, 2012.

[9] Y. Lu, D. Zhao, S. Yao et al., "Mitochondrial tRNA genes are hotspots for mutations in a cohort of patients with exercise intolerance and mitochondrial myopathy," *Journal of the Neurological Sciences*, vol. 379, pp. 137–143, 2017.

[10] P. F. Chinnery, D. J. Taylor, D. T. Brown, D. Manners, P. Styles, and R. Lodi, "Very low levels of the mtDNA A3243G mutation associated with mitochondrial dysfunction in vivo," *Annals of Neurology*, vol. 47, no. 3, pp. 381–384, 2000.

33

Vagus Nerve Stimulation (VNS) in Super Refractory New Onset Refractory Status Epilepticus (NORSE)

Mohankumar Kurukumbi,[1] James Leiphart,[1] Anam Asif,[2] and Jing Wang[3]

[1]*Department of Neurology, Inova Fairfax Hospital, Falls Church, VA, USA*
[2]*VCU School of Medicine, Inova Campus, Falls Church, VA, USA*
[3]*Department of Neurocritical Care, Inova Fairfax Hospital, Falls Church, VA, USA*

Correspondence should be addressed to Mohankumar Kurukumbi; mohan311@gmail.com

Academic Editor: Norman S. Litofsky

The treatment protocol of status epilepticus has many associated toxicities so there is interest in alternate nonmedicinal therapies for managing New Onset Refractory Status Epilepticus (NORSE) patients. Vagus nerve stimulation (VNS) is an FDA-approved therapy for refractory epilepsy that has been shown to decrease the frequency and severity of seizures. We present the case of a patient with new-onset refractory status epilepticus (NORSE) whose seizures were successfully treated with vagus nerve stimulation. A 25-year-old male with no history of epilepsy or other neurological disorders presented with altered mental status and generalized tonic-clonic seizures following a two-week history of an upper respiratory tract infection. Lumbar puncture showed neutrophilic pleocytosis, and he was treated for bacterial and viral meningoencephalitis. In spite of treatment, his seizures began increasing in frequency. On day three, the patient entered status epilepticus (SE) refractory to intensive pharmacotherapy with maximal doses of valproate, levetiracetam, and propofol. On day four, SE remained refractory, so pentobarbital was introduced with targeted burst suppression pattern on electroencephalography (EEG). Patient continued to be refractory to these measures, so a vagus nerve stimulator (VNS) was implanted (day eight). Following VNS implantation, EEG demonstrated significant reduction of seizure activity and subsequent magnet swiping continued aborting electrographic seizures. No SE or electrographic seizures were reported for seventy-two hours, but few occasional discharges were reported. Seizures eventually recurred on day fourteen and the patient succumbed to his multiple comorbidities on day seventeen. Due to the efficacy of VNS in refractory epilepsy, there was interest in using it in refractory status epilepticus. Multiple case reports have described a benefit from implantation of VNS in the treatment of SE. The successful use of VNS to acutely terminate status epilepticus for seventy-two hours in this critically ill patient adds to current evidence that there is utility in using VNS for refractory status epilepticus.

1. Introduction

New-onset refractory status epilepticus (NORSE) is a syndrome where status epilepticus manifests in patients who were previously healthy and lack a history of epilepsy or neurological disorders. The treatment protocol is intensive and includes benzodiazepines, anticonvulsants, and eventually anesthetics to medically induce coma when polypharmacy is exhausted [1]. If seizures continue or recur after 24 hours following treatment with anesthetics, it is termed superrefractory status epilepticus (SRSE). Because of high mortality with the polypharmacy and continuous anesthetic use, there has been great interest to use nonmedicinal devices like VNS in aborting a seizure. Here we present a case of super refractory NORSE treated with VNS.

2. Case Report

The patient was a 25-year-old male presenting with altered mental status and generalized tonic clonic seizures following a 2-week history of an upper respiratory tract infection. MRI of brain was negative for any acute pathology and nonlesional for seizures. *Results of a paraneoplastic antibody panel were negative but he was found to have neutrophilic pleocytosis on lumbar puncture. Cerebrospinal fluid cultures*

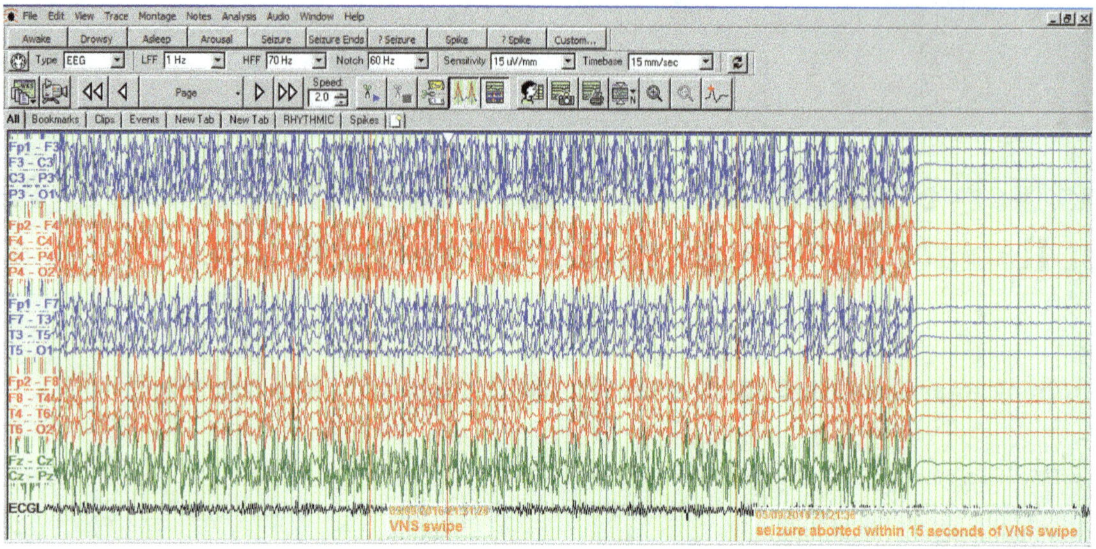

FIGURE 1: EEG demonstrated cessation of seizure activity within 15 seconds of magnet swiping.

were negative but he was empirically treated for bacterial and viral meningoencephalitis with ceftriaxone, vancomycin, and acyclovir. Seizures began increasing in frequency despite frequent treatment with benzodiazepines and, on day three, the patient worsened to have status epilepticus. Treatment with maximal doses of valproate, levetiracetam, and propofol was started but, by day four, the patient's seizures remained refractory. As a result, the patient was placed under a pentobarbital-induced coma with burst suppression pattern on electroencephalography (EEG). On day 8, five days after status and due to continued seizure activity as evidenced by EEG, a VNS was implanted. VNS was turned on with the settings: Output output current 1.5 milliamperes, Pulse Width 500 microseconds, Frequency 30, On time 30 seconds, and Time interval 3 minutes.

Magnet Output current 2 milliamperes, On time 60 seconds. *Three days after implantation of VNS, there was generalized suppression of EEG activity with continued use of pentobarbital; however, the patient continued to have electrographic seizures which were successfully aborted by the VNS magnet swiping (see Figure 1).* No other changes were made to the medical regimen. For the next 72 hours, no status epilepticus or electrographic seizures were reported, although few occasional discharges were seen. Unfortunately, seizures recurred on day 14 and the patient succumbed to his multiple comorbidities on day 17. However, VNS was successful in acutely terminating status epilepticus for 72 hours in this critically ill patient when the standard therapies failed.

3. Discussion

Status epilepticus is a medical emergency with seizure activity lasting five minutes or longer [2]. This can be either one continuous seizure or multiple repetitive seizures with no recovery of consciousness in between [3]. Status epilepticus can include both generalized and partial seizures and has a high potential to cause brain injury so it therefore requires immediate drug therapy. The treatment protocol is intensive and includes benzodiazepines, anticonvulsants, and eventually anesthetics to medically induce coma when polypharmacy is exhausted [1].

The pathophysiology of NORSE remains unclear, with one study of 130 patients finding 52% of cases (n=67) to be cryptogenic in origin. In cases with an identifiable etiology, the most common was nonparaneoplastic autoimmune, specifically an anti-NMDA receptor antibody, followed by paraneoplastic causes [4]. Analysis of cerebrospinal fluid in NORSE patients also commonly demonstrated inflammatory pleocytosis, with infectious etiology being the third most common identified, although often without an identifiable organism [4]. Furthermore, similar to our patient, NORSE often occurs in the background of a preceding upper respiratory tract infection so one hypothesis is it is initiated in response to increased proinflammatory molecules in the brain following a viral infection [5–7].

NORSE is seen most frequently in young adults, though all ages can be affected. It does share similarities with other seizure syndromes which occur mainly in children, including Febrile Illness-Related Epilepsy Syndrome (FIRES) and Idiopathic Hemiconvulsion-Hemiplegia and Epilepsy Syndrome (IHHES), so some hypothesize that all may be extensions of a common disorder afflicting younger populations [4]. It is difficult to estimate the incidence of NORSE since it is often underreported as status epilepticus attributed to encephalitis. However, one Finnish study on SRSE estimated an annual incidence of 0.7/100,000 and a mortality rate of 36% [7]. So although cases of refractory status epilepticus are rare, they are associated with significant mortality. Prognosis for NORSE survivors is poor as 50% of survivors develop a chronic cognitive or functional disability and often have epilepsy moving forward [4].

Seizures in NORSE do not respond to the standard status epilepticus medications; hence the majority of patients are treated with an anesthesia-induced coma and monitored in

ICUs [5]. One study estimates that nearly 40% of status epilepticus cases will be refractory to the first and second-line treatments of the aforementioned protocol [4]. The multiple toxicities of antiepileptic drugs have the potential to impart further damage to the already metabolically stressed brain. NORSE patients receive a median of five antiseizure medications during their treatment course yet 77% of cases culminate with administration of continuous anesthetics [4]. This trial-and-error approach may have deleterious effects; therefore, the high morbidity and mortality associated with NORSE may have an iatrogenic component rather than being entirely physiologic. Anesthetic use is particularly concerning since it is associated with poorer outcomes and increased mortality [4]. This relationship is not necessarily causal but still represents the need for alternative management strategies so there is great interest in aborting seizures with nonmedicinal devices.

One such option is vagus nerve stimulation (VNS), an FDA-approved therapy for refractory epilepsy that has been shown to decrease the frequency and severity of seizures [8, 9]. Unlike traditional antiepileptic drugs, VNS is hypothesized to control seizures by sending regular pulses to the brain through stimulation of the vagus nerve [8]. This different mechanism of action has a much lower side effect profile while still exerting a powerful antiseizure effect. One study reviewing seizure control in 65 patients with an implanted VNS found seizures decreased by 28% within 3 months of implantation [9]. This benefit extrapolates to long-term control with seizures decreasing by 36% within 6 months of implantation, 58% after 4 years, and 75% by 10 years [9].

Due to the efficacy of VNS in refractory epilepsy, there was interest in using it in refractory status epilepticus as an alternative nontoxic treatment option. We present the case of our patient with NORSE whose seizures were successfully controlled by VNS treatment.

This case report adds to current evidence on the effectiveness of using VNS for SRSE. Multiple case reports have described a benefit from implantation of VNS in the treatment of SRSE [10–15]. One such case report described a 24-year-old man with no history of epilepsy or neurological disorders presenting with delirium two days after onset of fever related to a mild upper respiratory tract infection [10]. On day 2 the patient developed left-sided clonic seizures which progressed to generalized tonic-clonic seizures. The frequency of seizures increased until patient entered status epilepticus. Status failed to be controlled by intravenous diazepam and phenytoin but eventually responded to intravenous propofol. The patient remained stable until day 14 when seizures recurred. Multiple therapies were tested, including thiopental, valproate, lamotrigine, steroid-pulse therapy, intravenous immunoglobulin, zonisamide, levetiracetam, topiramate, and midazolam but none provided lasting relief. Patient, presented 14 months later with refractory epilepsy and had deteriorated to the point of being bedridden, was incapable of verbal communication and required a feeding tube all while being treated with intravenous midazolam. Eventually a VNS was implanted in a final effort to control seizures. By day 10 the patient was successfully weaned off midazolam, and 2 months later he was seizure-free. The rapid modulation by VNS allowed reduction of intensive pharmacotherapy and contributed to seizure remission at one-year after implantation [10].

Another report described the case of a 30-year-old male with SRSE who could not remain on multiple antiepileptic medications including phenytoin, valproic acid, carbamazepine, and topiramate due to severe allergic reactions [13]. He was placed under a pentobarbital-induced coma without seizure control and after 9 days he underwent a VNS implantation. Within a day, EEG demonstrated resolution of seizures. During recovery the patient was able to be weaned off medications without triggering additional seizures and regained mental alertness and orientation with no residual compromise of his long-term memory [13].

Similarly, there was a case report of a 7-year-old girl with a history of thrombosis in the right internal cerebral vein and right thalamic bleeding 8 days after birth [11]. As a result of this early neurological insult, she developed epilepsy at 13 months of age. At 6 years she presented with refractory status epilepticus and spent 11 days in a medicine-induced coma. She subsequently underwent VNS placement with positive results. Her coma was withdrawn 3 days after implantation, her EEG normalized within 1 week, and at 13-month follow-up she was seizure-free and even her previous antiepileptic drugs were tapered. Although this is not a case of NORSE due to her history of epilepsy, this case shows the potential of VNS to acutely abort refractory status epilepticus, as well as impart a long-term benefit against seizures [11]. This is further demonstrated by the case report of a 23-year-old male who remained in SE for 3 weeks despite being on intravenous anesthetics. His SE terminated rapidly following VNS implantation and allowed anesthetics to be successfully weaned off and the patient fully recovered [9]. In another case report, a 13-year-old male had SRSE successfully aborted following VNS implantation [4]. Over the course of 1.5 years his seizures were better controlled in terms of both rate and severity [4].

One study reviewing current literature on all cases of VNS use in SRSE identified 17 studies in which a total of 28 patients were treated [15]. In patients with generalized SRSE, 76% displayed termination of SRSE with VNS use. Patients with focal SRSE demonstrated a less robust response, but 25% still responded to VNS insertion. Few adverse effects related to these VNS insertions were described. Despite a small sample size limiting the power of the study, this demonstrates strong evidence exists that there is improvement in seizure control with the use of VNS in generalized SRSE.

In most of these cases, like in our case, VNS was utilized late in the treatment plan, often following more than a week of status epilepticus and after multiple antiepileptic medications failed. However, the evidence shows that VNS has the capability to rapidly resolve status epilepticus within days of implantation. This discrepancy between the effectiveness of VNS and when it is to be employed must be studied with more cases.

We propose that VNS be considered earlier in the treatment course for SRSE as it is both efficacious and nontoxic. Despite our patient case being complicated by multiple confounding comorbidities, the case reports reviewed demonstrate a positive prognosis amongst patients treated with VNS which may offset the high mortality rates of SRSE syndromes. Furthermore, it would reduce the iatrogenic burden associated with status epilepticus polypharmacy treatments. In addition to having utility in halting the status, VNS has been shown to counteract the morbidity associated with SRSE. Patients receive the benefit of prophylaxis against future seizures and thereby require less long-term medications since epilepsy is common sequelae of SRSE disorders.

4. Conclusion

The medications used to control SRSE have several potential side effects which can further damage the brain so there is interest in finding an alternative treatment. VNS has been demonstrated by numerous case reports, including our case to be a safe and effective treatment for status epilepticus refractory to traditional treatment. Its lower side effect profile compared to antiepileptic medications reduces the toxicities vulnerable patients are exposed to, while offering a lasting protective effect against future seizures. Since there is typically extensive additional therapy complicating the complete assessment of VNS in status epilepticus, additional prospective study is warranted.

Abbreviations

NORSE: New Onset Refractory Status Epilepticus
FDA: Food and Drug Administration
SE: Status epilepticus
SRSE: Super Refractory Status Epilepticus
EEG: Electroencephalography
MRI: Magnetic resonance imaging
VNS: Vagus nerve stimulation
FIRES: Febrile Illness-Related Epilepsy Syndrome
IHHES: Idiopathic Hemiconvulsion-Hemiplegia and Epilepsy Syndrome.

References

[1] D. A. Greenberg, M. J. Aminoff, and R. P. Simon, *Clinical Neurology*, McGraw-Hill Education, New York, NY, USA, 9th edition, 2015.

[2] S. A. Mayer, J. Claassen, J. Lokin, F. Mendelsohn, L. J. Dennis, and B. F. Fitzsimmons, "Refractory status epilepticus: frequency, risk factors, and impact on outcome," *JAMA Neurology*, vol. 59, no. 2, pp. 205–210, 2002.

[3] R. D. Kilbride, A. S. Reynolds, J. P. Szaflarski, and L. J. Hirsch, "Clinical outcomes following prolonged refractory status epilepticus (PRSE)," *Neurocritical Care*, vol. 18, no. 3, pp. 374–385, 2013.

[4] N. Gaspard, B. P. Foreman, V. Alvarez et al., "New-onset refractory status epilepticus," *Neurology*, vol. 85, no. 18, pp. 1604–1613, 2015.

[5] E. P. Wilder-Smith, E. C. Lim, H. L. Teoh et al., "The NORSE (new-onset refractory status epilepticus) syndrome: defining a disease entity," *Annals of the Academy of Medicine Singapore*, vol. 34, pp. 417–420, 2005.

[6] R. Nabbout, A. Vezzani, O. Dulac, and C. Chiron, "Acute encephalopathy with inflammation-mediated status epilepticus," *The Lancet Neurology*, vol. 10, no. 1, pp. 99–108, 2011.

[7] A.-M. Kantanen, M. Reinikainen, I. Parviainen et al., "Incidence and mortality of super-refractory status epilepticus in adults," *Epilepsy & Behavior*, vol. 49, pp. 131–134, 2015.

[8] R. H. Howland, "Vagus Nerve Stimulation," *Current Behavioral Neuroscience Reports*, vol. 1, no. 2, pp. 64–73, 2014.

[9] R. E. Elliott, A. Morsi, O. Tanweer et al., "Efficacy of vagus nerve stimulation over time: review of 65 consecutive patients with treatment-resistant epilepsy treated with VNS >10 years," *Epilepsy & Behavior*, vol. 20, no. 3, pp. 478–483, 2011.

[10] T. Yamazoe, T. Okanishi, A. Yamamoto, T. Yamada et al., "New-onset refractory status epilepticus treated with vagus nerve stimulation: A case report," *Seizure*, vol. 47, pp. 1–4, 2017.

[11] V. De Herdt, L. Waterschoot, K. Vonck et al., "Vagus nerve stimulation for refractory status epilepticus," *European Journal of Paediatric Neurology*, vol. 13, no. 3, pp. 286–289, 2009.

[12] K. R. Winston, P. Levisohn, B. R. Miller, and J. Freeman, "Vagal nerve stimulation for status epilepticus," *Pediatric Neurosurgery*, vol. 34, no. 4, pp. 190–192, 2001.

[13] R. V. Patwardhan, J. Dellabadia Jr., M. Rashidi, L. Grier, and A. Nanda, "Control of refractory status epilepticus precipitated by anticonvulsant withdrawal using left vagal nerve stimulation: A case report," *World Neurosurgery*, vol. 64, no. 2, pp. 170–173, 2005.

[14] B. R. O'Neill, J. Valeriano, A. Synowiec et al., "Refractory status epilepticus treated with vagal nerve stimulation: Case report," *Neurosurgery*, vol. 69, no. 5, pp. E1172–E1175, 2011.

[15] F. A. Zeiler, K. J. Zeiler, J. Teitelbaum, L. M. Gillman, and M. West, "VNS for refractory status epilepticus," *Epilepsy Research*, vol. 112, pp. 100–113, 2015.

34

Endoscopic Endonasal Resection of Meckel's Cave Epidermoid Cysts: Case Discussion and Literature Review

Jehad Zakaria,[1] Pravesh Saini,[1] Mariya Yanovskaya,[1] John T. Tsiang,[1] Krishnan Ravindran,[1] Stephen Johans,[1] Chirag R. Patel,[2] and Anand V. Germanwala[1,2]

[1]*Department of Neurological Surgery, Stritch School of Medicine, Loyola University Medical Center, Maywood, IL, USA*
[2]*Department of Otolaryngology-Head and Neck Surgery, Stritch School of Medicine, Loyola University Medical Center, Maywood, IL, USA*

Correspondence should be addressed to Anand V. Germanwala; agermanwala@gmail.com

Academic Editor: Isabella Laura Simone

Meckel's cave (MC) epidermoid cysts are relatively uncommon lesions. In cases where surgical excision is indicated, resection is often carried out via a frontosphenotemporal craniotomy from an anterolateral approach or a temporal craniotomy with or without a petrosectomy for a lateral corridor; both of these routes are associated with brain retraction and potential neurovascular injury. The anterior location of MC in the middle cranial fossa makes safe access via posterior fossa-based approaches—such as the retrosigmoid approach—challenging as well. Here, we present the cases of two patients diagnosed with epidermoid cysts in MC who underwent surgical resection via an endoscopic endonasal transpterygoid approach. Near-total resection was achieved in both cases, with only mild transient neurologic disturbances postoperatively. Radiographically, no evidence of residual disease was noted in either patient. We further review the nuances of an extended endoscopic endonasal approach to these lesions.

1. Introduction

Epidermoids are cystic lesions that are generally considered to be benign lesions that occupy the CSF space. On magnetic resonance imaging (MRI), they characteristically appear hypointense on T1-weighted and hyperintense on T2-weighted sequences [1, 2]. Notably, these lesions restrict diffusion of water and thus appear hyperintense on diffuse-weighted imaging. Advocated treatment of epidermoids of MC depends on the extent of symptom profile [3]. Open surgical approaches, including extradural exposure via a pterional or temporal craniotomy (with or without a petrosectomy), require significant retraction and place at risk a number of critical neurovascular structures [4]. Posterior fossa approaches, such as the retrosigmoid corridor, are challenging given the anterior extent of MC within the middle fossa and the resultant long working corridor. Novel extension of the endoscopic endonasal approach to the middle cranial fossa carries significant promise to reach these and other lesions within MC with minimal brain retraction [5, 6]. Here, we describe the successful use of the endoscopic endonasal approach to treat two patients with epidermoid cysts in MC.

2. Case Presentations

2.1. Case 1. A 64-year-old woman was sent to our clinic for evaluation of a 2-year history of right-sided facial numbness. Her symptoms involved all divisions of the trigeminal nerve. She had initially presented to our institution 12 years prior with an MRI of the brain revealing both a large right cerebellopontine angle mass, suggestive of a vestibular schwannoma, as well as a right middle cranial fossa lesion radiographically consistent with an epidermoid cyst. She underwent resection of the vestibular schwannoma at our institution and remained asymptomatic during several years of clinical follow-up. Ten years following resection of the vestibular schwannoma, she began to experience progressive right-sided facial numbness, which persisted for two years. MRI of the brain at this time revealed mild radiographic progression of her known right-sided MC lesion, measuring 2.1 × 1.3 cm in greatest dimensions (Figure 1). Given the lesion growth and the progressive neurologic deficit, surgical intervention was considered and discussed with the patient. She underwent an endoscopic endonasal right transpterygoid approach to the cyst. CN VI was thought to be displaced medially and superiorly by the lesion and was not encountered. Successful evacuation of the cyst contents was achieved with histopathologic confirmation of an epidermoid. A CSF leak was encountered and closed in layers with a collagen-based duraplasty graft followed by a free mucosal graft. The patient's postoperative course was notable for intermittent pain in the right V2 distribution that gradually resolved over a period of several weeks. She was seen in the clinic after six weeks with continued improvement in her symptoms and remains stable from a clinical and imaging standpoint after one year.

2.2. Case 2. A 26-year-old woman with a history of congenital bilateral sensorineural hearing loss was found to have a large right-sided cerebellopontine angle mass extending anteriorly to the middle cranial fossa into the region of MC. The patient had previously undergone a right temporal and petrosal craniotomy for resection of this mass; histopathological analysis at that time demonstrated an epidermoid lesion. Given technical difficulties in resecting the anterior most aspect of the epidermoid via an open craniotomy, an endoscopic endonasal right transpterygoid approach to the remaining epidermoid cyst in MC was undertaken (Figures 2–4). CN VI was visualized directly over the cyst capsule requiring evacuation of cyst contents through windows both superomedial and inferolateral to it (Figures 5–7). Intermittent EMG activity was noted during the procedure, and the nerve stimulated normally at the end of the surgery. Visualization of the resection cavity within MC following the resection revealed the temporal lobe superolaterally and the lateral wall of the cavernous sinus medially (Figure 8). The defect was reconstructed in layers with a collagen-based duraplasty graft followed by a nasoseptal flap from the contralateral nasal cavity. Her postoperative course was notable for a transient partial abducens palsy that had resolved upon six-week follow-up. She remains stable from a clinical and imaging standpoint after one year.

2.3. Technical Note. The endoscopic endonasal transpterygoid approach has been well described previously and is beyond the scope of this paper [7]. Both patients underwent a standard right transpterygoid approach with neuromonitoring of somatosensory evoked potentials (SSEPs), electroencephalogram (EEG), and electromyography (EMG) of the masseter and lateral rectus muscle for trigeminal and abducens nerve monitoring, respectively.

3. Discussion

MC is a dural recess in the posteromedial portion of the middle cranial fossa. Lesions in this region are uncommon overall and can be varied in their etiologies [8]. Space-occupying lesions in this CSF-containing subarachnoid space can present with a variety of signs and symptoms, related to neurovascular structures within the cave and adjacent to it. Namely, compression of the gasserian ganglion or any of the trigeminal nerve branches in this region can readily lead to trigeminal distribution pain, numbness, or diminished sensation [9–11]. Additionally, extension of the compressive lesions beyond MC can cause compression of other cranial nerves, causing, among others, facial nerve palsy and oculomotor nerve palsy.

The PubMed electronic database was searched from inception until December 2019 for English language studies using the search terms "Meckel's" and "epidermoid." A total of 25 peer-reviewed articles were identified, reviewed, and included in our analysis. No articles were excluded. Only one of these 25 articles describes one patient with an epidermoid in a series of 8 patients with Meckel's cave tumors undergoing the endoscopic endonasal approach, substantiating the limited literature available on this topic [12]. Epidermoid cysts in MC are exceedingly rare and to our knowledge have only been described by a handful of case reports, with symptom profiles ranging from completely asymptomatic to severe compression causing trigeminal neuralgia [8, 13–15]. Indeed, in one of the largest series to date evaluating outcomes following surgical excision of MC tumors, out of twelve patients, only one epidermoid cyst was diagnosed [16]. The most common intrinsic lesions known to occur in MC are trigeminal schwannomas and meningiomas, among others [2, 6, 16]. Intracranial epidermoid cysts, on the other hand, are generally located extra-axially, with a predilection for the cerebellopontine angle and suprasellar regions, though intraparenchymal epidermoid cysts have also been described [13, 16].

The most commonly used surgical approach to MC has been the pterional approach, providing anterolateral access to MC but concomitantly associated with risk of damage to traversing neurovascular structures along a narrow operative corridor bounded by the internal carotid artery, the petrous apex, geniculate ganglion, and trigeminal nerve branches, amongst others [17, 18]. Furthermore, adequate exposure of MC may be limited with certain subtemporal/petrosal approaches, notwithstanding the need for temporal lobe retraction [19]. Other frequently used surgical approaches include the retrosigmoid approach. Safain et al. reported use of an endoscopic-assisted retrosigmoid approach to an epidermoid cyst at the cerebellopontine angle with extension into MC [20]. Although this technique is commonly used on tumors found at the cerebellopontine angle and allows proper exposure to the space, it should be noted that long working corridor to MC through the retrosigmoid approach adds to the risk of neurovascular injury [21].

The endoscopic endonasal approach to the cranial base has undergone a tremendous transformation over the past few decades, heralded by the advent of newer more sophisticated tools and instruments to allow access to the region. Careful consideration of anatomic corridors along with appropriate patient selection continues to allow surgeons to expand the use of the endoscope in addressing more complex regions in the anterior cranial fossa [22, 23]. The

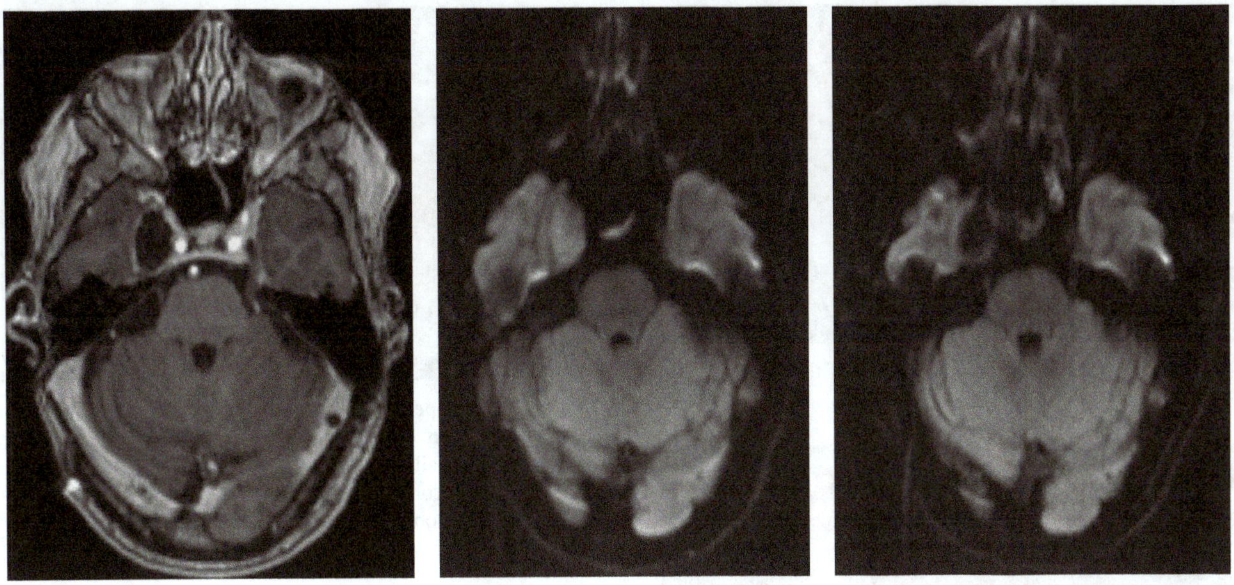

(a) (b) (c)

FIGURE 1: Imaging of patient 1. (a) Preoperative contrast-enhanced axial T1 MRI showing peripheral enhancement of the cyst wall. (b) Diffusion restriction noted in the lesion preoperatively. (c) Postoperative resolution of diffusion restriction within the lesion.

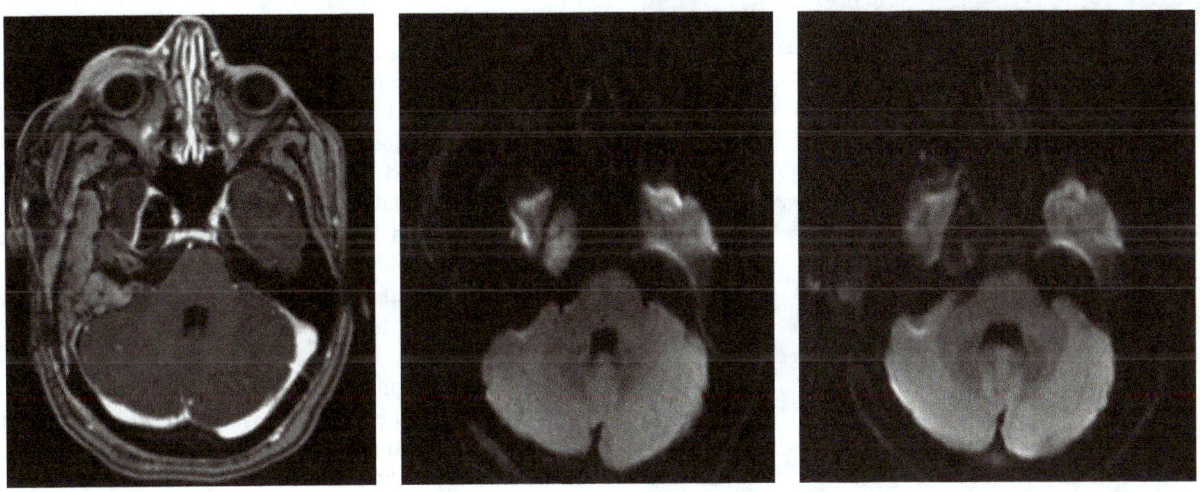

(a) (b) (c)

FIGURE 2: Imaging of patient 2. (a) Preoperative contrast-enhanced axial T1 MRI, showing peripheral enhancement of the cyst wall. (b) Diffusion restriction noted in the lesion preoperatively. (c) Postoperative resolution of diffusion restriction within the lesion.

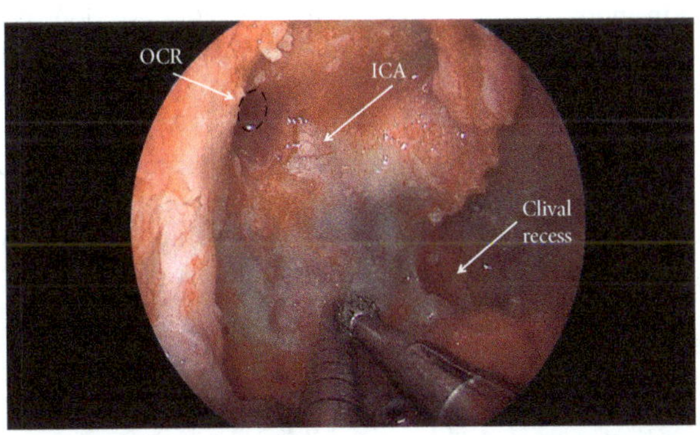

FIGURE 3: Intraoperative photo demonstrating drilling of the skull base through the endoscopic endonasal transpterygoid corridor.

lateral location of MC provides technical challenges to the endoscopic approach, given the difficult working trajectory as opposed to the straight endoscopic trajectory of approaches to the sellar region. Additional working corridors, such as the transmaxillary corridor via Caldwell-Luc, can be considered for access to more lateral structures [24].

An endoscopic endonasal approach, importantly, provides an anteromedial corridor to the trigeminal ganglion with reduced need for trigeminal nerve manipulation required to maximize operative views (Figure 9). Several expanded variations of the endoscopic endonasal approach to MC have been described with varying success, including the transpterygoid and transmaxillary approaches [12]. Particularly for trigeminal schwannomas in MC, the endoscopic

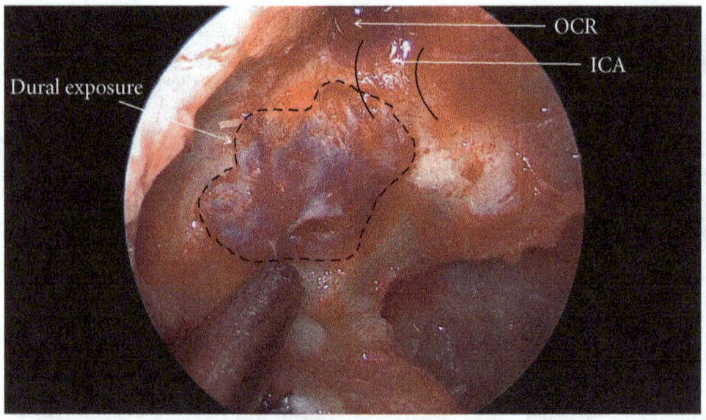

FIGURE 4: Exposure and opening of the dura.

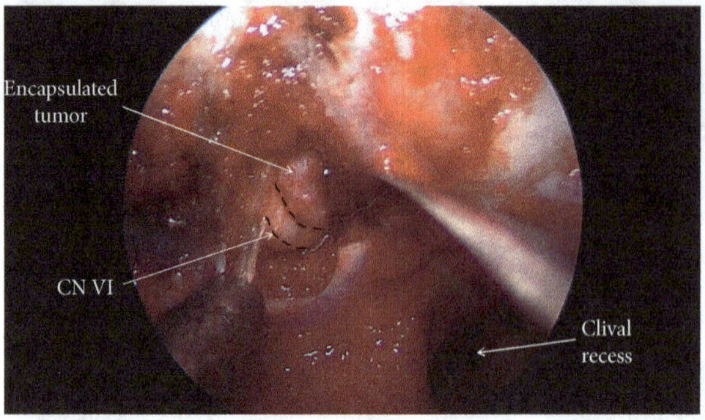

FIGURE 5: Visualization of the encapsulated epidermoid in a corridor superomedial to the abducens nerve.

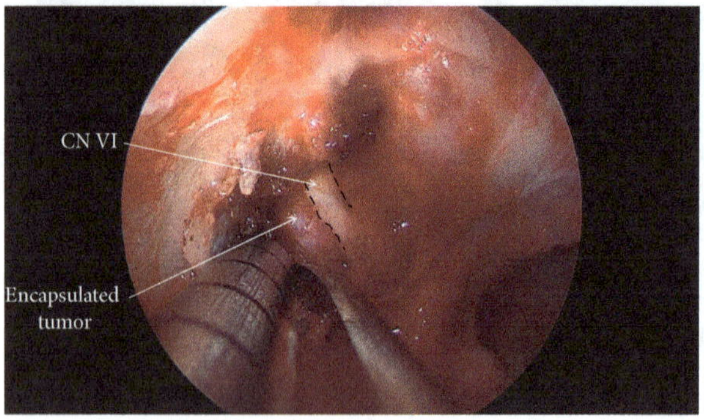

FIGURE 6: Visualization of the encapsulated epidermoid in a corridor inferolateral to the abducens nerve.

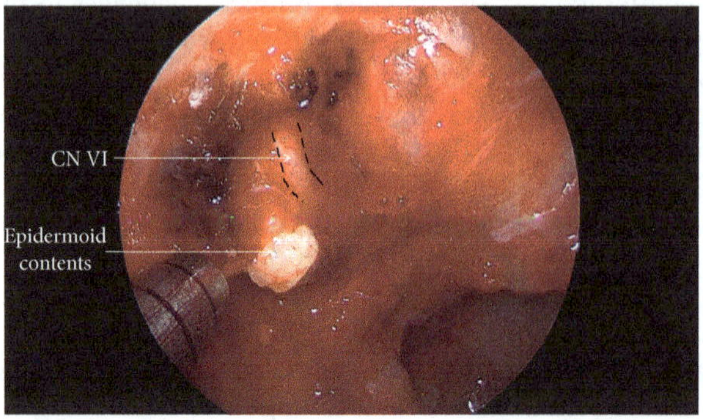

FIGURE 7: Visualization of the typical epidermoid contents following capsular opening inferolateral to the abducens nerve.

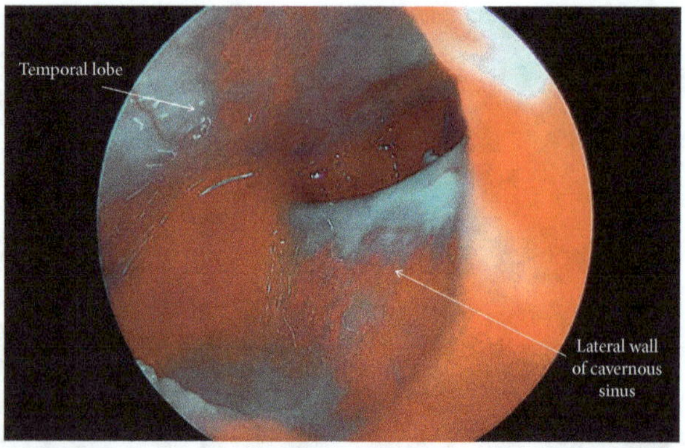

FIGURE 8: Intraoperative photo of Meckel's cave following epidermoid resection. The endoscope was advanced into the dural opening for visualization of Meckel's cave. The medial wall of Meckel's cave is contiguous with the lateral wall of the cavernous sinus. Temporal lobe is noted superolaterally.

endonasal transpterygoid approach has shown promising ability to achieve complete resection with minimal morbidity [25]. Alternatively, a transmaxillary route provides a safe working angle in conjunction with the transphenoidal route [23]. The feasibility of this transmaxillary approach to MC has moreover been substantiated in cadaveric specimens. Notably, as the endonasal approach is laterally extended, the contents of the infratemporal fossa begin to encroach on the operative corridor, making visualization and instrumentation more difficult [12, 26].

As epidermoid cysts are exceedingly rare intracranial lesions, documentation of successful operation on them in Meckel's cave via an endoscopic endonasal approach is limited. Endoscopic-assisted techniques have been shown to be useful in the visualization of epidermoid tumors in several studies [27, 28]. In addition, the endoscopic endonasal corridor has been utilized to resect epidermoid cysts from other locations along the cranial base [29–32]. However, to our knowledge, there have only been two reports of this approach for the successful resection of an epidermoid cyst in MC by a purely endoscopic endonasal approach, each describing just one adult patient [12, 33]. According to Best et al., this minimally invasive approach for removal of a cyst in the middle cranial fossa (that involved Meckel's cave) may also have potentially easier surveillance of future epidermoid recurrence [33].

In both of our cases, near-complete resection was achieved based on intraoperative impression and neuronavigational confirmation. Minor residual epidermoid remained in both cases, but postoperative MRI completed within 48 hours of surgery revealed no appreciable residual. Both patients were discharged from the hospital on postoperative day three without any major complications. Minor, transient neurologic deficits/symptoms relating to CN V (V2 pain) and VI (mild abducens palsy) were noted in patients 1 and 2, respectively. Transient V or VI deficits have commonly been described following resection of MC tumors through craniotomy approaches [8], likely due to trigeminal and abducens nerve manipulation, respectively, during the resection. These symptoms were resolved at six-week follow-

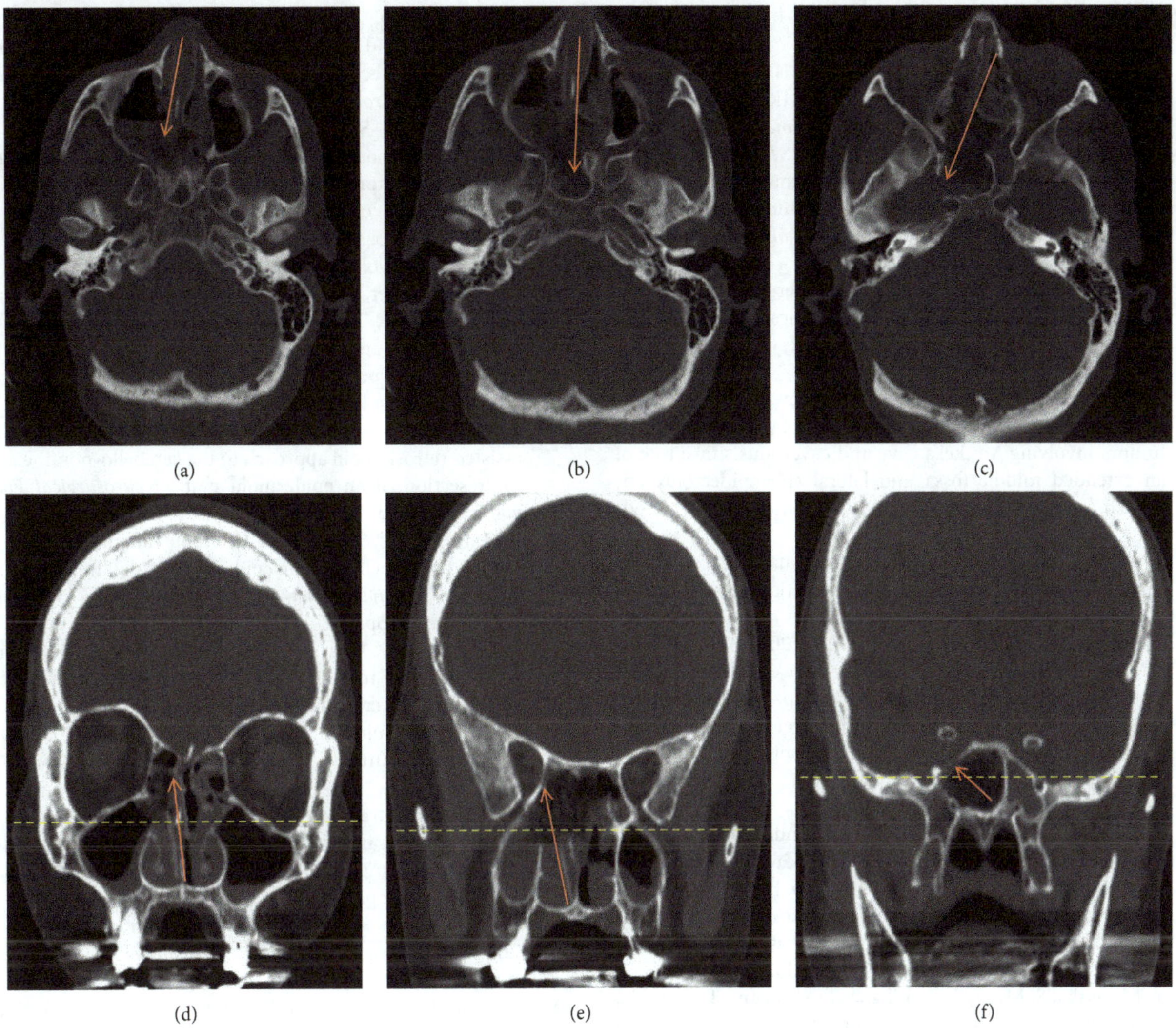

FIGURE 9: CT maxillofacial with sequential cuts to demonstrate the overall trajectory of an endoscopic endonasal right transpterygoid approach. (a–c) Axial views of the anterior skull base. (d–f) Coronal views of the same region. Red arrows estimate the working trajectory. Note the bony opening in the anteromedial aspect of the middle cranial fossa to expose the contents of MC in axial (c) and coronal views (f). This corresponds to the intraoperative view in Figure 4 with the internal carotid artery located superior and medial to the bony opening.

up in both patients, and one-year follow-up reveals continued clinical and radiographic stability. Our plan for the immediate future is to continue to follow these patients with annual MR imaging and clinical examination to evaluate for recurrence.

While only limited to two cases, our results suggest that the endoscopic endonasal approach to MC utilizing a transpterygoid approach may represent a safe alternative to open surgical approaches for epidermoid cysts at this region. Particularly, in our second case, an open craniotomy approach would have likely been associated with a lower rate of resection, given the marked anterior extension of the epidermoid and narrow working corridor. Given the proximity of the cranial nerve III through VI and the carotid artery, there is still potential for neurovascular injury with the endonasal approach. Utilization of image guidance to confirm intraoperative findings, the usage of neurophysiological monitoring to provide real-time feedback, judicious use of intraoperative ultrasound, and careful review of the preoperative imaging can help minimize such injuries. Additionally, such cases should only be considered and performed by multidisciplinary teams of neurosurgeons and otolaryngologists that are very experienced with endoscopic endonasal skull base surgery.

4. Conclusion

The endoscopic endonasal approach can be utilized for the safe and effective resection of MC epidermoid cysts. Intraoperative neurophysiological monitoring is very helpful in these particular cases. These approaches should only be considered by experienced, multidisciplinary teams following careful review of preoperative imaging. Additional follow-up and studies will be needed to determine long-term outcomes.

References

[1] D. F. Kallmes, J. M. Provenzale, H. J. Cloft, and R. E. McClendon, "Typical and atypical MR imaging features of intracranial epidermoid tumors," *American Journal of Roentgenology*, vol. 169, no. 3, pp. 883–887, 1997.

[2] W. Yuh, D. Wright, T. Barloon, D. Schultz, Y. Sato, and C. Cervantes, "MR imaging of primary tumors of trigeminal nerve and Meckel's cave," *American Journal of Roentgenology*, vol. 151, no. 3, pp. 577–582, 1988.

[3] F. Zhou, Z. Yang, W. Zhu et al., "Epidermoid cysts of the cavernous sinus: clinical features, surgical outcomes, and literature review," *Journal of Neurosurgery*, vol. 129, no. 4, pp. 973–983, 2018.

[4] D. Q. Sun, A. H. Menezes, M. A. Howard, B. J. Gantz, D. M. Hasan, and M. R. Hansen, "Surgical management of tumors involving Meckel's cave and cavernous sinus: role of an extended middle fossa and lateral sphenoidectomy approach," *Otology & Neurotology*, vol. 39, no. 1, pp. 82–91, 2017.

[5] J. M. González-Darder, V. Quilis-Quesada, and L. Botella-Maciá, "Abordaje pterional transcigomático. Parte 2: experiencia quirúrgica en la patología de base de cráneo," *Neurocirugía*, vol. 23, no. 3, pp. 96–103, 2012.

[6] J. Muto, T. Kawase, and K. Yoshida, "Meckel's cave tumors," *Operative Neurosurgery*, vol. 67, no. 3, pp. 291–299, 2010.

[7] R. F. Schmidt, O. J. Choudhry, J. Raviv et al., "Surgical nuances for the endoscopic endonasal transpterygoid approach to lateral sphenoid sinus encephaloceles," *Neurosurgical Focus*, vol. 32, no. 6, p. E5, 2012.

[8] T. Nadkarni, K. Dindorkar, D. Muzumdar, and A. Goel, "Epidermoid tumor within Meckel's cave: case report," *Neurologia Medico-Chirurgica*, vol. 40, no. 1, pp. 74–76, 2000.

[9] S. Furtado and A. Hegde, "Trigeminal neuralgia due to a small Meckel's cave epidermoid tumor: surgery using an extradural corridor," *Skull Base*, vol. 19, no. 5, pp. 353–357, 2009.

[10] Y. Miyasaka, S. Morii, S. Tachibana, T. Saito, and T. Ohwada, "Paratrigeminal epidermoid originated in the Meckel's cave (author's transl)," *No Shinkei Geka*, vol. 4, no. 5, pp. 483–488, 1976.

[11] K. Grahnke, D. Burkett, D. Li, C. Szujewski, J. Leonetti, and D. Anderson, "Cranial nerve preservation following surgical treatment for epidermoid cysts of the posterior and middle fossae," *Journal of Neurological Surgery Part B: Skull Base*, vol. 79, no. 5, pp. 445–450, 2018.

[12] M. Zoli, S. Ratti, F. Guaraldi et al., "Endoscopic endonasal approach to primitive Meckel's cave tumors: a clinical series," *Acta Neurochirurgica*, vol. 160, no. 12, pp. 2349–2361, 2018.

[13] P. Podeur, I. Okhremchuk, J. B. Morvan et al., "Multiple intracranial epidermoid cysts: case report," *Revue de Laryngologie—Otologie—Rhinologie*, vol. 136, no. 4, pp. 159–162, 2015.

[14] A. Arai, T. Sasayama, J. Koyama, A. Fujita, K. Hosoda, and E. Kohmura, "Epidermoid cyst in Meckel's cave with unusual computed tomography and magnetic resonance imaging findings," *Neurologia Medico-Chirurgica*, vol. 50, no. 8, pp. 701–704, 2010.

[15] H. Ohta, M. Ottomo, T. Nakamura, and A. Yokota, "A case of epidermoid tumor inside the Meckel's cave," *No Shinkei Geka*, vol. 25, no. 10, pp. 943–947, 1997.

[16] D. W. Beck and A. H. Menezes, "Lesions in Meckel's cave: variable presentation and pathology," *Journal of Neurosurgery*, vol. 67, no. 5, pp. 684–689, 1987.

[17] A. Nanda, D. Patra, A. Savardekar, N. Mohammed, V. Narayan, and S. Bir, "Surgery of tuberculum sellae meningioma: a technical purview on pterional approach," *Journal of Neurological Surgery Part B: Skull Base*, vol. 79, no. 3, pp. S265–S266, 2018.

[18] A. Tayebi Meybodi, A. Benet, R. Rodriguez Rubio, S. Yousef, and M. T. Lawton, "Comprehensive anatomic assessment of the pterional, orbitopterional, and orbitozygomatic approaches for basilar apex aneurysm clipping," *Operative Neurosurgery*, vol. 15, no. 5, pp. 538–550, 2018.

[19] C. P. Hofstetter, A. Singh, V. K. Anand, A. Kacker, and T. H. Schwartz, "The endoscopic, endonasal, transmaxillary transpterygoid approach to the pterygopalatine fossa, infratemporal fossa, petrous apex, and the meckel cave," *Journal of Neurosurgery*, vol. 113, no. 5, pp. 967–974, 2010.

[20] M. G. Safain, W. C. Dent, and C. B. Heilman, "An endoscopic assisted retrosigmoid approach to the cerebello-pontine angle for resection of an epidermoid cyst," *Neurosurgical Focus*, vol. 36, no. 1, p. 1, 2014.

[21] A. Farhoud, W. Khedr, and H. Aboul-Enein, "Surgical resection of cerebellopontine epidermoid cysts: limitations and outcome," *Journal of Neurological Surgery Part B: Skull Base*, vol. 79, no. 2, pp. 167–172, 2017.

[22] H. Q. Truong, X. Sun, E. Celtikci et al., "Endoscopic anterior transmaxillary "transalisphenoid" approach to Meckel's cave and the middle cranial fossa: an anatomical study and clinical application," *Journal of Neurosurgery*, vol. 130, no. 1, pp. 227–237, 2018.

[23] Y. Gu, Y. Yu, X. Zhang et al., "Endoscopic endonasal transmaxillary transpterygoid approach to Meckel cave: anatomical study and preliminary clinical results," *Journal of Neurological Surgery Part A: Central European Neurosurgery*, vol. 76, no. 3, pp. 205–210, 2015.

[24] M. Loyo-Varela, R. Del Valle Robles, T. Herrada, and J. Barges Coll, "Endoscopic endonasal transmaxillary approach," *World Neurosurgery*, vol. 80, no. 5, pp. 502–504, 2013.

[25] L. Yang, L. Hu, W. Zhao, H. Zhang, Q. Liu, and D. Wang, "Endoscopic endonasal approach for trigeminal schwannomas: our experience of 39 patients in 10 years," *European Archives of Oto-Rhino-Laryngology*, vol. 275, no. 3, pp. 735–741, 2018.

[26] N. Komune, S. Komune, K. Matsushima, and A. L. Rhoton, "Comparison of lateral microsurgical preauricular and anterior endoscopic approaches to the jugular foramen," *The Journal of Laryngology & Otology*, vol. 129, no. 2, pp. S12–S20, 2015.

[27] A. Tuchman, A. Platt, J. Winer, M. Pham, S. Giannotta, and G. Zada, "Endoscopic-assisted resection of intracranial epidermoid tumors," *World Neurosurgery*, vol. 82, no. 3-4, pp. 450–454, 2014.

[28] J. Krass, Y. Hahn, K. Karami et al., "Endoscopic assisted resection of prepontine epidermoid cysts," *Journal of Neurological Surgery Part A: Central European Neurosurgery*, vol. 75, no. 2, pp. 120–125, 2014.

[29] E. D. McCoul, S. Chow, D. L. Y. Lee, V. K. Anand, and T. H. Schwartz, "Endoscopic endonasal approach for resection of ventral skull base keratinaceous cysts," *International Forum of Allergy & Rhinology*, vol. 2, no. 3, pp. 258–263, 2012.

[30] R. K. Chandra and J. N. Palmer, "Epidermoids of the paranasal sinuses and beyond: endoscopic management," *American Journal of Rhinology*, vol. 20, no. 4, pp. 441–444, 2006.

[31] F. Esposito, D. P. Becker, J. P. Villablanca, and D. F. Kelly, "Endonasal transsphenoidal transclival removal of prepontine epidermoid tumors: technical note," *Operative Neurosurgery*, vol. 56, no. 4, pp. 1–443, 2005.
[32] S. Chivukula, M. Koutourousiou, C. H. Snyderman, J. C. Fernandez-Miranda, P. A. Gardner, and E. C. Tyler-Kabara, "Endoscopic endonasal skull base surgery in the pediatric population," *Journal of Neurosurgery: Pediatrics*, vol. 11, no. 3, pp. 227–241, 2013.
[33] J. Best, J. S. Schneider, and J. H. Turner, "Endoscopic endonasal resection of a giant middle fossa epidermoid cyst," *Allergy & Rhinology*, vol. 6, no. 3, pp. 195–197, 2015.

35

Malignant Ischemic Stroke in a Young Female: A Rare Primary Manifestation of Takayasu Arteritis

Bhupendra Shah and Roshan Chhetri

Department of Internal Medicine, B.P. Koirala Institute of Health Sciences, Dharan, Nepal

Correspondence should be addressed to Bhupendra Shah; bhupendra.shah@bpkihs.edu

Academic Editor: Peter Berlit

Takayasu arteritis is a rare chronic progressive granulomatous necrotizing large vessel panvasculitis mainly involving aorta and its main branches. It commonly affects the female in second to third decades. Common clinical features of Takayasu arteritis are hypertension, claudication, dizziness, headache, or fever. Takayasu arteritis is diagnosed with clinical history of claudication, absent pulse, discordant blood pressure, bruit over aorta, and typical angiographic findings. Stroke as a primary manifestation of Takayasu arteritis is rarely reported in the medical literatures. We are reporting a 16-year-old female who had malignant ischemic stroke as a first manifestation of Takayasu arteritis.

1. Introduction

Takayasu arteritis, named after Japanese professor of Ophthalmology Mikito Takayasu [1], is a chronic progressive large vessel necrotizing granulomatous panvasculitis mainly involving aorta and its main branches [2]. It commonly affects the female of second to third decade. Mwipatayi et al. reported that the common clinical features of Takayasu arteritis were hypertension, cardiac failure, deranged renal function, cerebrovascular diseases, claudication, or gangrene [3]. Of neurological manifestations, dizziness, visual disturbances, headache, seizure, or ischemic stroke are common manifestations [4]. Hwang J et al. reported that the prevalence of stroke among patient with Takayasu arteritis was 11.1% [5]. However, stroke as a primary manifestation of Takayasu arteritis is a rare event. Hence, we report a case of 16-year-old girl who had malignant left hemispheric ischemic stroke as a first manifestation of Takayasu arteritis.

2. Case Reports

A 16-year-old girl presented to emergency room with complaints of weakness of right upper limb and lower limb for an 18-hour duration. She also had facial deviation towards left side. She had inability to produce and comprehend the speech. There was no history of fever, head trauma, and seizure. She had no significant past medical history and family history. She was nonsmoker and never consumed alcohol. At emergency room, her Glasgow coma scale score (GCS) was 11/15(E4V1M6). Her blood pressure was 110/80 mmHg, pulse rate 80 beat per minute in left radial artery and absent pulse in right brachial and radial artery, respiratory rate -16 cycle per minute, temperature -98°F. Central nervous system examination revealed right sided hemiplegia, global aphasia, and upper motor neuron type facial nerve paralysis. Other central nervous examination and systematic examination findings were normal. The baseline investigation reports were illustrated in Table 1. Computed tomography of head showed hypodensity at left frontotemporoparietal region along with middle cerebral artery dot sign (Figure 1). Patient was admitted with provisional diagnosis of ischemic malignant lobar stroke with modified ranking scale of 5/6. Ultrasonography Doppler revealed thickening of right common carotid, right internal carotid, right external carotid, and right subclavian artery with significant lumen obstruction. Computed tomographic aortogram revealed circumferential thickening of arch of aorta, brachiocephalic trunk, and right common carotid (Figure 2). Electrocardiogram, Chest

TABLE 1: Baseline laboratory reports of the patient.

Laboratory parameters	Values	Normal range
Haemoglobin	9.5 gm/dl	11-16 gm/dl
Total leucocyte count	14300	4000-11000 cell/mm3
Platelet count	430000 cell/mm3	150000-400000 cell/mm3
Glucose	122 mg/dl	<140 mg/dl
Urea	11 mg/dl	10-50 mg/dl
Creatine	0.2	0.5-1.4 mg/dl
Sodium	138 mmol/L	136-145 mmol/L
Potassium	4.4 mmol/l	3.5-5 mmol/l
ANA	5.68 U/ml	<10.00 IU/ml
Anti ds DNA	0.24	<0.9 IU/ml

Abbreviations. ANA-antinuclear antibody, Anti ds DNA: anti-double stranded deoxyribonucleic acid.

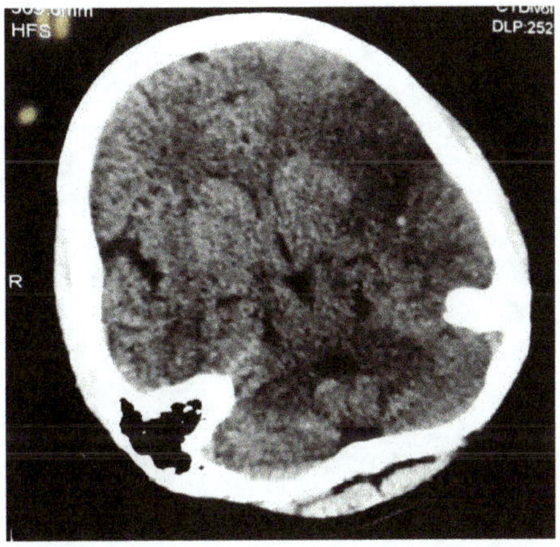

FIGURE 1: Computed tomography of head showed hypodensity at left frontotemporoparietal region along with middle cerebral artery dot sign.

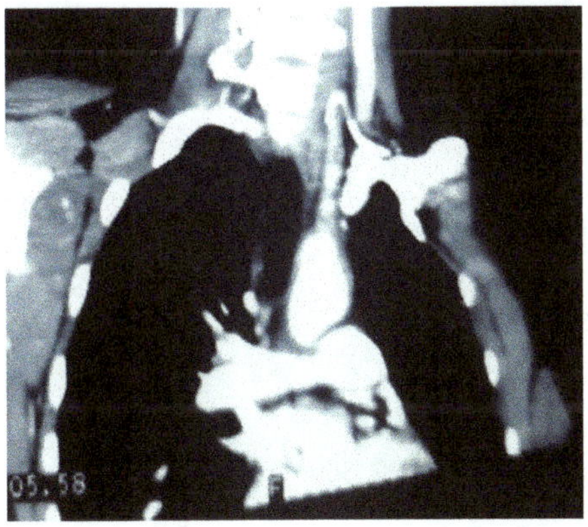

FIGURE 2: Computed tomographic aortogram revealed circumferential thickening of arch of aorta, brachiocephalic trunk, and right common carotid.

X-RAY, Ultrasound abdomen and Echocardiography was normal. We made final diagnoses of malignant ischemic stroke secondary to Takayasu arteritis. She was treated with tablet aspirin 75 mg once daily, tab, and prednisolone 40 mg once daily. Physiotherapy was initiated on second day of admission. She was discharged from hospital on tenth day of admission on prednisolone and aspirin. At the time of discharge her stroke disability modified ranking scale was 3/5.

TABLE 2: American Rheumatology Criteria for diagnosing Takayasu arteritis.

1.	Age at disease onset ≤40 years
2.	Claudication of extremities
3.	Decreased arterial pulse
4.	Blood pressure difference >10 mmHg
5.	Bruits over subclavian or aorta
6.	Arteriogram abnormality

To diagnose the Takayasu arteritis patient should fulfill at least 3 criteria. Our patient had fulfilled criteria 1, 3, 4, 5, and 6.

3. Discussion

We report a case of 16-year-old girl who had left hemispheric ischemic stroke. She had absent pulse in the right brachial artery, discordant blood pressure in two arms, and aortogram abnormality; hence we diagnose her as a case of Takayasu arteritis presenting as ischemic stroke based on American Rheumatology Criteria as illustrated in the Table 2 [6].

Our patient had ischemic stroke as a first presentation of the Takayasu arteritis. Similar case report of ischemic stroke in a patient with Takayasu arteritis was done by Gao S et al. from China [7] and Silver M et al. [8] while Hwang J et al. reported that the most common form of stroke in Takayasu arteritis was large lobar [5] stroke similar to our case. Most of the published literatures showed that stroke can occur as one of multiple manifestations of the Takayasu arteritis; however, the stroke as sole and primary presentation of Takayasu arteritis is rarely reported in the medical literatures; hence, the malignant ischemic stroke in our patient was a rare manifestation of Takayasu arteritis. Despite hypertension, traditional risk factor of stroke is reported in up to 77% in a patient with Takayasu arteritis as by Mwipatayi BP et al. [3] our patient had normal blood pressure. The other risk factors of stroke were absent in our case.

Our patient had new onset of stroke, decreased pulse volume in brachial artery, and elevated ESR and CRP which suggest the active form of Takayasu arteries as reported by the Direskeneli H et al. [9]. Kesar G et al. in their systematic review on management of Takayasu arteritis reported that corticosteroids and immunosuppressive like methotrexate, cyclophosphamide, azathioprine, and leflunomide are commonly prescribed medication for active Takayasu arteritis [10]. Ito I reported that the corticosteroids alone were effective in 20 to 75% patient with active Takayasu arteritis [11]. Hence, we managed our patient with Takayasu arteritis with malignant ischemic stroke with prednisolone and aspirin. This case report highlights the significance of measuring pulse volume and blood pressure in two arms in a young patient with ischemic stroke which may lead to suspicion of Takayasu arteritis. Diagnosing the Takayasu arteritis and treating it with immunosuppressive might differ in the outcome of the patient.

Acknowledgments

The authors acknowledge Dr. Mukesh Sah, the Head of the Department of Radiology, for reporting the aortogram, Dr. Achyut bhakta acharya for English language editing, and Professor Sanjib Sharma, the Head of the Department of Internal Medicine for constantly motivating them to write the case report.

References

[1] C. Terao, "History of Takayasu arteritis and Dr. Mikito Takayasu," *International Journal of Rheumatic Diseases*, vol. 17, no. 8, pp. 931–935, 2014.

[2] J. B. Wolfe, "Report of the committee on nomenclature of the american society for the study of arterio-sclerosis," *Circulation*, vol. 12, p. 1065, 1955.

[3] B. P. Mwipatayi, P. C. Jeffery, S. J. Beningfield et al., "Takayasu arteritis: Clinical features and management: Report of 272 cases," *ANZ Journal of Surgery*, vol. 75, no. 3, pp. 110–117, 2005.

[4] L.-X. Zhou, J. Ni, S. Gao, B. Peng, and L.-Y. Cui, "Neurological manifestations of Takayasu arteritis," *Chinese Medical Sciences Journal*, vol. 26, no. 4, pp. 227–230, 2011.

[5] J. Hwang, S. J. Kim, O. Y. Bang et al., "Ischemic stroke in takayasu's arteritis: lesion patterns and possible mechanisms," *Journal of Clinical Neurology*, vol. 8, no. 2, pp. 109–115, 2012.

[6] W. P. Arend, B. A. Michel, D. A. Bloch et al., "The american college of rheumatology 1990 criteria for the classification of takayasu arteritis," *Arthritis & Rheumatology*, vol. 33, no. 8, pp. 1129–1134, 1990.

[7] S. Gao and R. Wang, "Takayasu arteritis presenting with massive cerebral ischemic infarction in a 35-year-old woman: a case report," *Journal of Medical Case Reports*, vol. 7, pp. 1–5, 2013.

[8] M. Silver, "Takayasu's arteritis - an unusual cause of stroke in a young patient," *Western Journal of Emergency Medicine*, vol. 13, no. 6, pp. 484–487, 2012.

[9] H. Direskeneli, S. Z. Aydin, and P. A. Merkel, "Assessment of disease activity and progression in Takayasu's arteritis," *Magn Reson Imaging*, vol. 31, pp. 477–479, 2013.

[10] G. Keser, H. Direskeneli, and K. Aksu, "Management of Takayasu arteritis: a systematic review," *Rheumatology*, vol. 53, no. 5, Article ID ket320, pp. 793–801, 2014.

[11] I. Ito, "Medical treatment of Takayasu's arteritis," *Heart and Vessels*, vol. 7, pp. 133–137, 1992.

36

Neurosarcoidosis Presentation as Adipsic Diabetes Insipidus Secondary to a Pituitary Stalk Lesion and Association with Anti-NMDA Receptor Antibodies

Jose Gabriel Solis,[1] Arturo Olascoaga Lugo,[1] Marco Antonio Rodríguez Florido,[2] Bayron Alexander Sandoval Bonilla,[3] and Jose Malagón Rangel[1]

[1]*Department of Internal Medicine, Hospital de Especialidades "Dr. Bernardo Sepúlveda Gutiérrez", Centro Médico Nacional Siglo XXI, Instituto Mexicano del Seguro Social, Ciudad de México, Mexico*
[2]*Department of Pathology, Hospital de Pediatría Centro Médico Nacional Siglo XXI, Instituto Mexicano del Seguro Social, Ciudad de México, Mexico*
[3]*Department of Neurosurgery, Hospital de Especialidades "Dr. Bernardo Sepúlveda Gutiérrez", Centro Médico Nacional Siglo XXI, Instituto Mexicano del Seguro Social, Ciudad de México, Mexico*

Correspondence should be addressed to Jose Gabriel Solis; gabrielsolismd@gmail.com

Academic Editor: Majaz Moonis

Sarcoidosis is a multisystemic inflammatory disease of unknown cause. It is characterized by the presence of noncaseating granuloma on a biopsy specimen. Clinical presentation varies across case report series with myriad of symptoms ranging from fever, respiratory symptoms, and skin lesions, or atypical symptoms like heart block or neurological symptoms. Hence, we report the case of a 22-year-old woman with encephalitis, a pituitary mass, and adipsic diabetes insipidus. The diagnostic approach did not end on the biopsy of the lesion, which reported noncaseating granulomas; on the contrary, it was the beginning of a path to exclude other causes of the central nervous system granulomas that ended with the diagnosis of the isolated central nervous system sarcoidosis. Also, we report the first proven association between anti-NMDA receptor antibodies and sarcoidosis.

1. Introduction

Sarcoidosis is a multisystemic inflammatory disease of unknown cause, whose primary feature is the presence of noncaseating granulomas [1]. It has an incidence of less than 10 cases per 100,000 people, with a predilection to the ages of 20–40 years. There is evidence of lung involvement in 95% of the cases [2]; however, neurosarcoidosis is present only in 5–15% of the cases, of which in 50% is the initial manifestation. Isolated neurosarcoidosis is very rare, and up to a third of the patients will develop systemic features in the future [3].

We report the case of a patient who presented with adipsic diabetes insipidus secondary to a pituitary stalk lesion, with the final diagnosis of neurosarcoidosis. Also, the patient had neuropsychiatric symptoms and anti-NMDA antibodies detected in cerebrospinal fluid, an association that has never been reported.

2. Case Presentation

A 22-year-old woman, resident of Acapulco, Mexico, presented to our unit with a two-month clinical picture of headache, incoherent language, aggressive behavior, inappropriate conducts of disinhibition, and visual-auditory hallucinations. The previous day, the patient had gradually developed a diminished state of awareness. Her medical history was unremarkable. She had two uncomplicated previous pregnancies. Her mother denied any animal contact, recent traveling, ingestion of drugs, or exposure to toxics. She referred a lack of water and food intake in the previous days.

On physical examination, her blood pressure was normal, and she was tachycardic with a weak pulse, dry mucous membranes, and prolonged capillary refill time. In the neurological sphere, she was disoriented and presented retrograde amnesia, impairment in judgment, and loss of abstract thinking. Her chest X-ray and head computed tomography (CT) were normal. Laboratory results revealed severe hypernatremia (Na 180 mEq/L) and acute kidney injury (AKI) (measured creatinine 2 mg/dl–baseline creatinine 0.6 mg/dl). Serum electrolytes, liver tests, blood count, urinalysis, and toxicologic screen were normal. Her spot urinary electrolytes showed a urinary sodium of 20 mEq/L, with a fractional excretion of sodium (Fe_{Na}) of 0.5% suggesting hypovolemia. Her calculated water deficit was of 7.5 liters. However, her calculated electrolyte-free water excretion was of 805 ml within a 24-hour urinary volume of 1,000 ml, a value that was inappropriately elevated.

We initiated treatment with enteral administration of free water and hypotonic intravenous solutions for restitution of intravascular volume. During her hospital stay, the patient presented a partial clinical response, with optimization of volemia and resolution of (AKI). A new electrolyte profile showed persistence of hypernatremia (Na 157 mEq/L) and mild hypokalemia (K 3.2 mEq/L). She had a urinary sodium level of 8 mEq/L, with a calculated urine osmolarity of 85 mEq/L, in the context of a 24-hour urinary volume of 4 liters and electrolyte-free water excretion of 3.3 liters. The documented aqueous polyuria and hypernatremia suggested diabetes insipidus. The water deprivation test, that is normally the next step in the diagnosis, was contraindicated, so we ordered a brain magnetic resonance imaging (MRI), which showed a pituitary stalk lesion with chiasmatic and hypothalamic extension (Figure 1(a)).

Treatment with desmopressin was initiated, with progressive normalization of her sodium level, urinary volume, and volemia status (Table 1) (Figure 2). The hormonal profile was compatible with panhypopituitarism, so we initiated treatment with thyroid and glucocorticoid hormones. The cerebrospinal fluid (CSF) analysis showed an elevated protein level of 75 mg/dl, normal glucose, a cell count of zero, and negative Gram and India ink stains. An electroencephalogram documented diffuse cerebral dysfunction without the epileptiform activity. Her blood, urine, CSF, and bone marrow cultures were all negative. A CSF polymerase chain reaction (PCR) for the detection of viral agents and *Mycobacterium tuberculosis* was negative. The determination of anti-N-methyl-D-aspartate (NMDA) receptor antibodies in CSF was positive. Diverse imaging studies such as thoraco-abdominopelvic CT, endovaginal ultrasound, and whole-body scintigraphy showed no significant abnormalities.

Considering the characteristic clinical behavior of the patient, we decided to order a stereotactic biopsy of the pituitary mass. The pathology report revealed noncaseating granulomatous inflammation and gliosis (Figures 1(b)–1(d)). The periodic acid Schiff stain (PAS), Ziehl–Neelsen stain, and Grocott stain of the tissue were all negative. Immunohistochemical markers CD1a and langerin to rule out Langerhans cell histiocytosis were negative. Serological tests for Epstein–Barr, hepatitis B, hepatitis C, cytomegalovirus, toxoplasma, and *Brucella spp* were all negative. A PCR for the detection of *Rickettsia spp*, *Ehrlichia spp*, *Anaplasma spp*, and *Borrelia burgdorferi* were also negative. A nested PCR in biopsy tissue for the detection of *Mycobacterium tuberculosis* was also negative. The angiotensin converting enzyme serum level was in the normal range.

Based on the pathology findings and the 2018 consensus diagnostic criteria [4], we concluded the final diagnosis of isolated neurosarcoidosis. She received treatment with prednisone and showed significant improvement of the neuropsychiatric symptoms. The patient was discharged from our unit to continue ambulatory treatment; however, she was lost at the follow-up.

3. Discussion

Neurosarcoidosis can infiltrate practically any structure of the central nervous system. The most frequent manifestation is cranial neuropathy; however, aseptic meningitis, cauda equina syndrome, diffuse encephalopathy, focal neurological symptoms, hypothalamic and pituitary disfunction, intracranial hypertension, peripheral neuropathy, and vascular syndromes have all been described [5].

We report the case of a 22-year-old female patient with a pituitary granulomatous infiltrative lesion. This is the most frequent and characteristic form of the disease and is present in 15–25% of the cases. This can produce symptoms related to the mass effect or endocrine dysfunction [3, 6]. The patient had multiple endocrine manifestations of the disease, which are reported with the following frequencies: hypogonadotropic hypogonadism (38.5%), diabetes insipidus (37%), amenorrhea (29%, 58.7% of women), panhypopituitarism (23%), visual defects (22%), headache (7.7%), and psychoaffective changes (7.7%) [7]. Hyperprolactinemia has been considered as a predictor of hypothalamic involvement [8].

Polyuria-polydipsia syndrome in these patients is usually multifactorial and can be secondary to central diabetes insipidus, primary polydipsia, nephrogenic diabetes insipidus secondary to hypercalcemia, or less frequently dysfunction of the thirst control mechanism [9]. The latter is a very rare type of diabetes insipidus, in which there is a deficient or absent thirst response to hypernatremia and is associated with more morbidity and mortality. Descriptions of neurosarcoidosis as a cause of this variety of diabetes insipidus has been anecdotal [10]. Central diabetes insipidus in sarcoidosis has been described in case reports or series of cases [11, 12]; however, this as a form of presentation is extremely rare and has only been reported in a 10-year-old girl [13]. The only published follow-up study including patients with sarcoidosis and diabetes insipidus found a clinical profile very similar to that of our patient. Those patients started at ages between 18 and 33 years and had associated neurological symptoms and endocrine defects. Peculiarly, the polyuria in these patients did not respond to treatment with steroids [12].

The initial clinical features of our patient were associated with hypovolemia and severe hypernatremia. We can deduce

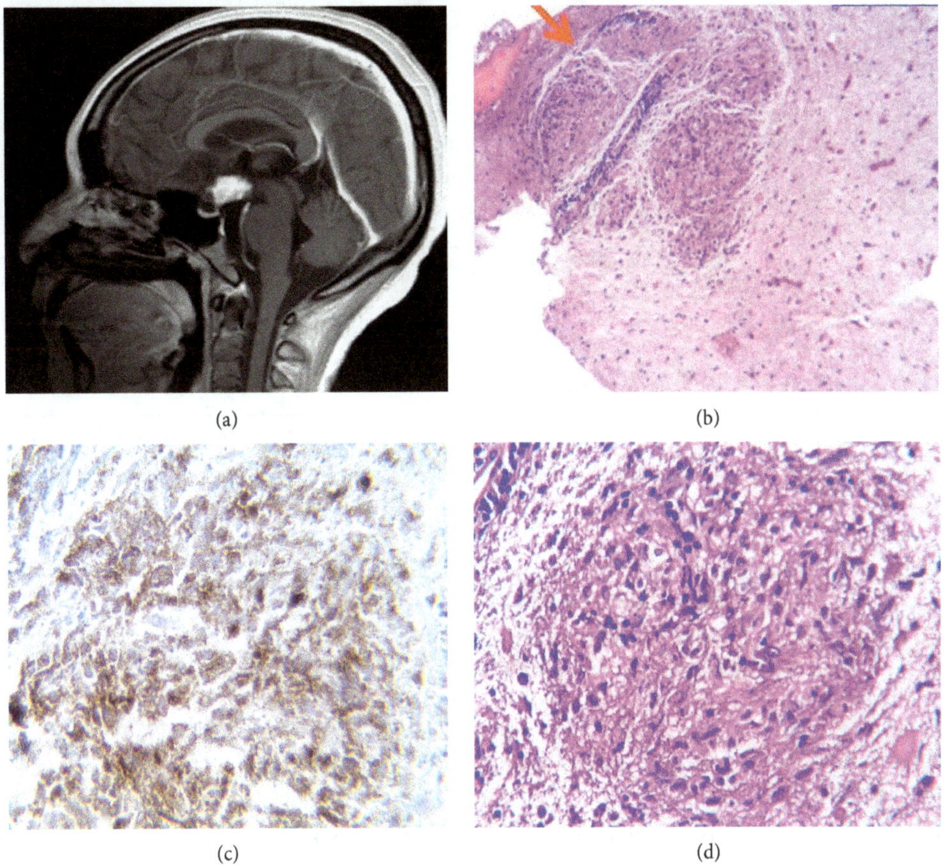

Figure 1: (a) MRI T1-weighted sequence showing a pituitary stalk lesion with marked reinforcement and chiasmatic and hypothalamic extension. (b) Perivascular granulomas HE 10x. (c) CD 68 positive in epithelioid cells. IHQ 40x. (d) Granuloma composed by epithelioid cells and reactive gliosis at the periphery. HE 40x. MRI, magnetic resonance imaging. IHQ, immunohistochemistry. HE, hematoxylin and eosin.

Table 1: Serum and urinary sodium levels, osmolarity, urinary volume, and calculated electrolyte-free water excretion during hospitalization. Desmopressin was administered from day 5 according to requirements.

	Day 1	Day 2	Day 3	Day 4	Day 5	Day 7	Day 9	Day 11	Day 13	Day 15	Day 17	Day 20	Day 23	Day 25
Serum Na (mEq/L)	180	170	165	163	157	164	156	151	147	152	149	139	142	135
Urinary Na (mEq/L)	20	17	5	9	8	33	17	113	50	170	127	29	65	188
Serum osm (mOsm/l)	366	345	336	331	326	337	317	307	299	308	306	284	272	276
Urinary osm (mOsm/l)	219	342	380	225	85	574	339	580	305	512	750	144	290	474
Urinary volume (lts)	1	1.25	2	3	4	1.85	2.5	1.8	1.5	1.9	2	2.8	2	1.5
EFWE (lts)	0.805	0.888	1.468	2.52	3.3	−0.56	1.21	−0.239	0.613	−0.42	−1	2	1.09	−1.16

Na, sodium; Osm, osmolarity; EFWE, electrolyte-free water excretion.

that these were masking the polyuria expected in diabetes insipidus and were exacerbated by the dysfunction of the thirst mechanism and neuropsychiatric manifestations. In the context of neurosarcoidosis, the diagnosis of diabetes insipidus can be hard because it can be masked by hypovolemia, adrenal insufficiency [14], or hypothyroidism [15], which are contraindications to perform a water deprivation test.

Pituitary stalk lesions have a broad differential diagnosis. Turcu et al. published a retrospective description of patients with pituitary stalk lesions conducted at the Mayo Clinic. In this study, neurosarcoidosis was the most common inflammatory etiology, and it was found in 11 of 92 patients [16]. The most frequent MRI finding was a thickened pituitary stalk [16]. Other possible findings include an intrasellar well-defined lesion with hyperintense behavior in the T1 sequence, which can have suprasellar extension, a cystic component, or leptomeningeal reinforcement, although the findings can be nonspecific [17]. In the CSF analysis, an elevated protein level is the most frequent finding present in 63% of the patients. An elevated angiotensin converting enzyme is relatively rare, only observed in 35% of the patients, which is the reason we did not consider its normal value relevant in our case [18].

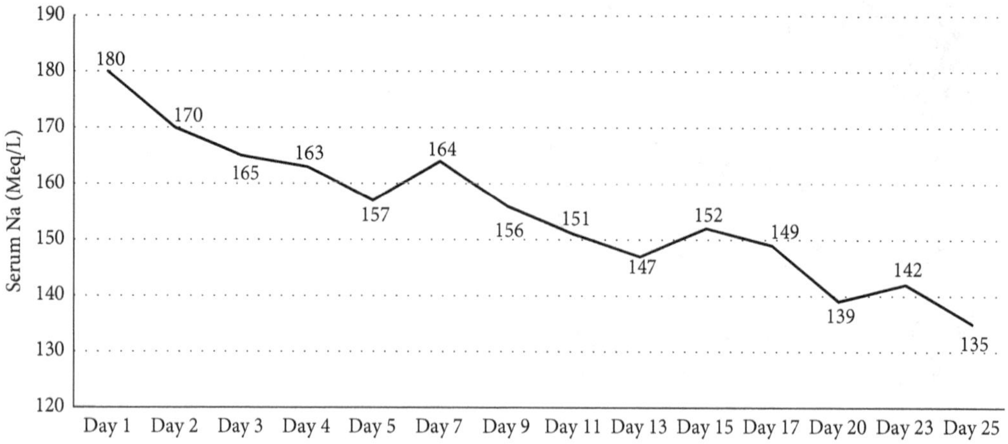

FIGURE 2: Graphical representation of serum sodium levels behavior during hospitalization. Desmopressin was administered from day 5 according to requirements.

Diagnostic criteria were proposed by the neurosarcoidosis consortium consensus group in 2018, although they have not been prospectively validated [4]. Our patient fulfilled the diagnostic criteria for definite neurosarcoidosis, which includes a clinical presentation and diagnostic evaluation compatible with the disease, the central nervous system pathology consistent with neurosarcoidosis, and rigorous exclusion of other causes [4].

An important clinical feature in our patient was the presence of psychiatric and encephalopathic symptoms. These types of symptoms in neurosarcoidosis are considered secondary to granulomatous inflammation, although this has not been confirmed. Remarkably, our patient had anti-NMDA receptor antibodies detected in CSF, an association that has never been reported in medical literature. Limbic encephalitis secondary to neurosarcoidosis was present in a case report, in which it was considered secondary to direct infiltration of the disease; however, in this case, anti-NMDA receptor antibodies were not measured [19]. This could imply that there is an autoimmune component of neuropsychiatric symptoms in patients with neurosarcoidosis. There is a case report of anti-NMDA receptor encephalitis in a 3-year-old boy secondary to microdeletion of the chromosome 6p21.32 that includes the HLA-DPB1 y HLADPB2 genes [20], which have been also associated with the development of sarcoidosis [21]. This could also be related to a B cell-mediated encephalopathy [22].

In conclusion, we report the case of a very rare presentation of neurosarcoidosis whose almost unique clinical features have only been described in case reports. The etiologic diagnosis of pituitary stalk lesions is difficult, which highlights the need of performing a biopsy and a histopathologic diagnosis, especially in atypical cases. This has fundamental therapeutic implications. To our knowledge, this is the first report of documented anti-NMDA antibodies in a definite case of neurosarcoidosis. This may be a reason for future research.

Acknowledgments

The authors had no funding, but the study was performed in ¨Department of Internal Medicine¨, Hospital de Especialidades. "Dr. Bernardo Sepúlveda Gutiérrez", Centro Médico Nacional Siglo XXI, Instituto Mexicano del Seguro Social, Ciudad de México.

References

[1] E. Hoitsma, C. G. Faber, M. Drent, and O. P. Sharma, "Neurosarcoidosis: a clinical dilemma," *The Lancet Neurology*, vol. 3, no. 7, pp. 397–407, 2004.

[2] P. Ungprasert, C. S. Crowson, and E. L. Matteson, "Influence of gender on epidemiology and clinical manifestations of sarcoidosis: a population-based retrospective cohort study 1976-2013," *Lung*, vol. 195, no. 1, pp. 87–91, 2017.

[3] B. J. Stern, A. Krumholz, C. Johns, P. Scott, and J. Nissim, "Sarcoidosis and its neurological manifestations," *Archives of Neurology*, vol. 42, no. 9, pp. 909–917, 1985.

[4] B. J. Stern, W. Royal, J. M. Gelfand et al., "Definition and consensus diagnostic criteria for neurosarcoidosis," *JAMA Neurology*, vol. 75, no. 12, pp. 1546–1553, 2018.

[5] R. T. Ibitoye, A. Wilkins, and N. J. Scolding, "Neurosarcoidosis: a clinical approach to diagnosis and management," *Journal of Neurology*, vol. 264, no. 5, pp. 1023–1028, 2017.

[6] K. Nozaki and M. A. Judson, "Neurosarcoidosis: clinical manifestations, diagnosis, and treatment," *La Presse Médicale*, vol. 41, pp. e331–e348, 2012.

[7] G. Murialdo and G. Tamagno, "Endocrine aspects of neurosarcoidosis," *Journal of Endocrinological Investigation*, vol. 25, no. 7, pp. 650–662, 2002.

[8] R. W. Turkington and J. H. MacIndoe, "Hyperprolactinemia in sarcoidosis," *Annals of Internal Medicine*, vol. 76, no. 4, pp. 545–549, 1972.

[9] C. Stuart, F. Neelson, and H. Levovitz, "Disordered control of thirst in hypothalamic-pituitary sarcoidosis," *New England Journal of Medicine*, vol. 323, no. 16, pp. 1120–1123, 1990.

[10] R. K. Crowley, M. Sherlock, A. Agha, D. Smith, and C. J. Thompson, "Clinical insights into adipsic diabetes insipidus: a large case series," *Clinical Endocrinology*, vol. 66, no. 4, pp. 475–482, 2007.

[11] K. Loh, A. Green, P. Fitzgerald, N. Weidner, J. Tyrrell, and J. B. Tyrrell, "Diabetes insipidus from sarcoidosis confined to the posterior pituitary," *European Journal of Endocrinology*, vol. 137, no. 5, pp. 514–519, 1997.

[12] R. P. Tabuena, S. Nagai, T. Handa et al., "Diabetes insipidus from neurosarcoidosis: long-term follow-up for more than eight years," *Internal Medicine*, vol. 43, no. 10, pp. 960–966, 2004.

[13] D. Konrad, M. Gartenmann, E. Martin, and E. J. Schoenle, "Central diabetes insipidus as the first manifestation of neurosarcoidosis in a 10-year-old girl," *Hormone Research in Paediatrics*, vol. 54, no. 2, pp. 98–100, 2000.

[14] L. Non, D. Brito, and C. Anastasopoulou, "Neurosarcoidosis-associated central diabetes insipidus masked by adrenal insufficiency," *BMJ Case Report*, vol. 2015, pp. 1–4, 2015.

[15] V. Sanghi and A. Kapoor, "Unusual presentation of central diabetes insipidus in a patient with neurosarcoidosis," *Journal of Investigative Medicine High Impact Case Reports*, vol. 4, no. 3, pp. 0–5, 2016.

[16] A. F. Turcu, B. J. Erickson, E. Lin et al., "Pituitary stalk lesions: the mayo clinic experience," *The Journal of Clinical Endocrinology & Metabolism*, vol. 98, no. 5, pp. 1812–1818, 2013.

[17] K. M. Lury, J. K. Smith, M. G. Matheus, and M. Castillo, "Neurosarcoidosis-review of imaging findings," *Seminars in Roentgenology*, vol. 39, no. 4, pp. 495–504, 2004.

[18] D. Fritz, D. van de Beek, and M. C. Brouwer, "Clinical features, treatment, and outcome in neurosarcoidosis: systematic review and meta-analysis," *BMC Neurology*, vol. 16, no. 1, pp. 1–8, 2016.

[19] M. Taoudou-Daouda, H. Assadeck, and B. Efared, "Sarcoidosis limbic encephalitis. a case report," *Iranian Journal of Neurology*, vol. 16, no. 3, pp. 156–158, 2017.

[20] H. Verhelst, P. Verloo, K. Dhondt et al., "Anti-NMDA-receptor encephalitis in a 3-year-old patient with chromosome 6p21.32 microdeletion including the HLA cluster," *European Journal of Paediatric Neurology*, vol. 15, no. 2, pp. 163–166, 2011.

[21] P. A. Lympany, M. Petrek, A. M. Southcott, A. J. N. Taylor, K. I. Welsh, and R. M. d. Bois, "HLA-Dpb polymorphisms: glu 69 association with sarcoidosis," *International Journal of Immunogenetics*, vol. 23, no. 5, pp. 353–359, 1996.

[22] J. Dalmau, "Looks can be deceiving," *Neurology—Neuroimmunology Neuroinflammation*, vol. 5, no. 3, p. e461, 2018.

37

Acute Partial Brown-Séquard Syndrome Secondary to Intraforaminal Disc Prolapse and Spinal Cord Infarction

Athanasios Astreinidis,[1] **Stephanos Finitsis,**[1] **Xanthippi Mavropoulou,**[2] **Elisavet Psoma,**[2] **and Panagiotis Prassopoulos**[2]

[1]*Department of Endovascular Surgery, AHEPA Hospital, Aristotle University of Thessaloniki, Panepistimioupoli, 54124 Thessaloniki, Greece*
[2]*Department of Radiology and Medical Imaging, AHEPA University Hospital, Panepistimioupoli, 54124 Thessaloniki, Greece*

Correspondence should be addressed to Athanasios Astreinidis; astrinthan@protonmail.ch

Academic Editor: Dominic B. Fee

We report the case of a 45-year-old female who presented with acute left abdominal pain and subsequently developed a left partial Brown-Séquard syndrome. Spinal fluid, inflammatory and prothrombotic tests were unremarkable. Magnetic resonance showed a left intraforaminal disc prolapse at the T9–T10 level and a hyperintense lesion on T2-weighted images in the left postero-lateral cord at the T8–T9 level with restricted diffusion on DWI imaging. A diagnosis of spinal cord infarction due to compromise of the left T8 thoracic radicular artery was made. The patient was managed conservatively and at the 3 months follow-up, she was ambulant and able to walk small distances without a walker.

1. Introduction

A 45-year-old female with no prior medical history and a body mass index of 25 abruptly developed left abdominal pain while seated. She subsequently developed left lower limb weakness and contralateral paraesthesia.

Admitted 24 hours post ictus, hyperreflexia and severe paresis was found involving all muscle groups of the left lower limb with minimally preserved extension of the thigh (grade 2/5) and foot (grade 2/5). Left kinaesthesia was slightly reduced. Profound sensory loss was noted below the T9–T10 level on the left. Pain sensation was diminished in the right lower limb, while pyramidal function was normal. Proprioception and vibration were symmetrical.

Blood tests including levels of CRP, RF, immunoglubolin, protein electrophoresis and immunofixation, prethrombotic tests including Factor V-Leiden, prothrombin mutations, levels of AT3, quantity of protein C, lupus anticoagulation and homocysteine levels, as well as CSF examination including biochemical examination, levels of glucose, protein ANA, AMA, ANCA, ASMA autoantibodies and cultures were negative.

MRI of the head and cervical spinal cord, cardiac echo, and abdominal echo were unremarkable.

The signs and symptoms are consistent with a partial BSS on the left at the level of T9–T10. Thoracolumbar MRI demonstrates a left intraforaminal disc protrusion at T9–T10 with no significant compression of the spinal cord (Figure 1). On T2 weighted sequences, there is a high intensity lesion in the left postero-lateral spinal cord extending from T8 to T9 (Figure 2). On DWI the lesion has a reduced ADC value (Figure 3).

The patient was managed conservatively with intravenous administration of glucocorticoids (methylprednisolone 1 gr/day for 3 days, tapered for another 3 days), mannitol (400 mg/day for 4 days), and subcutaneous enoxaparin 75 mg/12 hours for 1 week. Three months later, the patient was ambulant and could walk small distances without a walker. No further clinical improvement was observed after 6 months and 12 months. Control MRI showed no residual lesion on T2-weighted sequences without restriction on DWI images, while the disc prolapse had resolved completely.

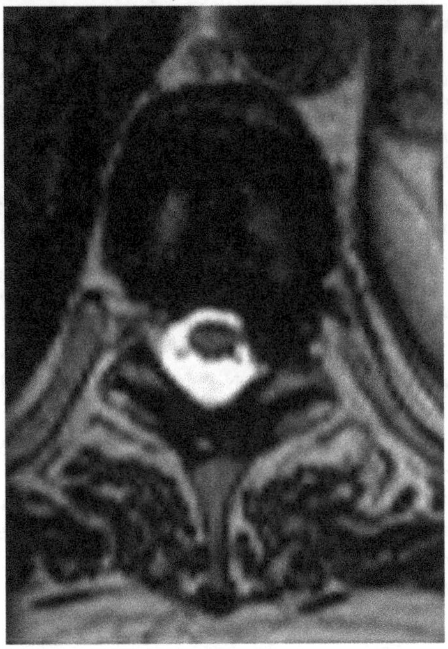

FIGURE 1

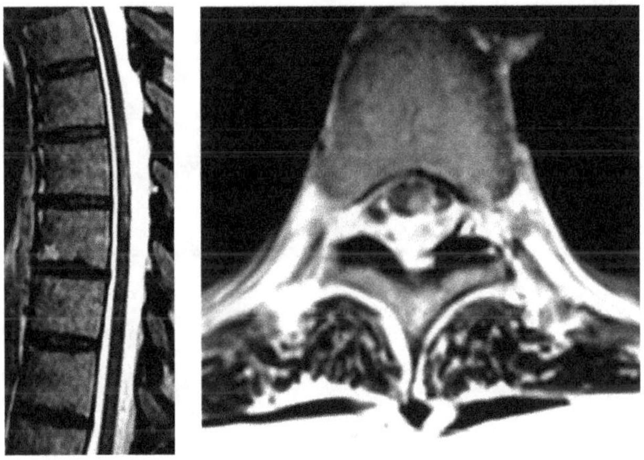

(a) (b)

FIGURE 2

The protruding thoracic disk produced an acute partial Brown-Séquard syndrome most probably either by direct compression or by disk fragment embolization of the left T8 radicular artery. This is the third case of partial Brown-Séquard syndrome secondary to disc protrusion reported in the literature. In the first case, the artery of Adamkiewicz was intraoperatively demonstrated to be compressed, while in the second case FCE was probably the aetiology of ischemia because of coexisting ischemic changes in the neighbouring vertebral body [5]. Our case also highlights the use of DWI in the acute setting of SCI to establish the ischemic nature of a spinal cord lesion when adjacent vertebral bone marrow ischemic changes are lacking.

2. Discussion

SCI is rare among younger patients and its aetiology often remains unexplained in more than 50% of cases. Differential diagnoses which have to be considered are spinal contusion,

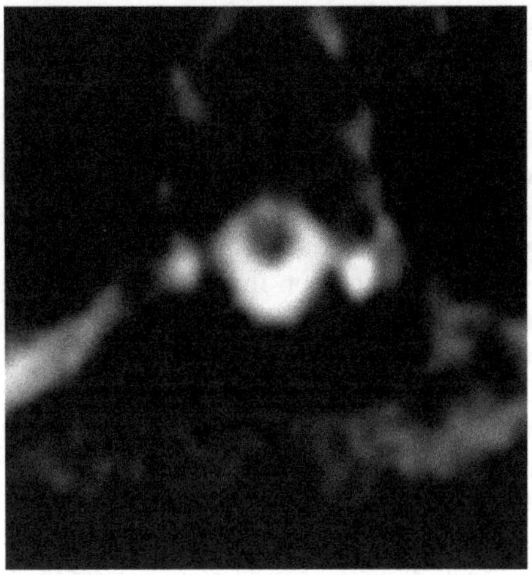

FIGURE 3

spinal hypoperfusion, acute transverse myelitis, and cord compression subsequent to medial disc herniation or tumour growth [1].

The typical BSS comprises a unilateral spinal lesion, resulting in ipsilateral loss of motor function, interruption of the ascending fibres in the posterior white column resulting in ipsilateral loss of tactile discrimination, and of vibratory and positional sensation. Additionally, BSS is characterized by spinothalamic tract dysfunction resulting in contralateral loss of pain and temperature sensation. The syndrome is most frequently observed in association with traumatic injuries to the spinal cord and extramedullary spinal cord tumours [2].

The entire spinal column and its structures receives their blood supply from 31 pairs of segmental arteries derived mainly from vertebral arteries or the aorta. The intraspinal branches of the segmental arteries which enter the spinal canal through the intervertebral foramina are called radicular arteries. They accompany the exiting nerves and veins and have an ascending course from caudal to cranial. Each radicular artery supplies the nearby bone and soft tissues, and divides into an anterior and posterior branch. Concerning the spinal cord, the anterior two-thirds and the centre are supplied by the ASA that runs superficially to the anterior median fissure and gives of sulcocomissural arteries that penetrate the fissure. The posterior third of the spinal cord is supplied by the paired PSAs. Both ASA and PSAs extend from the medulla to the conus medullaris [3]. The ASA is supplied by 2 radicular arteries through their anterior branch, while the PSA is formed by 10–23 radicular arteries through their posterior branch. A radicular branch suppling the spinal cord is called a radiculomedullary artery. The artery of Adamkiewicz is the largest anterior radiculomedullary artery and usually supplies a large portion of the thoracolumbar spinal cord. Besides supplying the ASA and PSAs, the radiculomedullary branches supply the vasa corona, a fine arterial network that gives perforators to the circumference of the cord.

The diagnosis of acute spinal cord ischemia is often clinical based on an abrupt presentation of a neurological deficit and back pain in 70% of cases. The most common artery involved is the ASA, resulting in an ASA syndrome. The PSA syndrome is relatively infrequent, while total transverse spinal cord ischemia involving both ASA and PSA has rarely been described. The rare cases of incomplete Brown-Séquard syndrome are thought to be secondary to involvement of sulcocomissural arteries.

Acute SCI may manifest on MRI as an intramedullary hyperintensity on T2-weighted images with cord enlargement. However, these signs are visible in approximately 45% of patients. When the occlusion involves vessels supplying the vertebrae, vertebral body infarction adjacent to a cord abnormality may be found on MRI in 4%–35% of cases and is a confirmatory sign of ischemia. Vertebral body infarctions are usually seen in the thoracolumbar region and are often associated with aortic disease. The bone marrow abnormality of the vertebra tends to appear earlier and be more exaggerated compared to the cord. DWI is more sensitive than T2 weighted images and may show ischemic lesions earlier than conventional MRI. When an infarction of the vertebral body is not observed, as in our case, DWI may be used to confirm the diagnosis of cord ischemia. Another important role of MRI is to rule out compressive myelopathies, vascular malformations, infective myelitis, demyelinating disorders, and tumours.

Atherosclerosis, aortic dissection (3%–5% risk), and aortic surgery (1%–10% risk) are the most common causes of acute SCI. Other rare causes include cardiac embolism, decompression sickness, coagulopathy, spinal arteriovenous malformations, systemic hypotension, epidural anaesthesia, trauma, and vasculitis. However, in 50% of patients, the aetiology remains unclear. Rarely, SCI may be due to mechanical compromise of a radicular artery following minor trauma. It is postulated that a sudden change of intervertebral disc pressure, especially in a degenerative disc may lead to rupture and penetration of cartilaginous material into neighbouring spinal vessels. FCE is thought to be a rarely recognized but important cause of SCI [4]. However, FCE lacks definitive diagnostic criteria.

Usually there is acute severe pain and the neurological deficit appears 15 min to 48 hours or later. MRI should be compatible with SCI, the cerebrospinal fluid is normal and inflammatory or autoimmune causes of myelopathy should be excluded. Different treatments options like intravenous steroids, plasma exchange, iv heparin, and emergent decompressive surgery have been tried without much success. The functional outcome varies from moderate to severe disability or even death if the cervical region is involved.

In the present case, control MRI at 3 months failed to show persisting T2 signal changes though the patient had a clear neurological deficit, while the disk prolapse had resolved completely. We suspect that the remaining spinal cord lesion was beyond the spatial resolution of the MRI equipment. The complete resolution of the disk prolapse in such a short time span attests to the dynamic nature of the lesion.

Abbreviations

SCI: Spinal cord ischemia
FCE: Fragment cartilage embolization
BSS: Brown-Séquard syndrome
ASA: Anterior spinal artery
PSA: Posterior spinal artery.

References

[1] J. Thöne, A. Hohaus, A. Bickel, and F. Erbguth, "Severe spinal cord ischemia subsequent to fibrocartilaginous embolism," *Journal of the Neurological Sciences*, vol. 263, no. 12, pp. 211–213, 2007.

[2] D. Gill, S. Ifthikharuddin, and L. M. Samkoff, "Acute Brown-Sequard Syndrome," *Archives of Neurology*, vol. 61, no. 1, p. 131, 2004.

[3] A. C. M. Amato and N. A. G. Stolf, "Anatomy of spinal blood supply," *Jornal Vascular Brasileiro*, vol. 14, no. 3, pp. 248–252, 2015.

[4] F. J. Mateen, P. A. Monrad, A. N. Leep Hunderfund, C. E. Robertson, and E. J. Sorenson, "Clinically suspected fibrocartilaginous embolism: clinical characteristics, treatments, and outcomes," *European Journal of Neurology*, vol. 18, no. 2, pp. 218–225, 2011.

[5] H. Mansour, F. Hammoud, and B. Vlahovitch, "Brown-Séquard syndrome caused by foramen and calcified disk herniation, responsible for direct compression of Adamkiewicz's artery," *Neurochirurgie*, vol. 33, no. 6, pp. 478–481, 1987.

38

Primary Angiitis of the Central Nervous System: From Psychiatry to Neurology

Joel Leonardi,[1] Christian Saleh ,[1] Phillip Jaszczuk,[1] Kristine A. Blackham,[2] Sabrina Zechel,[3] Stefanie Wilmes,[1] and Margret Hund-Georgiadis[1]

[1]*REHAB Basel, Clinic for Neurorehabilitation and Paraplegiology, Basel, Switzerland*
[2]*Department of Radiology, Division of Diagnostic and Interventional Neuroradiology, University Hospital Basel, Basel, Switzerland*
[3]*Institute of Neuropathology, University Medical Center Göttingen, Göttingen, Germany*

Correspondence should be addressed to Christian Saleh; chs12us75010@yahoo.com

Academic Editor: Norman S. Litofsky

We present a case of a 54-year-old man with primary angiitis of the central nervous system (PACNS) who was initially admitted to a psychiatric clinic with a diagnosis of delirium. We discuss the difficulty in establishing the diagnosis of PACNS and provide the reader with some recommendations on how to promptly and correctly diagnose this disease in order to avoid potentially lethal outcomes.

1. Introduction

Primary angiitis of the central nervous system (PACNS) is a vasculitis of unknown origin confined to the brain and spinal cord [1]. PACNS was first described in the late 1950s by Cravioto and Feigin [2]. Histopathology is characterized by segmental granulomatous inflammation of small- and medium-sized arteries and veins of the CNS. Definitive diagnosis is made by biopsy.

All the vasculitides that affect the central nervous system (CNS) are characterized by inflammation and necrosis of blood vessels and may be primary or secondary. They may cause tissue ischemia, which can have a variety of clinical presentations. Isolated CNS vasculitis is a known, rare disease entity with a variety of presentations; headache, dementia, lethargy, seizures, or multifocal neurological deficits [3]. Incidence rate of 2.4 person-years was reported by Salvarani et al. [4].

The clinical presentation is highly unspecific ranging from psychiatric to neurological symptoms, therefore, frequently delaying a prompt diagnosis and treatment with potentially lethal consequences. We describe a patient initially admitted to a psychiatric hospital, but diagnosed subsequently with PACNS. In addition, we provide a brief review of the literature.

2. Case Presentation

A 54-year-old Caucasian man presented with agitation and confusion. Glasgow coma score (GCS) was 14 out of 15. The patient was reported to be in his baseline state (of generally good health) when his family last saw him one week prior. The initial working diagnosis was delirium. The clinical picture worsened rapidly when the patient developed hypertension, tremor, meningism, and an increase in C-reactive protein (CRP 143 mg/l, reference: 0–1), without fever. MRI FLAIR—sequences presented abnormal but nonspecific bilateral hyper-intensities supra- and infratentorially in the gray and white matter (periventricular and subcortical white matter), the basal ganglia, the thalamus, the middle cerebellar peduncle, and in the brainstem (Figures 1(a)–1(c)). A lumbar puncture showed a leukocytosis $9\times10–/l$ (reference: 0–5), a total protein 789 mg/l (reference: 200–400), a lactate level of 3.2 mmol/l (reference: 1.2–2.1). Intravenous antibiotic (ceftriaxone 2 g/day) and antiviral (acyclovir 750 mg/day) treatment was started, but once infection-screening and biochemistry results showed no evidence of infection it was stopped. Over the following weeks, the patient developed a progressive tetraparesis, rigidity, and mutism, with a GCS fluctuating between 6 and 10. Repeated autoimmune, vasculitis, viral, prion, and bacterial screenings were negative. Digital subtraction angiography (DSA) showed no specific evidence of

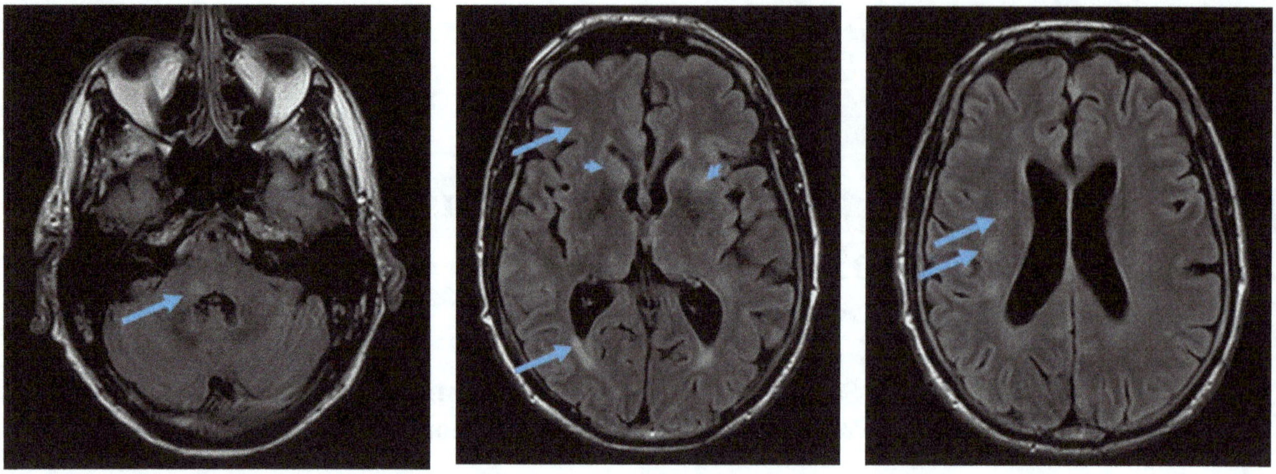

(a) (b) (c)

FIGURE 1: Initial MRI brain, FLAIR transversal images with multifocal abnormal hyperintensities (arrows). (a) Middle cerebellar peduncle. (b) Periventricular and subcortical white matter, right caudate nucleus, and left lentiform nucleus. (c) Deep white matter.

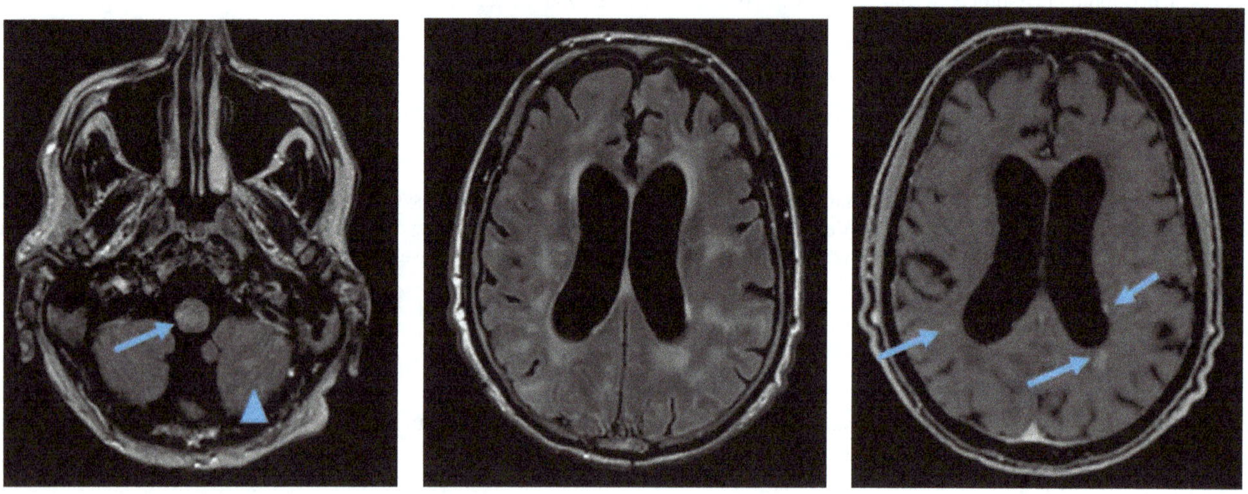

(a) (b) (c)

FIGURE 2: MRI brain 4 months after presentation. FLAIR transversal images (a and b) and post contrast image (c) demonstrating marked brain atrophy and new abnormal hyperintensities in the spinal cord (arrow, a) and cerebellum (arrowhead, a) , throughout the periventricular and subcortical white matter (b) and new enhancement (arrows, c).

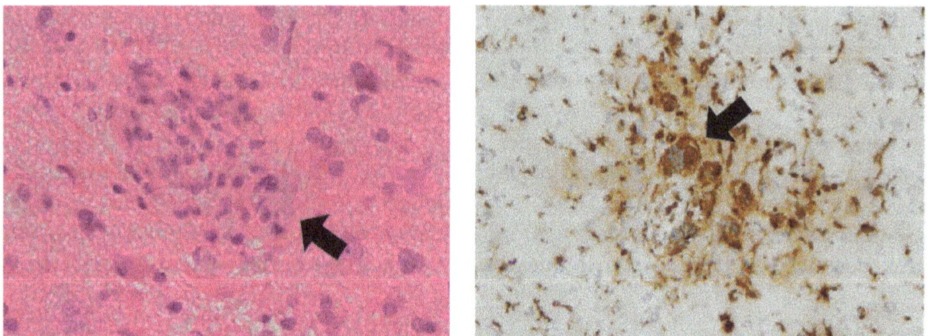

(a) (b)

FIGURE 3: (a) HE staining of brain biopsy showing a nearly obliterated vessel with perivascular lymphocytes and a giant cell (arrow points ta the giant cell). Scale bar: 100 μm. (b) Immunostaining against Kim1P positive monocytes and monocytic giant cells (arrow points at giant cells, counterstaining of nuclei with hemalum). Scale bar: 100 μm vasoconstriction or vasculitis. A follow up brain MRI showed progressive patchy and confluent T2w signal hyperintensities, again supra- and infratentorially and, again, of the gray and white matter. There were new lesions in the upper cervical spinal cord and new small areas of parenchymal enhancement as well as marked brain atrophy, indicating a progressive and prolonged disease process (Figures 2(a)–2(c)). In the absence of infection and even in the absence of vasculopathy on DSA, these findings were consistent with vasculitis. Brain biopsy (Figures 3(a) and 3(b)) from the right frontal lobe revealed perivascular and transmural leukocyte infiltration of small vessels composed of CD8 positive cytotoxic T cells, macrophages, and giant Langerhans type cells. CD20 positive B cells were almost absent. Moreover, reactive astrogliosis as well as microglial activation were found. There was no vessel wall fibrinoid necrosis. A biopsy of the dura mater showed no abnormalities. A diagnosis of suspected primary central nervous system angiitis was made. The etiology of inflammation could not be precisely determined despite vast immunohistological screening. Treatment with methylprednisone 1 g/d i.v., intravenous immunoglobulin (IVIG) 27.5 g/daily over 4 days and i.v. cyclophosphamide (three cycles of 15 mg/kg) was started. The patient recovered gradually with slight improvement of neurological deficits.

3. Discussion

Despite a large volume of literature on PACNS definitive diagnosis is frequently delayed resulting in potentially lethal consequences. One major reason is the unspecific clinical presentation ranging from recurrent headaches, altered consciousness, seizures, stroke, and a lack of high clinical suspicion (Table S1). Imaging findings of PACNS are variable and nonspecific [14]. Although MRI examinations are sensitive (abnormal in 90% to 100% of patients), the typical findings are nonspecific. The lesions seen include discrete or diffuse supra- and infratentorial lesions most commonly involving the superficial white matter, followed by the deep gray matter, the deep white matter, and the cerebral cortex, in decreasing order of frequency [5]. Infarctions may be seen in approximately 50% of cases and mass lesions in as many as 15% of cases. These imaging characteristics can be mistaken for malignancy, multiple sclerosis, small vessel ischemic disease, and atherosclerosis among others. Gadolinium enhancement may occur in as many as one-third of cases [5]. The overall sensitivity of angiography in detecting PACNS has been estimated to be between 50% and 90%. Angiograms have a limited specificity as there is a range of noninflammatory vasculopathies, which can cause angiographic findings similar to those seen with PACNS [6]. In a recent systematic review of 127 articles including 701 patients, only 248 patients had both angiography and biopsy performed. Of those, only 32 patients (4.6%) had the classic angiographic appearance of vasculitis with concurrent histopathological vasculitis [7].

4. Conclusion

A high degree of clinical suspicion is needed for a prompt diagnosis of PACNS in patients manifesting with (transient) multi-focal symptoms associated with encephalopathy [13]. Vasculitis screening, imaging (MRA, DSA) to consider prompt initiation of immune-modulatory treatment is mandatory.

Additional Points

(i) PACNS is to be suspected with an array of symptoms ranging from psychiatric to neurologic manifestations (especially when associated with encephalopathy) that cannot be clearly localized.

(ii) Prompt diagnostic work up including vasculitis screening and MR-Angiography is recommended by suspicion of PACNS.

(iii) Brain biopsy is considered the gold standard investigation in establishing the diagnosis of PACNS; however, it will confirm the diagnosis only in circa 60% of patients [13].

(iv) PACNS should be treated as a diagnosis of exclusion using a broad differential diagnosis. When there is a high degree of certainty of PACNS, immune-modulatory treatment should be started promptly.

References

[1] C. Salvarani, R. D. BrownJr., K. T. Calamia et al., "Primary central nervous system vasculitis: analysis of 101 patients," *Annals of Neurology*, vol. 62, no. 5, pp. 442–451, 2007.

[2] H. Cravioto and I. Feigin, "Noninfectious granulomatous angiitis with a predilection for the nervous system," *Neurology*, vol. 9, pp. 599–609, 1959.

[3] T. R. Cupps, P. M. Moore, and A. S. Fauci, "Isolated angiitis of the central nervous system. Prospective diagnostic and therapeutic experience," *The American Journal of Medicine*, vol. 74, no. 1, pp. 97–105, 1983.

[4] C. Salvarani, R. D. BrownJr, T. Christianson et al., "An update of the mayo clinic cohort of patients with adult primary central nervous system vasculitis: description of 163 patients," *Medicine (Baltimore)*, vol. 94, no. 21, p. e738, 2015.

[5] J. Birnbaum and D. B. Hellmann, "Primary angiitis of the central nervous system," *JAMA Neurology*, vol. 66, no. 6, pp. 704–709, 2009.

[6] A. A. K. Abdel Razek, H. Alvarez, S. Bagg, S. Refaat, and M. Castillo, "Imaging spectrum of CNS vasculitis," *Radiographics*, vol. 34, no. 4, pp. 873–894, 2014.

[7] F. McVerry, G. McCluskey, P. McCarron, K. W. Muir, and M. O. McCarron, "Diagnostic test results in primary CNS vasculitis: a systematic review of published cases," *Neurology Clinical Practice*, vol. 7, no. 3, pp. 256–265, 2017.

[8] H. Pourmahmoodian, H. A. Ghelichnia Omrani, M. H. Harrirchian, M. Ghabaee, B. Zamani, and M. Ghaffarpour, "Primary angiitis of the central nervous system," *Acta Medica Iranica*, vol. 50, no. 3, pp. 216–221, 2012.

[9] S. Singh, T. Soloman, G. Chacko, and T. P. Joseph, "Primary angiitis of the central nervous system: an ante-mortem diagnosis," *Journal of Postgraduate Medicine*, vol. 46, no. 4, pp. 272–274, 2000.

[10] N. Coronel-Restrepo, F. Bonilla-Abadia, O. A. Cortes et al., "Primary angiitis of the central nervous system: a report of three cases from a single colombian center," *Case Reports in Neurological Medicine*, vol. 2013, Article ID 940438, 4 pages, 2013.

[11] H. Ay, G. Sahin, I. Saatci, F. Soylemezoglu, and O. Saribas, "Primary angiitis of the central nervous system and silent cortical hemorrhages," *American Journal of Neuroradiology*, vol. 23, no. 9, pp. 1561–1563, 2002.

[12] M. J. Faer, J. H. Mead, and R. D. Lynch, "Cerebral granulomatous angiitis: case report and literature review," *American Journal of Roentgenology*, vol. 129, no. 3, pp. 463–467, 1977.

[13] P. Berlit and M. Kraemer, "Cerebral vasculitis in adults: what are the steps in order to establish the diagnosis? red flags and pitfalls," *Clinical and Experimental Immunology*, vol. 175, no. 3, pp. 419–424, 2014.

[14] C. Beuker, A. Schmidt, D. Strunk et al., "Primary angiitis of the central nervous system: diagnosis and treatment," *Therapeutic Advances in Neurological Disorders*, vol. 9, 2018.

39

Effect of Zolpidem in the Aftermath of Traumatic Brain Injury: An MEG Study

Praveen Sripad,[1] **Jessica Rosenberg**,[1,2,3] **Frank Boers**,[1] **Christian P. Filss**,[1,4] **Norbert Galldiks**,[5,6,7] **Karl-Josef Langen**,[1,4,7,9] **Ralf Clauss**,[8] **N. Jon Shah**,[1,2,3,9] **and Jürgen Dammers**[1]

[1]*Institute of Neuroscience and Medicine (INM-4), Medical Imaging Physics, Forschungszentrum Jülich GmbH, 52425 Jülich, Germany*
[2]*Institute of Neuroscience and Medicine (INM-11), JARA, Forschungszentrum Jülich GmbH, 52425 Jülich, Germany*
[3]*Department of Neurology, RWTH Aachen University, Aachen, Germany*
[4]*Department of Nuclear Medicine, RWTH Aachen University, Aachen, Germany*
[5]*Institute of Neuroscience and Medicine (INM-3), Forschungszentrum Jülich, Jülich GmbH, 52425 Jülich, Germany*
[6]*Department of Neurology, University of Cologne, Cologne, Germany*
[7]*Center of Integrated Oncology (CIO), Universities of Cologne and Bonn, Cologne, Germany*
[8]*Nuclear Medicine Department, Royal Surrey County Hospital, Guildford, Surrey GU2 7XX, UK*
[9]*JARA - BRAIN - Translational Medicine, Aachen, Germany*

Correspondence should be addressed to Praveen Sripad; p.sripad@fz-juelich.de

Academic Editor: Dennis J. Rivet

In the past two decades, many studies have shown the paradoxical efficacy of zolpidem, a hypnotic used to induce sleep, in transiently alleviating various disorders of consciousness such as traumatic brain injury (TBI), dystonia, and Parkinson's disease. The mechanism of action of this effect of zolpidem is of great research interest. In this case study, we use magnetoencephalography (MEG) to investigate a fully conscious, ex-coma patient who suffered from neurological difficulties for a few years due to traumatic brain injury. For a few years after injury, the patient was under medication with zolpidem that drastically improved his symptoms. MEG recordings taken before and after zolpidem showed a reduction in power in the theta-alpha (4–12 Hz) and lower beta (15–20 Hz) frequency bands. An increase in power after zolpidem intake was found in the higher beta/lower gamma (20–43 Hz) frequency band. Source level functional connectivity measured using weighted-phase lag index showed changes after zolpidem intake. Stronger connectivity between left frontal and temporal brain regions was observed. We report that zolpidem induces a change in MEG resting power and functional connectivity in the patient. MEG is an informative and sensitive tool to detect changes in brain activity for TBI.

1. Introduction

Zolpidem is a short-acting nonbenzodiazepine hypnotic that is commonly used to treat insomnia [1] and has been shown to be highly selective for the GABA-A receptor [2]. To the best of our knowledge, Daniele and colleagues were the first to report a seemingly paradoxical therapeutic effect on a patient with Parkinson's disease [3]. They reported a 61-year-old woman with a 25-year history of Parkinson's who showed antiparkinsonian improvements in akinesia and rigidity, instead of drowsiness upon a 10 mg dosage of zolpidem. Findings stemming from a case study of a patient in the persistent vegetative state followed, where a patient woke up from his semi-coma and could recognize and talk to his mother after the intake of zolpidem [4]. Since then, there have been many reports where zolpidem has been used to treat a variety of neurological disorders of consciousness [5–10]. In a systematic review, Bomalaski and colleagues discussed the literature regarding the potential of zolpidem to treat a variety of neurological disorders and concluded that more research is needed to interrogate the complex underlying neurophysiological mechanisms involved and in order to understand zolpidem's usefulness as a therapeutic drug [11].

It is well known that resting state magnetoencephalography (MEG) is a useful tool in understanding function and dysfunction in the human brain [12]. Slow and fast oscillatory changes in the resting state functional connectivity during MEG have been shown to reflect various brain disorders such as stroke, epilepsy [13], traumatic brain injury (TBI) [14], Alzheimer's disease [15], and autism spectrum disorders [16]. Thus, looking at large-scale MEG resting state networks may give us an insight into the functional organisation of the injured brain and the effects of various drugs on it. It has been shown that MEG can pick up changes in GABA function in the brain and that zolpidem has an influence on changes in GABA action [17]. This makes the analysis of resting state brain oscillations using MEG particularly relevant to understanding the effects of zolpidem.

Unfortunately, there are only a limited number of studies using MEG or electroencephalogram (EEG) to observe changes in brain activity following treatment with zolpidem to relieve neurological symptoms. However, one study conducted by Hall and colleagues used MEG (along with fMRI, MRS, and SPECT) (functional magnetic resonance imaging, magnetic resonance spectroscopy, and single-photon emission computed tomography) to observe coincidental sensorimotor and cognitive improvements in a stroke patient [18]. The authors reported reduced MEG signal power in the theta (4–10 Hz) and beta (15–30 Hz) bands after zolpidem uptake. Subsequently, Williams and colleagues investigated the resting state brain using EEG in order to identify a possible mechanism underlying zolpidem response after brain injury and reported reduced EEG power and coherence at low frequencies (6–10 Hz) [19]. A number of other studies using EEG reported incomplete or inconclusive results [20–22]. In a structured study, Whyte and Myers investigated 84 participants with disorders of consciousness and reported that 4.8% of the participants were responsive to zolpidem [23]. The relative rarity of such cases and a lack of understanding of the mechanisms involved are a strong motivation for continued research.

Here we report differences in the spectral power and MEG functional connectivity at the source level using weighted phase lag index (WPLI) [24] in the resting state brain recordings of the patient before and after intake of zolpidem.

2. Case Presentation

The subject (male, 35), henceforth referred to as W, suffered from a severe traumatic brain injury to the left side of his brain in a major car accident in 2005. Based on computerized tomography (CT) scans of the brain, W suffered from intraventricular hemorrhage that was resolved within 19 days of the accident. A very small left fronto-temporal collection not causing obvious mass effect was suspected along with some atrophic change in the inferior aspect of the left frontal lobe with sulcal prominence inferiorly. Figure 1 shows the CT scans of the patient brain immediately after the accident and 19 days later. After the accident, he remained in a coma for a few weeks, progressing to a vegetative state, and eventually gained full consciousness three months after the accident. After a phase of hospital rehabilitation, he returned home after a year. The accident left him disabled with difficulty walking and a limp. His coordination, short-term memory, and speech (particularly pronunciation of consonants) were also affected, leading to lack of confidence in performing daily activities. In 2011, it was discovered that these deficits markedly improved following the administration of a 10 mg dose of zolpidem. At this stage, a neurological examination showed that W was right-handed, normally oriented in time, place, and person. W had a severe dysarthria and an impaired uvula elevation, but no dysphagia. The left biceps and brachoradialis reflexes were absent, and the left triceps reflex impaired. There was a bilateral brady-dysdiadochokinesia, more pronounced left, and dysmetria in the finger-to-nose and heel-to-shin tests. There was a broad-based gait, impaired tandem walking, an abnormal postural response, and a broad-based stance. The Romberg test was abnormal. The unified Parkinson's disease rating scale (UPDRS) measured 10, and the Tinetti and Barthel scores were 21 and 10, respectively [25–27]. After intake of zolpidem, W's speech, movement, coordination, and gait showed drastic improvements. The improvements started approximately 30 minutes after ingestion and lasted up to 4 hours, with a maximum effect after around 1 hour. While W's Barthel index remained normal before and after zolpidem, his ability on the Tinetti Falls Efficacy Scale improved from 21/100 to 15/100. A baseline ^{99m}Tc-HMPAO brain SPECT scan in 2011 showed a decreased cerebral perfusion in the left fronto-parietal and temporal regions and the left thalamus, which improved after zolpidem intake. Upon starting 10 mg of zolpidem daily, W's speech, movement, coordination, and gait improved, leading to him being able to lead a near normal life. After two years, along with the MEG measurements, ^{18}F-FDG and ^{11}C-flumazenil PET scans were performed before and after zolpidem intake and showed no abnormalities in W's brain. A 99m Tc-HMPAO brain SPECT scan repeated in 2014 appeared normal and showed no changes upon zolpidem intake. At the time of the MEG measurement (used in this study) in November 2013, W was under 10 mg of zolpidem daily. The MEG measurements were obtained during a no-task resting condition with eyes open (EO) and eyes closed (EC) for three minutes. The first measurement was taken without W having taken zolpidem for 24 hours. Subsequently, 10 mg of zolpidem was administered and measurements were taken an hour later. Thus W was measured under two conditions: without any zolpidem (NOZO) and with zolpidem (ZO). Voluntary consent from the subject was obtained before performing the measurement, and the measurement was conducted in the presence of the subject's supervising physician.

3. Results

Previously in 2011, following intake of zolpidem, W had shown marked improvements in speech, movement, gait,

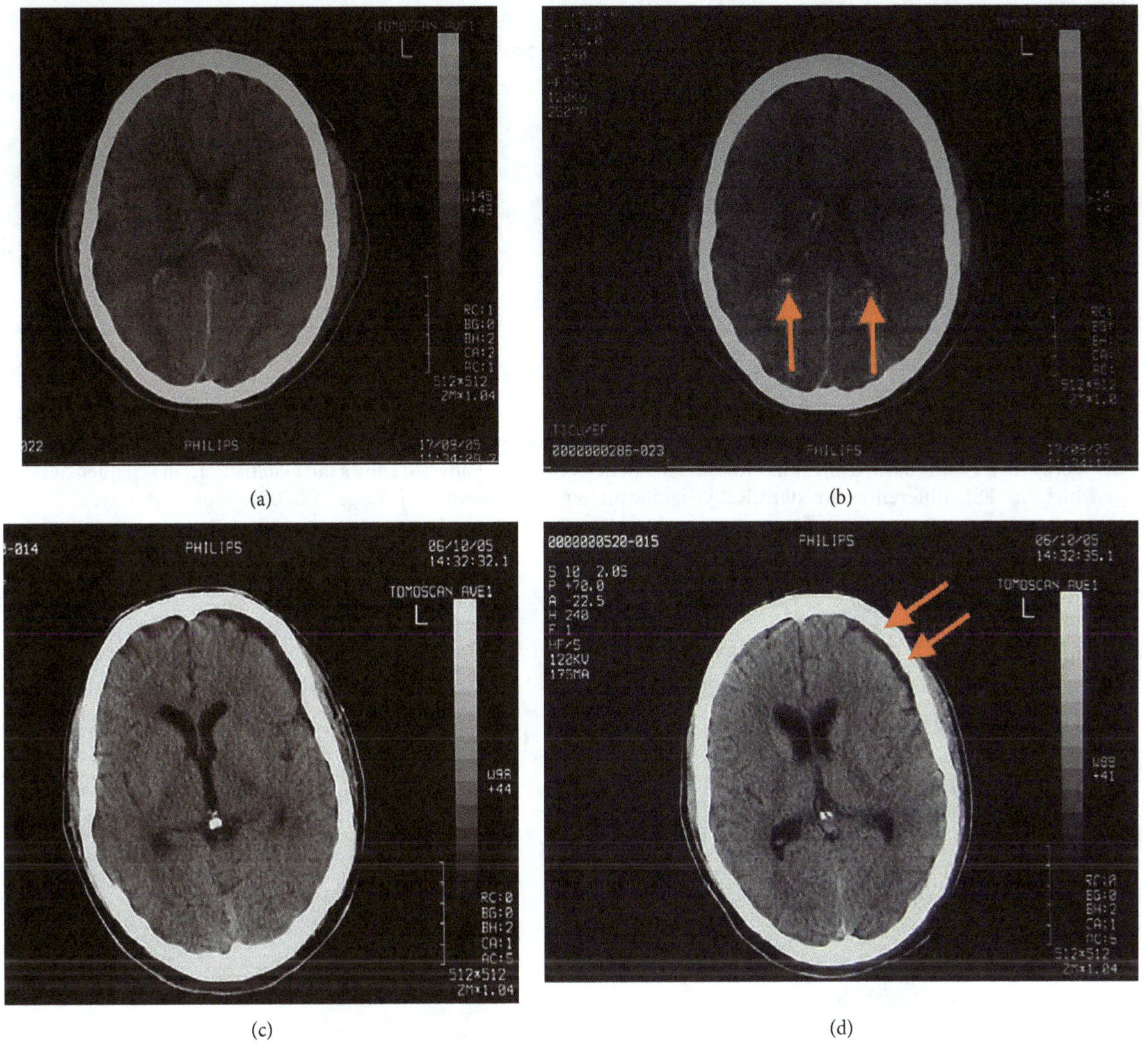

FIGURE 1: CT scans of the patient brain immediately after (a and b) and 19 days after accident (c and d). The images (a) and (b) above show some intraventricular hemorrhage (arrows show intraventricular hemorrhage in the posterior horns of the lateral ventricles) after accident. In the images (c) and (d), the intraventricular hemorrhage has resolved completely. Arrows show suspected new discrete atrophic changes in the left frontal lobe with sulcal prominence that was not present in the initial scans.

and coordination. However, at the time of measurement in 2013, upon neurological examination, the patient showed no clinical effects following intake of zolpidem and only minor subjective improvements were reported. For example, W's family felt that he functioned better when on zolpidem. A structural MR scan performed at the time of MEG measurement showed no major structural abnormalities.

MEG power spectral densities at the sensor level analysis were computed to identify differences, if any, in the subject before and after zolpidem intake. As shown in Figure 2, a permutation cluster test [28] showed a significant decrease ($p < 0.01$) in power in the frequency range of 4–12 Hz and 15–20 Hz, whereas an increase can be observed above 20 Hz up to 43 Hz (see Figure 3).

Sensor level topomaps computed across the frequency bands of interest before and after intake of ZO shows how the power is distributed across the sensors. A clear decrease in power is observed after ZO for the frequency band 4–12 Hz. The 15–43 Hz frequency bands show an increase in power, especially in the sensors above the left frontal areas of the brain.

Connectivity analysis was performed on representative time courses from different brain regions [29] obtained from MEG data projected onto the source space using minimum norm estimates (MNE) [30]. WPLI was used to quantify the connectivity strength between brain regions. In Figure 4 a circle plot shows the contrast of WPLI strength between NOZO and ZO conditions for different brain areas in the 15–43 Hz frequency band. The areas, corresponding to the 68 anatomical labels, are grouped according to cortical regions and color-coded accordingly. The strength of connectivity (WPLI) is indicated using the color of the lines connecting various areas. Differences in connections between the frontal and temporal regions that are absent in NOZO show up strongly (blue lines) in the ZO condition, particularly in the left hemisphere.

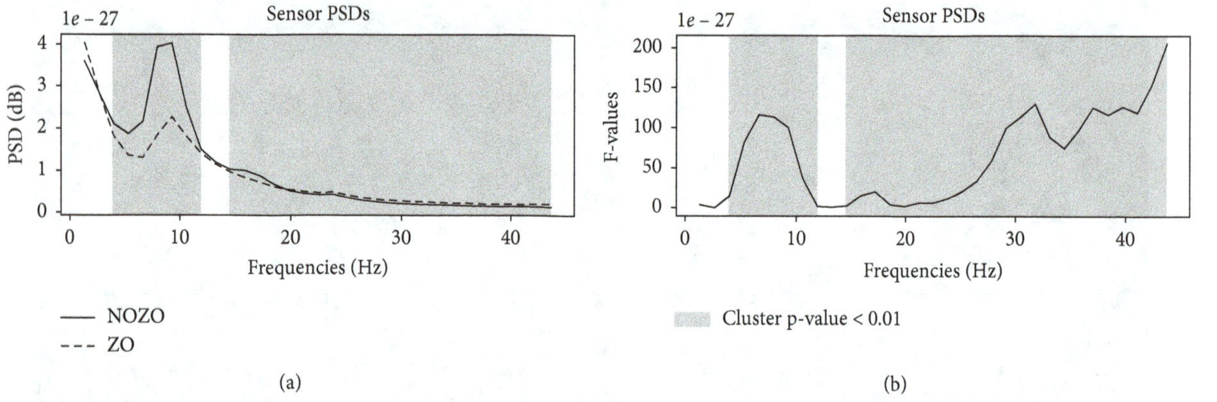

Figure 2: Significant differences in the sensor level PSDs in the subject with (ZO) and without (NOZO) zolpidem drug. Panel (a) shows average PSDs across trials with (dashed line) and without zolpidem (solid line). Panel (b) shows the F-statistic across frequencies. Frequency clusters for which the PSD differences are statistically significant across trials with a p value of 0.01 as shown in gray.

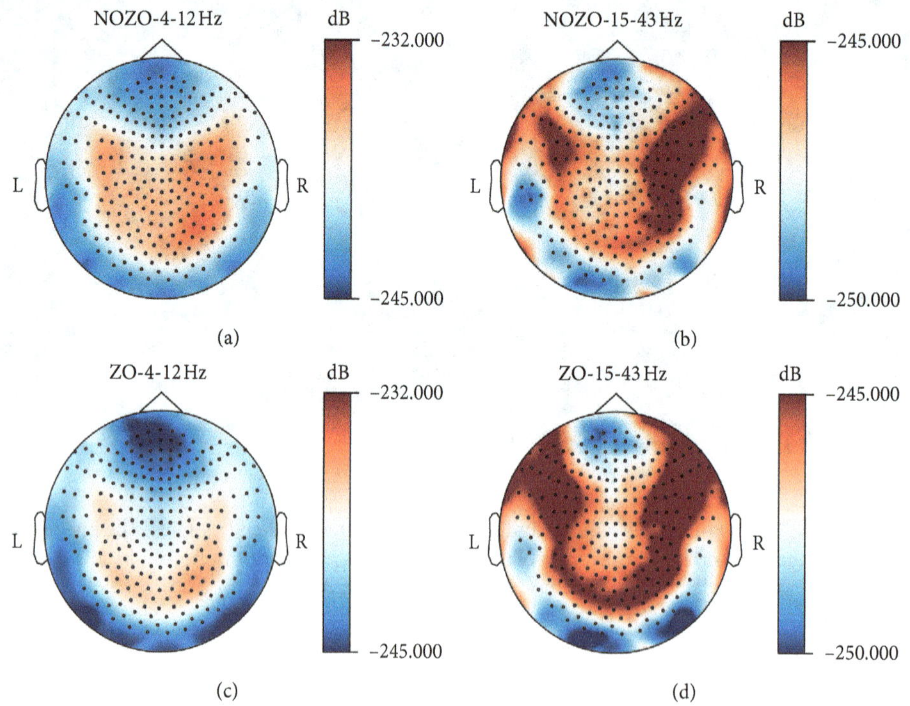

Figure 3: Power spectral densities across the sensor topography for 4–12 Hz and 15–43 Hz frequency bands for the patient with (ZO) and without Zolpidem (NOZO). Differences in PSD values in the left frontal areas (neurological orientation) before and after ZO under frequency 15–43 Hz can be seen.

4. Discussion

W, suffering from several neurological disabilities as an aftermath of TBI showed drastic improvement in speech and motor function after the intake of zolpidem in low doses. This transient counterintuitive effect of zolpidem, a commonly used hypnotic, has been observed in many people with a variety of neurological disorders. While this effect has been well documented in the literature, much still remains to be understood [11].

In this case study, we have measured the resting state brain activity in W using ME and have documented the differences in source power and functional connectivity before and after intake of zolpidem.

Strong differences in power were found at the sensor level. A spectral permutation clustering between trials showed a significant reduction in power after intake of zolpidem between 4 and 12 Hz, and from 15 to 20 Hz that includes the theta, alpha, and lower beta range. We find that this is in agreement with previous studies using MEG and EEG [18, 19]. In a case report describing the paradoxical effects of zolpidem in a patient in a persistent vegetative state, Hall and colleagues demonstrated high theta (4–10 Hz) and beta (15–30 Hz) MEG power that decreased upon zolpidem uptake. This was also coupled with improvements in cognitive and motor function in the patient [18]. Williams and colleagues reported a similar reduction in 6–10 Hz EEG

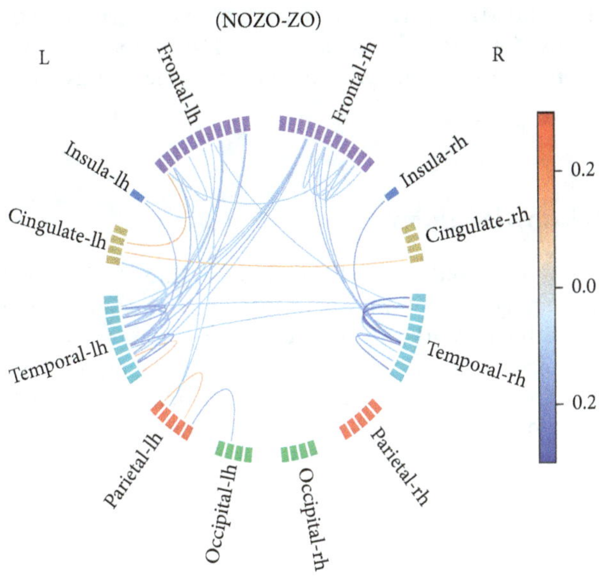

FIGURE 4: Connectivity difference before (NOZO) and after the intake of zolpidem (ZO) in the 15–43 Hz frequency band. The 50 strongest connections are visualized, where reddish lines indicate stronger connections without zolpidem and bluish lines indicate stronger connections with zolpidem.

power in several subjects with brain injury [19]. The effect has also been observed in healthy subjects in both M/EEG [2, 17] and in functional magnetic resonance imaging (fMRI) [31]. It is particularly relevant that among other regions, Licata and colleagues also report a strong increase in the resting state blood oxygen level-dependent (BOLD) response after zolpidem intake in the occipital area [31]. The anticorrelation between MEG power and BOLD, especially in the occipital cortex is well documented [32, 33]. Our results also show an increase in power in the lower gamma range that has not been reported thus far. The topomaps show asymmetrically stronger power in the right hemisphere before zolpidem intake that disappears after zolpidem. This may be explained by the fact that W suffered from a left-sided head TBI, with some dormancy of function observed in the left fronto-parietal, temporal, and thalamic regions (as reported by the ^{99m}Tc-HMPAO brain SPECT scans from his physician).

The functional connectivity analysis results show variation in connectivity after zolpidem intake with the frontal and temporal regions of the left hemisphere being most prominent. Studies on healthy subjects using MEG show that frontal and temporal areas are actively involved in the resting state [34]. Furthermore, zolpidem is a well-known positive modulator of γ-aminobutyric acid$_A$ (GABA$_A$) receptors [1, 35], and studies on healthy populations have shown that GABA levels are correlated to functional connectivity [36]. Zolpidem increased functional connectivity in the resting state networks of healthy participants measured using fMRI BOLD time-series [31]. A number of hypotheses have been proposed to understand the mechanism of the action of zolpidem and to explain the functional significance of its effects in clinical observations [37–39].

It is important to note that, at the time of measurement, the patient was on a daily dose of zolpidem for two years and was zolpidem free for a period of 24 hours before start of the experiment, raising the possibility that the results are confounded due to tolerance effects. The half-life of zolpidem is around 2.4 hours. A 24 hours zolpidem free period translates to ten half lives which is enough time for the effects of the previous dose to wash out of the system. As far as the long-term tolerance effects of zolpidem are concerned, the current body of literature is not very clear. A meta-analysis from 1999 has shown that zolpidem produces only a minimum tolerance in the long run [40]; however, the analysis did not include a contradictory study where tolerance to the hypnotic effects of zolpidem was reported [41]. A later study from 2012 reports no tolerance on insomnia to zolpidem after a year of use [42]. When W was first introduced to zolpidem medication in 2011, a ^{99m}Tc-HMPAO brain SPECT scan showed decreased cerebral perfusion with transient improvement after zolpidem. A subsequent scan in 2014 showed a normal perfusion with no significant change after zolpidem. Positron emission tomography (PET) measurements with ^{18}F-FDG and ^{11}C-Flumazenil conducted in 2013 around the same time as the MEG measurements showed normal glucose metabolism and benzodiazepine receptor distribution without significant changes after zolpidem. These unpublished results from the SPECT and PET scans suggest that W may have shown secondary long-term improvement parallel to that of daily transient improvements induced by zolpidem. Considering that the literature is unclear in terms of tolerance caused by zolpidem, we hypothesize that the patient has undergone a partial healing over the years rather than develop a tolerance to the drug. Therefore, there is a possibility that a part of the changes observed would be expected to occur in the healthy brain as well. This gradual process of natural recovery has also been observed in other patients with TBI too [43].

Furthermore, it has to be considered that the changes in spectral power and functional connectivity analysis of MEG data after administration of zolpidem could not be substantiated by the neurological examination. Previous studies have shown that MEG is a very sensitive method to detect functional changes in the brain of TBI patients as compared to EEG, SPECT, and MRI [44–46]. In their 1999 study, Lewine and colleagues have shown MEG abnormalities even in an asymptomatic patient with a history of mild TBI as compared to controls. Similarly, Tarapore and colleagues show disrupted MEG functional connectivity in patients years after TBI, even in patients with normal MRI findings [46]. Based on these observations, it is reasonable to assume that the functional changes observed with MEG in our study are real, even though they are not directly substantiated by the neurological examination. In this context, we consider the subjective improvements reported by the patient and his family as confirmation, but not as proof of the functional changes.

From the above findings we may state that zolpidem produces a transient change in the MEG resting state spectral power and functional connectivity in the patient. We hypothesize that although damage to the brain has slowly healed over the time; there may remain decreased cortical network activity that is improved upon zolpidem intake. The extent of zolpidem-induced changes observed may be a function of time since injury, and therefore it is important to keep this in mind when interpreting the results and in comparing different studies. Abnormally reduced connectivity in TBI, observed via resting state MEG has been shown to improve over time [46]. Longitudinal studies involving the effect of zolpidem on an injured brain would also help further understanding whether daily doses of zolpidem would have any long-term influence in aiding recovery. Studies with a larger cohort looking at the influence of zolpidem on healthy subjects using resting state MEG would also greatly help understand the mechanisms involved.

5. Conclusion

We have reported findings from a case of traumatic brain injury where zolpidem produced transient paradoxical improvements in a patient with neurological disabilities. We report a reduction in MEG power in the theta-alpha band (4–12 Hz) and an increase in the frequency band (20–43 Hz) after zolpidem intake. Changes in the cortico-cortical functional connectivity after zolpidem intake were also observed. Our findings support the assumption that zolpidem has an effect on the neuronal activity. However, this needs to be evaluated further in a larger cohort in order to be helpful for the future treatment of patients affected by such neurological disorders. We also highlight the efficacy of resting state MEG as an investigative tool for TBI.

Consent

A written letter of consent has been obtained from the patient and can be made available upon request.

Authors' Contributions

Praveen Sripad is an MEG expert and was involved in data acquisition, analysis, design of the study, and in writing and revision of the manuscript. Jessica Rosenberg is a clinical expert and was involved in revising the manuscript. Frank Boers was responsible for the data acquisition and experimental setup and contributed to revising the manuscript. Karl-Josef Langen is a clinical and PET expert and was involved in the revision of the manuscript. Christian P. Filss is a clinical expert and was responsible for PET measurements. Norbert Galldiks is a neurological and clinical expert and was involved in examining the patient during the course of the study. Ralf Clauss is a neurological and clinical expert and was involved in clinical monitoring of the patient and writing and revision of the manuscript. N. Jon Shah is an MEG and MR expert and was involved in the revision of the manuscript. Jürgen Dammers is an MEG expert and was involved in study design and revision of the manuscript.

Acknowledgments

The authors would like to thank Andrea Muren for help with conducting the MEG measurements. The authors would also like to thank Markus Lang and Johannes Ermert for technical assistance in radiosynthesis of 11C-Flumazenil and Silke Frensch, Suzanne Schaden, Natalie Judov, and Kornelia Frey for technical assistance in performing the PET measurements.

References

[1] H. D. Langtry and P. Benfield, "Zolpidem," *Drugs*, vol. 40, no. 2, pp. 291–313, 1990.

[2] S. de Haas, R. Schoemaker, J. van Gerven, P. Hoever, A. Cohen, and J. Dingemanse, "Pharmacokinetics, pharmacodynamics and the pharmacokinetic/pharmacodynamic relationship of zolpidem in healthy subjects," *Journal of Psychopharmacology*, vol. 24, no. 11, pp. 1619–1629, 2010.

[3] A. Daniele, A. Albanese, G. Gainotti, B. Gregori, and P. Bartolomeo, "Zolpidem in Parkinson's disease," *The Lancet*, vol. 349, no. 9060, pp. 1222-1223, 1997.

[4] R. P. Clauss, W. M. Güldenpfennig, H. W. Nel, M. M. Sathekge, and R. R. Venkannagari, "Extraordinary arousal from semi-comatose state on zolpidem. A case report," *South African Medical Journal*, vol. 90, no. 1, pp. 68–72, 2000.

[5] C. Brefel-Courbon, P. Payoux, F. Ory et al., "Clinical and imaging evidence of zolpidem effect in hypoxic encephalopathy," *Annals of Neurology*, vol. 62, no. 1, pp. 102–105, 2007.

[6] S. I. Cohen and T. T. Duong, "Increased arousal in a patient with anoxic brain injury after administration of zolpidem," *American Journal of Physical Medicine & Rehabilitation*, vol. 87, no. 3, pp. 229–231, 2008.

[7] N. E. Nyakale, R. P. Clauss, H. W. Nel, and M. M. Sathekge, "Blood-brain barrier integrity in a zolpidem-responder patient," *South African Medical Journal*, vol. 102, no. 10, pp. 790-791, 2012.

[8] C. Machado, M. Estévez, R. Rodríguez et al., "Zolpidem arousing effect in persistent vegetative state patients: autonomic, EEG and behavioral assessment," *Current Pharmaceutical Design*, vol. 20, no. 26, pp. 4185–4202, 2014.

[9] B. Du, A. Shan, X. Zhong, Y. Zhang, D. Chen, and K. Cai, "Zolpidem arouses patients in vegetative state after brain injury: quantitative evaluation and indications," *The American Journal of the Medical Sciences*, vol. 347, no. 3, pp. 178–182, 2014.

[10] R. P. Clauss and W. H. Nel, "Effect of zolpidem on brain injury and diaschisis as detected by ^{99m}Tc HMPAO brain

SPECT in humans," *Arzneimittelforschung*, vol. 54, no. 10, pp. 641-646, 2004.

[11] M. N. Bomalaski, E. S. Claflin, W. Townsend, and M. D. Peterson, "Zolpidem for the treatment of neurologic disorders," *JAMA Neurology*, vol. 74, no. 9, p. 1130, 2017.

[12] S. Baillet, "Magnetoencephalography for brain electrophysiology and imaging," *Nature Neuroscience*, vol. 20, no. 3, pp. 327–339, 2017.

[13] S. Ge, T. Wu, X. Xiao, K. Iramina, and W. Wu, "Coherence analysis for epilepsy patients: an MEG study," *World Academy of Science, Engineering and Technology*, vol. 80, no. 8, pp. 517–519, 2011.

[14] C. R. Gillebert and D. Mantini, "Functional connectivity in the normal and injured brain," *The Neuroscientist*, vol. 19, no. 5, pp. 509–522, 2013.

[15] T. Montez, S.-S. Poil, B. F. Jones et al., "Altered temporal correlations in parietal alpha and prefrontal theta oscillations in early-stage Alzheimer disease," *Proceedings of the National Academy of Sciences*, vol. 106, no. 5, pp. 1614–1619, 2009.

[16] S. Khan, A. Gramfort, N. R. Shetty et al., "Local and long-range functional connectivity is reduced in concert in autism spectrum disorders," *Proceedings of the National Academy of Sciences*, vol. 110, no. 8, pp. 3107–3112, 2013.

[17] D. Nutt, S. Wilson, A. Lingford-Hughes, J. Myers, A. Papadopoulos, and S. Muthukumaraswamy, "Differences between magnetoencephalographic (MEG) spectral profiles of drugs acting on GABA at synaptic and extrasynaptic sites: a study in healthy volunteers," *Neuropharmacology*, vol. 88, pp. 155–163, 2015.

[18] S. D. Hall, N. Yamawaki, A. E. Fisher, R. P. Clauss, G. L. Woodhall, and I. M. Stanford, "GABA (A) alpha-1 subunit mediated desynchronization of elevated low frequency oscillations alleviates specific dysfunction in stroke—a case report," *Clinical Neurophysiology*, vol. 121, no. 4, pp. 549–555, 2010.

[19] S. T. Williams, M. M. Conte, A. M. Goldfine et al., "Common resting brain dynamics indicate a possible mechanism underlying zolpidem response in severe brain injury," *Elife*, vol. 2, Article ID e01157, 2013.

[20] L. Cohen, B. Chaaban, and M.-O. Habert, "Transient improvement of aphasia with zolpidem," *New England Journal of Medicine*, vol. 350, no. 9, pp. 950–952, 2004.

[21] R. S. Calabrò, I. Aricò, S. De Salvo, V. Conti-Nibali, and P. Bramanti, "Transient awakening from vegetative state: is high-dose zolpidem more effective?" *Psychiatry and Clinical Neurosciences*, vol. 69, no. 2, pp. 122-123, 2015.

[22] M. E. Machado and Calixto. Faan, "a Cuban perspective on management of persistent vegetative state," *MEDICC Review*, vol. 14, no. 1, pp. 44–48, 2012.

[23] J. Whyte and R. Myers, "Incidence of clinically significant responses to zolpidem among patients with disorders of consciousness," *American Journal of Physical Medicine & Rehabilitation*, vol. 88, no. 5, pp. 410–418, 2009.

[24] M. Vinck, R. Oostenveld, M. van Wingerden, F. Battaglia, and C. M. A. Pennartz, "An improved index of phase-synchronization for electrophysiological data in the presence of volume-conduction, noise and sample-size bias," *Neuroimage*, vol. 55, no. 4, pp. 1548–1565, 2011.

[25] F. I. Mahoney and D. W. Barthel, "Functional evaluation: the barthel index," *Maryland State Medical Journal*, vol. 14, pp. 61–65, 1965.

[26] M. E. Tinetti, D. Richman, and L. Powell, "Falls efficacy as a measure of fear of falling," *Journal of Gerontology*, vol. 45, no. 6, pp. P239–P243, 1990.

[27] C. Ramaker, J. Marinus, A. M. Stiggelbout, and B. J. van Hilten, "Systematic evaluation of rating scales for impairment and disability in Parkinson's disease," *Movement Disorders*, vol. 17, no. 5, pp. 867–876, 2002.

[28] E. Maris and R. Oostenveld, "Nonparametric statistical testing of EEG- and MEG-data," *Journal of Neuroscience Methods*, vol. 164, no. 1, pp. 177–190, 2007.

[29] R. S. Desikan et al., "An automated labeling system for subdividing the human cerebral cortex on MRI scans into gyral based regions of interest," *NeuroImage*, vol. 31, no. 3, pp. 968–980, 2006.

[30] A. Gramfort, "MEG and EEG data analysis with MNE-Python," *Frontiers in Neuroscience*, vol. 7, p. 267, 2013.

[31] S. C. Licata, L. D. Nickerson, S. B. Lowen, G. H. Trksak, R. R. MacLean, and S. E. Lukas, "The hypnotic zolpidem increases the synchrony of BOLD signal fluctuations in widespread brain networks during a resting paradigm," *Neuroimage*, vol. 70, pp. 211–222, 2013.

[32] J. C. Pang and P. A. Robinson, "Neural mechanisms of the EEG alpha-BOLD anticorrelation," *Neuroimage*, vol. 181, pp. 461–470, 2018.

[33] R. I. Goldman, J. M. Stern, J. Engel, and M. S. Cohen, "Simultaneous EEG and fMRI of the alpha rhythm," *Neuroreport*, vol. 13, no. 18, pp. 2487–2492, 2002.

[34] M. J. Brookes, M. Woolrich, H. Luckhoo et al., "Investigating the electrophysiological basis of resting state networks using magnetoencephalography," *Proceedings of the National Academy of Sciences*, vol. 108, no. 40, pp. 16783–16788, 2011.

[35] K. G. Lloyd and B. Zivkovic, "Specificity within the GABAA receptor supramolecular complex: a consideration of the new ω1-receptor selective imidazopyridine hypnotic zolpidem," *Pharmacology Biochemistry and Behavior*, vol. 29, no. 4, pp. 781–783, 1988.

[36] F. A. Nasrallah, K. K. D. O. R. Singh, L. Y. Yeow, and K.-H. Chuang, "GABAergic effect on resting-state functional connectivity: dynamics under pharmacological antagonism," *Neuroimage*, vol. 149, pp. 53–62, 2017.

[37] R. Clauss, "Disorders of consciousness and pharmaceuticals that act on oxygen based amino acid and monoamine neurotransmitter pathways of the brain," *Current Pharmaceutical Design*, vol. 999, no. 999, pp. 9-10, 2013.

[38] N. D. Schiff, "Recovery of consciousness after brain injury: a mesocircuit hypothesis," *Trends in Neurosciences*, vol. 33, no. 1, pp. 1–9, 2010.

[39] E. J. Prokic, C. Weston, N. Yamawaki et al., "Cortical oscillatory dynamics and benzodiazepine-site modulation of tonic inhibition in fast spiking interneurons," *Neuropharmacology*, vol. 95, pp. 192–205, 2015.

[40] C. R. Soldatos, D. G. Dikeos, and A. Whitehead, "Tolerance and rebound insomnia with rapidly eliminated hypnotics," *International Clinical Psychopharmacology*, vol. 14, no. 5, pp. 287–304, 1999.

[41] J. C. Ware, J. K. Walsh, M. B. Scharf, T. Roehrs, T. Roth, and G. W. Vogel, "Minimal rebound insomnia after treatment with 10-mg zolpidem," *Clinical Neuropharmacology*, vol. 20, no. 2, pp. 116–125, 1997.

[42] T. A. Roehrs, S. Randall, E. Harris, R. Maan, and T. Roth, "Twelve months of nightly zolpidem does not lead to rebound insomnia or withdrawal symptoms: a prospective placebo-controlled study," *Journal of Psychopharmacology*, vol. 26, no. 8, pp. 1088–1095, 2012.

[43] J. T. Povlishock and D. I. Katz, "Update of neuropathology and neurological recovery after traumatic brain injury," *Journal of Head Trauma Rehabilitation*, vol. 20, no. 1, pp. 76–94, 2005.
[44] J. D. Lewine, J. T. Davis, E. D. Bigler et al., "Objective documentation of traumatic brain injury subsequent to mild head trauma," *Journal of Head Trauma Rehabilitation*, vol. 22, no. 3, pp. 141–155, 2007.
[45] J. D. Lewine, J. T. Davis, J. H. Sloan, P. W. Kodituwakku, and W. W. Orrison Jr, "Neuromagnetic assessment of pathophysiologic brain activity induced by minor head trauma," *Am. J. American Journal of Neuroradiology*, vol. 20, no. 5, 1999.
[46] P. E. Tarapore, A. M. Findlay, S. C. LaHue et al., "Resting state magnetoencephalography functional connectivity in traumatic brain injury," *Journal of Neurosurgery*, vol. 118, no. 6, pp. 1306–1316, 2013.

40

Subcutaneous EEG Monitoring Reveals AED Response and Breakthrough Seizures

Sigge Weisdorf[1,2] **Ivan C. Zibrandtsen,**[1] **and Troels W. Kjaer**[1,2]

[1]*Zealand University Hospital, Department of Neurology, Roskilde, Denmark*
[2]*University of Copenhagen, Department of Clinical Medicine, Copenhagen, Denmark*

Correspondence should be addressed to Sigge Weisdorf; siggewe@gmail.com

Academic Editor: Massimiliano Filosto

Unrecognized seizures are a common problem in temporal lobe epilepsy potentially leading to undertreatment. Objective seizure counting using EEG home monitoring for prolonged periods with a minimally invasive device has not been feasible until now. We present a case in which a novel, subcutaneous EEG device was utilized to provide an objective seizure count. This information revealed unrecognized breakthrough seizures and informed treatment response, prompting treatment adjustment. The case illustrates how objective seizure counting in epilepsy using new devices can completely change diagnosis and management.

1. Introduction

For patients with epilepsy, self-monitoring of disease activity most commonly relies on a seizure diary. Seizure diaries mostly depend on input from the patient and therefore cannot account for any unrecognized seizures. Unrecognized seizures are a common problem in temporal lobe epilepsy (TLE) [1] and can obscure the true effect of antiepileptic drugs (AEDs). Objective seizure counting based on electroencephalography (EEG) can reveal unrecognized seizures, but until now, such monitoring has usually been performed during hospital admission, which is impractical and expensive, and can therefore only be performed for a limited time. A novel subcutaneous EEG device has been developed for EEG home monitoring. In a previously published proof-of-concept paper, we showed that the new device records clinically relevant potentials reliably compared to scalp EEG [2]. Here, we present a case in which EEG home monitoring reveals essential information on breakthrough seizures and AED response that would otherwise have remained unknown.

2. Case Presentation

A 42-year-old woman known with left-sided temporal lobe epilepsy (TLE) and seizure onset at the age of 18 was referred to the outpatient epilepsy clinic due to recurrence of seizures after two decades of seizure-free remission. She lived with her husband, who reported 1-2 seizures/month, but most of these seizures went unrecognized by herself. In addition, she frequently felt unrefreshed after sleep, possibly indicating that unrecognized seizures also occurred at night. Clinically, three different epileptic seizure types were described:

(1) Focal onset seizure with severely impaired awareness. Behavioral arrest, frequently accompanied by manual automatisms. Duration 30–60 seconds.
(2) Focal onset seizure with only slightly impaired awareness. Behavioral slowing, but not arrest. Inappropriate behavior.
(3) Type 1 or 2 seizure with progression to bilateral tonic-clonic seizure (BTCS).

In addition to her seizures, the patient also reported memory difficulties of increasing severity.

Brain MRI (1, 5T) showed an old lacunar infarct (1 cm^3) in the anterior part of the left external capsule but no abnormalities in the temporal regions. A previous EEG recorded in her youth suggested an epileptic focus in the left temporal region. Due to the suspicion of unrecognized seizures, she underwent repeated short admissions (up to four days) in an epilepsy monitoring unit (EMU). These investigations confirmed the left temporal epileptic focus and revealed that unrecognized seizures occurred.

Treatment with valproate, levetiracetam, and lacosamide was apparently without major effect on seizure frequency or severity.

A year later, the patient was enrolled in a research study testing a novel subcutaneous EEG device. At this point, she was treated with lacosamide (200 mg × 2) and add-on treatment with lamotrigine was commenced during the study. Written informed consent was obtained from the patient prior to inclusion to the study. The study was approved by the regional ethical committee.

The subcutaneous EEG device, described in more details here [2], consists of two main parts, the implanted electrode and an external logging device for battery and data logging. The electrode and external logging device communicate via a transceiver at either device. The subcutaneous electrode has three leads for recording (a proximal (P), a distal (D), and a reference (R) in between), providing two bipolar channels (P-R; D-R). It was implanted over the left temporal region in local anesthesia through a small incision behind the ear without complications. After implantation there was some mild self-limiting tenderness. The proximal electrode was positioned approximately at T7 and the distal electrode approximately at F7. The approximate position of the implanted electrode is illustrated in Figure 1.

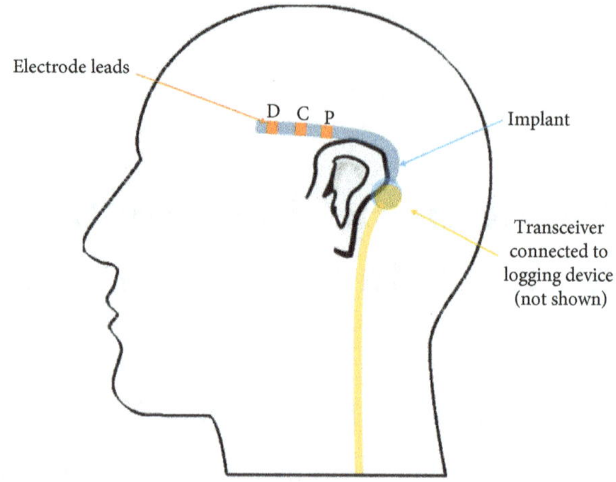

Figure 1: An illustration of the approximate position of the implanted electrode (blue) with the individual leads highlighted. The transceiver from the external logging device (orange) must be attached to the skin near the implanted electrode using double-sided glue pads.

The patient had the EEG device active for 76 days during which the actual usage was 63%. All recordings from the subcutaneous electrode was analyzed by an expert visual review of spectrograms using Nicolet Reader to identify electrographical seizures and these were compared to self-reported seizures from the patient's seizure diary. Candidate spectrographical seizure patterns were double-checked by an additional review in the time domain by a board-certified neurophysiologist. Due to the documented seizure unawareness, we regarded the electrographical seizures as the ground truth in this comparison. As such, any self-reported seizures without a corresponding electrographical seizure would be considered a false report. Figure 2 compares timing of self-reported and electrographic seizures and visualizes AED intake.

The EEG home monitoring revealed 16 electrographical seizures with three different seizure patterns well in line with the reported seizure types. None of the electrographical seizures were reported by the patient, including the seizures progressing to bilateral tonic-clonic seizures (BTCS). However, she reported two events with no corresponding electrographical seizures.

3. Discussion

The case exemplifies a situation where there is an important discrepancy between self-reported seizure counts and objective seizure counts, where the pattern of self-reported counts lead to an interpretation of inefficacy of lamotrigine whereas the objective seizure counts suggest a positive effect of lamotrigine add-on therapy. Figure 2 shows that the frequency of electrographical seizures seems to decrease as the dose of lamotrigine is increased. This hypothesis is weakened by the fact that only a single seizure occurs after permanent discontinuation of lamotrigine, but only approximately one week off lamotrigine was monitored. Regardless of the efficacy of add-on lamotrigine, the possible effect is not evident from the self-reported seizures at all. This case study highlights the pitfalls of basing decisions on self-reported information. With objective seizure quantification, a completely different picture of response to medication emerges that would otherwise have remained hidden. This suggests important advantages of ultralong-term monitoring for objective seizure counting in the management of epilepsy.

Figure 2 also informs on the relation between missed AED doses and breakthrough seizures. Qualitatively, there seems to be a tendency towards breakthrough seizures within a few days of a missed dose. Our dataset does not allow for proper testing of this hypothesis. Nonetheless, the data demonstrate that the continuous EEG monitoring enables such investigations, given enough events. However, it is unsurprising that missed AED doses could precipitate breakthrough seizures. The subcutaneous EEG device, however, offers a quantification of the problem based on an objective seizure count, making the results more reliable and reproducible.

The detection of BTCS is of particular interest to physicians and patients alike, as these seizures have the highest risk of secondary injuries and sudden unexplained death in epilepsy (SUDEP) [3] and a greater impact on life quality [4]. These factors often warrant more aggressive treatment of BTCS. Our dataset contained two BTCS. We used a slightly modified version of a method previously described [5] to investigate if the subcutaneous EEG recording contains enough seizure-related EMG activity to form the basis for a simple tonic-clonic seizure detection algorithm. We calculated the root mean square (RMS) within 4-second windows across a six-hour recording containing the two BTCS (Figure 3). Cooccurrence of the RMS peaks with the BTCS

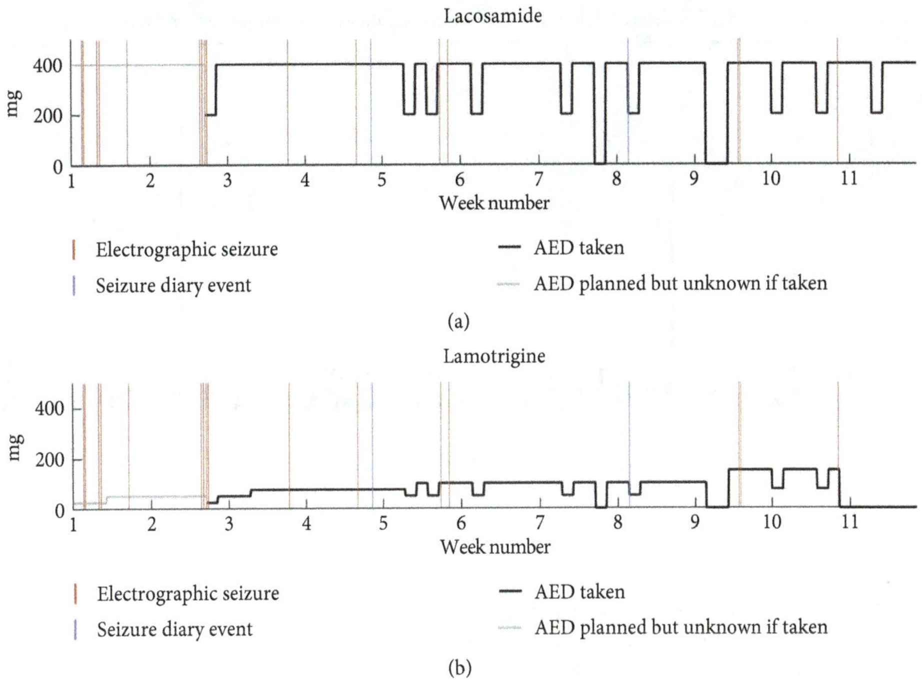

FIGURE 2: Overview of the monitoring period AED dosages plotted over time for lacosamide (a) and lamotrigine (b). Solid black line is the daily dose taken. It can drop 50% or 100% on some days indicating one or two missed doses. It is greyed out when no information about the dose taken was available. Red vertical lines indicate electrographical seizure. The two first seizures were focal to bilateral tonic-clonic seizures. Blue vertical lines indicate a patient event diary entry. These two do not overlap with any of the electroencephalographic seizures.

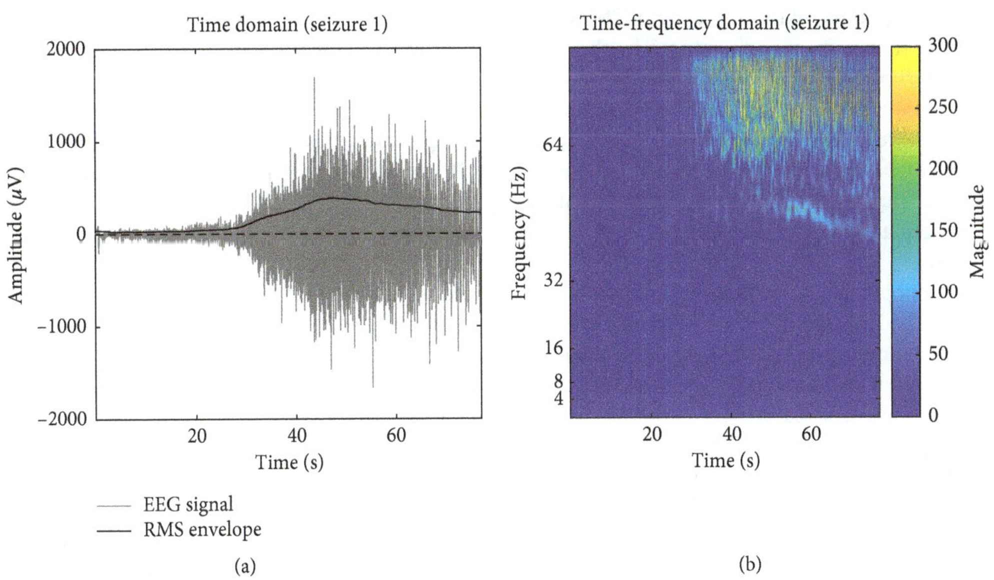

FIGURE 3: Continued.

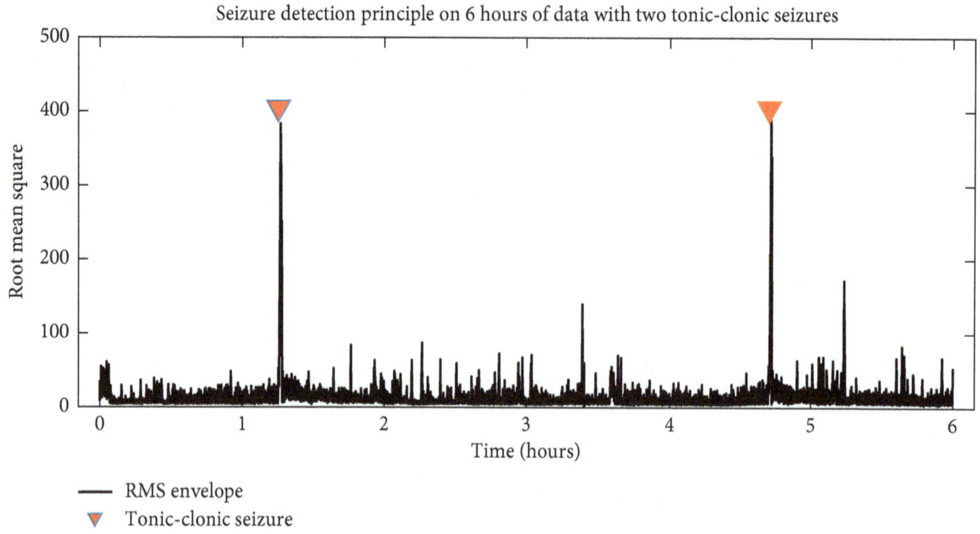

(c)

Figure 3: Detection of BTCS. (a) shows 80 seconds of a BTCS in the time domain. Superpositioned on the EEG signal, the bold black line shows the root mean square (RMS) envelope, which increases during the tonic-clonic phase of the seizure. (b) shows the time-frequency decomposition from a continuous wavelet transform of the same seizure. During the tonic-clonic phase, a high-frequency component can be observed, approaching the Nyquist frequency of the device (103.5 Hz). (c) shows the RMS envelope of a six-hour epoch containing two BTCS indicated with red triangles. The RMS shows an abrupt increase only in close relation to these seizures, providing proof-of-concept that the device can be used for the detection of BTCS.

events demonstrates that it was possible to identify BTCS using this method using simple thresholding. Tonic-clonic seizures, presumably regardless of focal or generalized onset, have very stereotypical and specific signatures in the time domain as has been shown in previous studies [6]. As we observe a similar signature, we can reasonably infer that the seizure event has a tonic-clonic component.

This is a promising basis for the use of the subcutaneous electrode for BTCS detection. A reliable differentiation between focal seizures and BTCS is an important piece of clinical information.

Temporal lobe epilepsy (TLE) is the most common type of focal onset epilepsies in adults [7]. Typical temporal lobe seizure semiology includes speech arrest, impaired awareness, automatisms, and a wide array of other features [8]. Impaired awareness during seizures increases the risk of unrecognized seizure and resulting under-reporting. This may lead to insufficient treatment and risk of additional seizures. Impaired awareness is frequent in temporal lobe epilepsy [1, 9], so while there is nothing unusual about our patient's problem, the solution is extraordinary. Using ultralong-term EEG home monitoring we have provided an example on the advantage of objective vs. subjective seizure quantification and how this can inform management. While the EEG monitoring allowed us to record many electrographical seizures, it also holds its own issues. In our single case, the electrographical seizures were identified by an expert visual review, which is prohibitively resource demanding for routine use of such monitoring. Implementation of long-term monitoring in clinical practice will therefore require automated seizure detection algorithms. We propose that the subcutaneous EEG device would be a well-tolerated platform to acquire data for such automated methods, as it offers the ability to obtain large amounts of data from single individuals, providing a solid basis for personalized algorithms. Evidence that seizure signatures appear unaffected by time, AED changes, and recording modality is important for the seizure detection algorithm design strategies. In a paper from 2017, Zibrandtsen et al. [10] proposed that personalized algorithms could take advantage of within subject seizure stereotopy. Figure 4 shows a comparison between two seizures recorded from the patient. One was recorded with the subcutaneous electrode and the other was recorded with scalp EEG one year before. A distinct spectrographical pattern (a "signature") is clearly present in both recordings.

For now, identification of focal seizures relies on an expert review of the data. In the future, this will be assisted by a software solution to identify rhythmic patterns for manual review, significantly decreasing the time needed to review ultralong-term recordings.

The novel device presented in this case does have some limitations. The limited spatial coverage resulting from the small size could lead to seizures from a contralateral seizure focus going undetected, resulting in false negatives. Due to the proximity of the device to the temporal muscle, false negatives could also occur in situations with high muscle activity, e.g., in hyperkinetic seizures. Such activity would cause EMG noise, possibly obscuring electrographical seizure patterns. Rhythmic noise and artifacts, whatever the cause, generally do not look like seizures, so overinterpretation resulting in false positives is less likely, if the reviewer is experienced. Video monitoring would have been helpful in revealing cases of false negative and/or positive seizures,

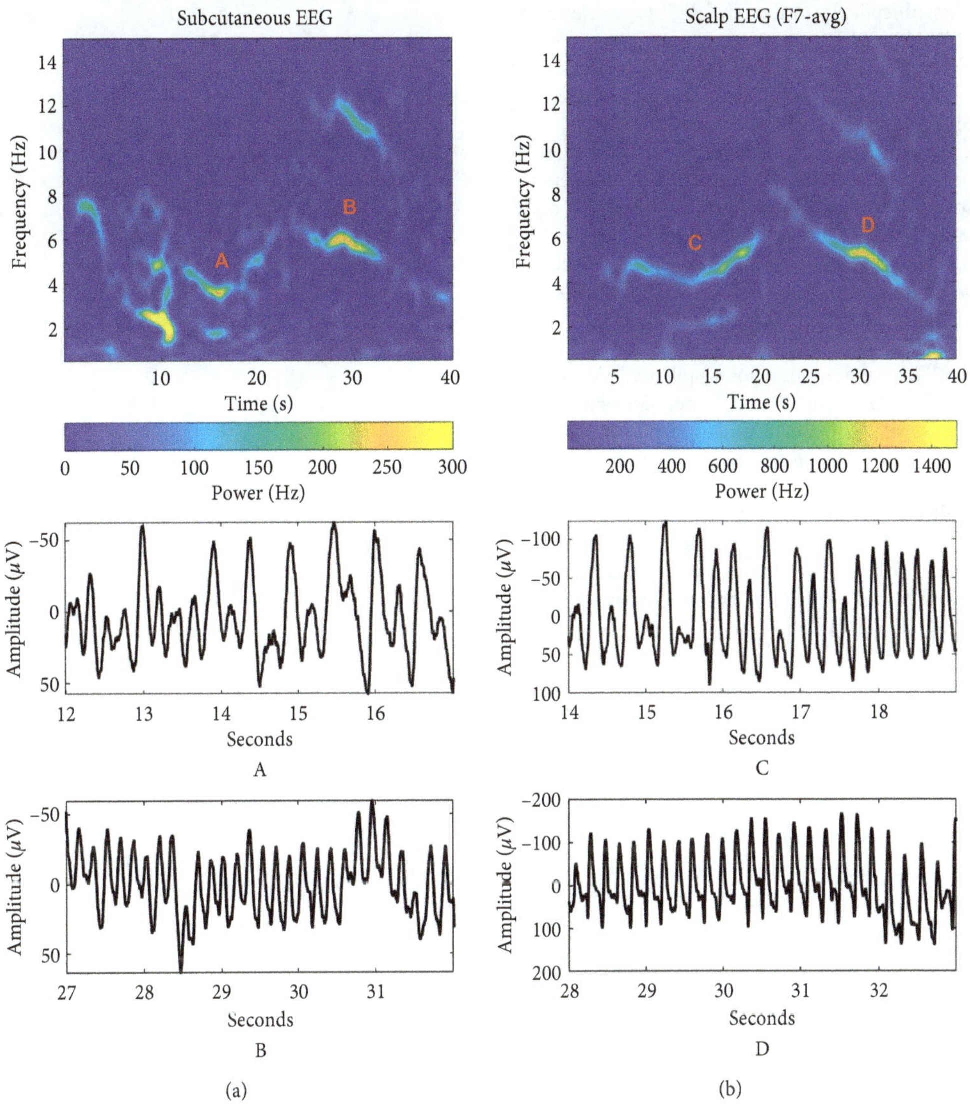

FIGURE 4: Persistent seizure signature. Comparison of two focal seizures recorded with one year in between from subcutaneous EEG (a) and scalp EEG (b). Time-frequency-power plots of 40 seconds are shown in the top. We see the same overall frequency dynamics between the two, but the subcutaneous device records with lower power and the seizure has more mixed frequencies in the early part. For each seizure, the letters designate different time-domain magnifications shown below for approximately the same corresponding part of the spectrographical signature. At around 15 seconds, 4-5 Hz activity can be observed. Around 30 seconds, 5-6 Hz activity with a sharper morphology in the time-domain is visible, mirrored by the higher-frequency subharmonic visible in this part of the spectrum.

but continuous video monitoring during daily life is neither achievable nor ethical.

In conclusion, this clinical case presents a scenario where the subcutaneous EEG provided a completely different picture of responsiveness to medication compared to seizure diaries, which could lead to a different conclusion about efficacy of add-on AED therapy. A wider use of this technology in clinical practice depends on the development of accurate seizure detection algorithms. We expect that this device and others like it will play a growing role in future epilepsy management.

References

[1] C. Hoppe, A. Poepel, and C. E. Elger, "Epilepsy: accuracy of patient seizure counts," *Archives of Neurology*, vol. 64, no. 11, pp. 1595–1599, 2007.

[2] S. Weisdorf, S. W. Gangstad, J. Duun-Henriksen, K. S. S. Mosholt, and T. W. Kjær, "High similarity between EEG from subcutaneous and proximate scalp electrodes in patients with temporal lobe epilepsy," *Journal of Neurophysiology*, vol. 120, no. 3, pp. 1451–1460, 2018.

[3] D. C. Hesdorffer, T. Tomson, E. Benn et al., "Do antiepileptic drugs or generalized tonic-clonic seizure frequency increase SUDEP risk? A combined analysis," *Epilepsia*, vol. 53, no. 2, pp. 249–252, 2012.

[4] A. Ring, A. Jacoby, G. Baker et al., "What really matters? A mixed methods study of treatment preferences and priorities

among people with epilepsy in the UK," *Epilepsy & Behavior*, vol. 95, pp. 181–191, 2019.

[5] I. C. Zibrandtsen, P. Kidmose, and T. W. Kjaer, "Detection of generalized tonic-clonic seizures from ear-EEG based on EMG analysis," *Seizure*, vol. 59, pp. 54–59, 2018.

[6] S. Beniczky, I. Conradsen, R. Pressler, and P. Wolf, "Quantitative analysis of surface electromyography: biomarkers for convulsive seizures," *Clinical Neurophysiology*, vol. 127, no. 8, pp. 2900–2907, 2016.

[7] J. F. Téllez-Zenteno and L. Hernández-Ronquillo, "A review of the epidemiology of temporal lobe epilepsy," *Epilepsy Research and Treatment*, vol. 2012, Article ID 630853, 5 pages, 2012.

[8] W. O. Tatum, "Mesial temporal lobe epilepsy," *Journal of Clinical Neurophysiology*, vol. 29, no. 5, pp. 356–365, 2012.

[9] D. E. Blum, J. Eskola, J. J. Bortz, and R. S. Fisher, "Patient awareness of seizures," *Neurology*, vol. 47, no. 1, pp. 260–264, 1996.

[10] I. C. Zibrandtsen, P. Kidmose, C. B. Christensen, and T. W. Kjaer, "Ear-EEG detects ictal and interictal abnormalities in focal and generalized epilepsy-a comparison with scalp EEG monitoring," *Clinical Neurophysiology*, vol. 128, no. 12, pp. 2454–2461, 2017.

41

Winging of Scapula due to a Sinister Etiology

Shania Niromi Gunasekera, Priyanka Yogananda, Harindra Karunatilaka, and Bimsara Senanayake

National Hospital of Sri Lanka, Colombo, Sri Lanka

Correspondence should be addressed to Shania Niromi Gunasekera; shania.g89@gmail.com

Academic Editor: Mehmet Turgut

Background. Scapular winging is a rare but disabling deformity, which is commonly caused by lesions of the long thoracic and spinal accessory nerves that innervate the serratus anterior and trapezius muscles, respectively. Across the literature, traumatic injury to the nerves account for the majority of cases. Less common, nontraumatic causes include viral illness, neuroinflammatory conditions, toxins, compressive lesions, and C7 radiculopathy. We present a case where an apical lung malignancy causes winging of scapula by infiltrating C5–C7 roots of brachial plexus, which has been reported only once in the literature. *Case.* A 54-year-old male presented with recent onset painful difficulty in raising his right arm. He had no respiratory or constitutional symptoms. On examination, winging of scapula on the right side was noted with wasting and fasciculation involving the ipsilateral shoulder girdle. Proximal muscle power of the right upper limb was of 3/5 with preserved distal muscle power. No sensory loss was noted. A patch of bronchial breathing was found in the upper zone of the right lung with multiple hard cervical lymphadenopathies. Chest X-ray and contrast-enhanced computerized tomography-chest revealed a large tumor in the upper lobe of the right lung, which was confirmed to be a carcinoma of the lung. Electromyogram revealed large motor unit potentials and poor activation of right serratus anterior and internal scapulae muscles, while nerve conduction studies concluded the presence of a compressive lesion involving C5–C7 nerve roots of brachial plexus. Histology of a biopsy of the cervical lymph node confirmed metastasis from a poorly differentiated adenocarcinoma of the lung. The patient denied further investigation with MRI cervical spine. He was transferred to the cancer institute for further treatment. *Conclusion.* This case highlights the value of considering a compressive lung pathology with infiltration in the differential diagnosis, when evaluating winging of scapula.

1. Introduction

Scapular winging is a disabling deformity caused by lesions of the long thoracic and spinal accessory nerves that innervate the serratus anterior and trapezius muscles, respectively [1]. Rarely, it can be caused by damage to the dorsal scapular nerve which innervates the rhomboid muscle [1]. The spinal accessory nerve is the XIth cranial nerve, while the long thoracic and dorsal scapular nerves originate from the cervical nerve roots, C5, 6, and 7, and C4, 5, and 6, respectively. Traumatic damage to these nerves causing neuropraxia accounts for the majority of the cases of scapular winging [2].

Apical lung tumors produce various neurological manifestations owing to its local infiltration or paraneoplastic effects. Reported cases of winging of scapula as the initial mode of presentation of an apical lung malignancy are extremely rare [3]. We present a case where an apical lung malignancy is manifested as winging of the ipsilateral scapula, by the infiltration of C5–C7 roots of the brachial plexus.

2. Case

A 54-year-old man presented with gradual onset slowly progressive weakness of the right arm over a period of 2 months. Weakness was preceded by pain in the right shoulder region which radiated down the right arm. Pain was present even at rest. Weakness was predominant in the proximal muscles of the right upper limb, with preserved fine movements of the right hand. He denied a sensory loss

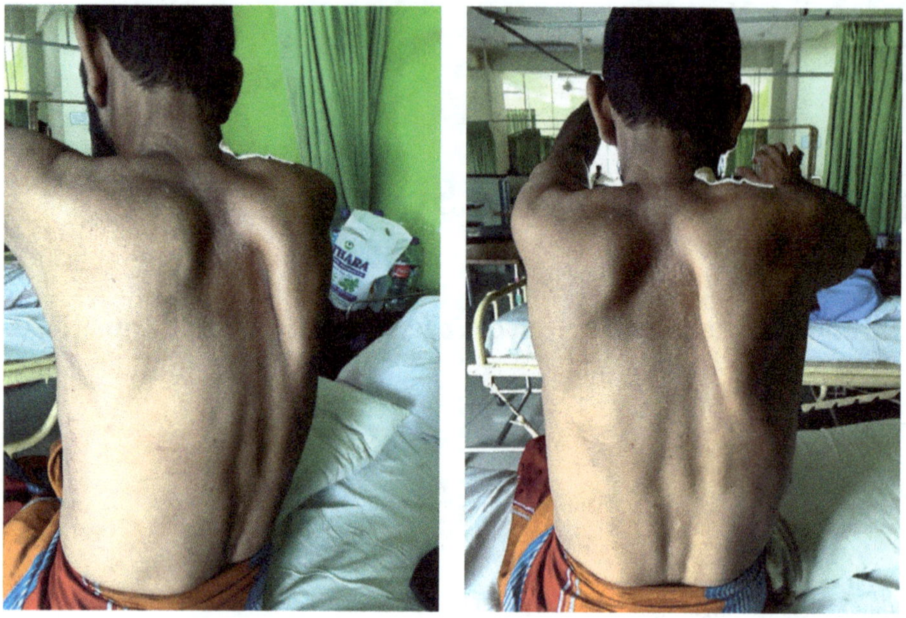

(a) (b)

Figure 1: Winging of scapula. (a) Winging of the right scapula posteriorly (lateral view). (b) Winging of the right scapula (posterior view).

involving the affected limb. His left upper limb and both the lower limbs were normal with regard to the power and sensation. He did not have dysphagia, dysarthria, diplopia, or unsteadiness. His higher functions were intact. He did not report any fever, loss of appetite or weight, chronic cough, or hemoptysis. There was no recent history of trauma. He was not a smoker and neither did he consume any illicit drugs.

On examination, enlarged, multiple, hard, and fixed lymph nodes were noted in right supraclavicular fossa and anterior triangle of the neck. There was no finger clubbing. Wasting and fasciculation were observed in the muscles of the shoulder girdle and proximal part of the right upper limb, sparing forearm, and the hand muscles. Proximal muscle power was of 3/5 with preserved distal power. Posterior winging of the right scapula was noted, which became more prominent up on pushing against resistance (Figures 1(a) and 1(b)). Rest of the examination including voice, cranial nerves, pupils, contralateral upper limb, and lower limbs was normal. Bronchial breathing was heard in the upper zone of the right lung, with trachea slightly deviated to the opposite side.

The electromyography (EMG) revealed large motor unit potentials with increasing amplitude and duration and poor activation of right serratus anterior and internal scapulae muscles. The nerve conduction studies (NCS) suggested a compressive lesion involving C5–C7 nerve roots of the brachial plexus. The chest radiograph revealed a large homogenous opacity involving the right apical region (Figure 2).

Subsequent contrast-enhanced computerized tomography (CECT) showed an ill-defined enhancing malignant lesion, obliterating the right upper bronchus, right upper lobe, pulmonary artery, and pleura (Figure 3). Probable stage was IV (T4N3M1a). Enlarged necrotic lymph nodes were seen in the mediastinum, with some in the right supraclavicular fossa. Histology and immunohistochemistry (Figure 4) of a cervical lymph node revealed metastatic deposits from a poorly differentiated carcinoma, most probably of pulmonary origin.

At bronchoscopy, right upper bronchus was seen to be completely obstructed by a tumor with endobronchial invasion. The histology (Figure 5) and immunohistochemistry from the tissue obtained by bronchoscopy confirmed a poorly differentiated adenocarcinoma of the lung. Magnetic resonant imaging (MRI) of cervical spine was planned, but the patient refused to undergo further investigation.

3. Discussion

Scapular winging is a disabling condition that hinders the ability to lift, pull, and push against objects. Winging of scapula results from paralysis of the muscles that keeps the scapula anchored to the chest wall. The commonest cause of scapular winging is isolated serratus anterior muscle (SAM) paralysis [2]. Long thoracic nerve (LTN) innervates the serratus anterior muscle. Due to its lengthy course and superficial location, LTN is susceptible to blunt and penetrating trauma [3]. The causes of nontraumatic injury to the LTN include viral infections such as poliomyelitis, drugs, exposure to toxins (herbicides and tetanus antitoxin), muscular dystrophies (fascio-scapulo-humeral dystrophy), C7 radiculopathy, and aortic coarctation [1]. Iatrogenic causes such as thoracotomies for lung or cardiac surgeries, hematomas secondary to anticoagulation therapy, are also identified as causes of SAM palsy [3].

An apical lung malignancy causing scapular winging has been reported only once in the literature [3]. In the case reported by Toshkezi et al., apart from the winging scapula,

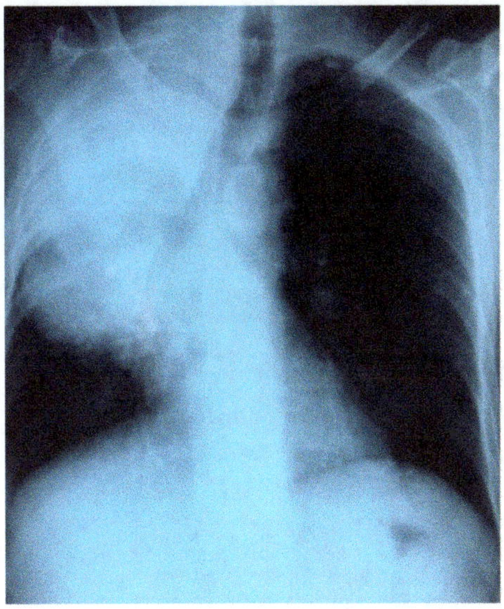

FIGURE 2: Chest radiograph—posterior-anterior view—right side apical ill-defined mass causing tracheal deviation to opposite side.

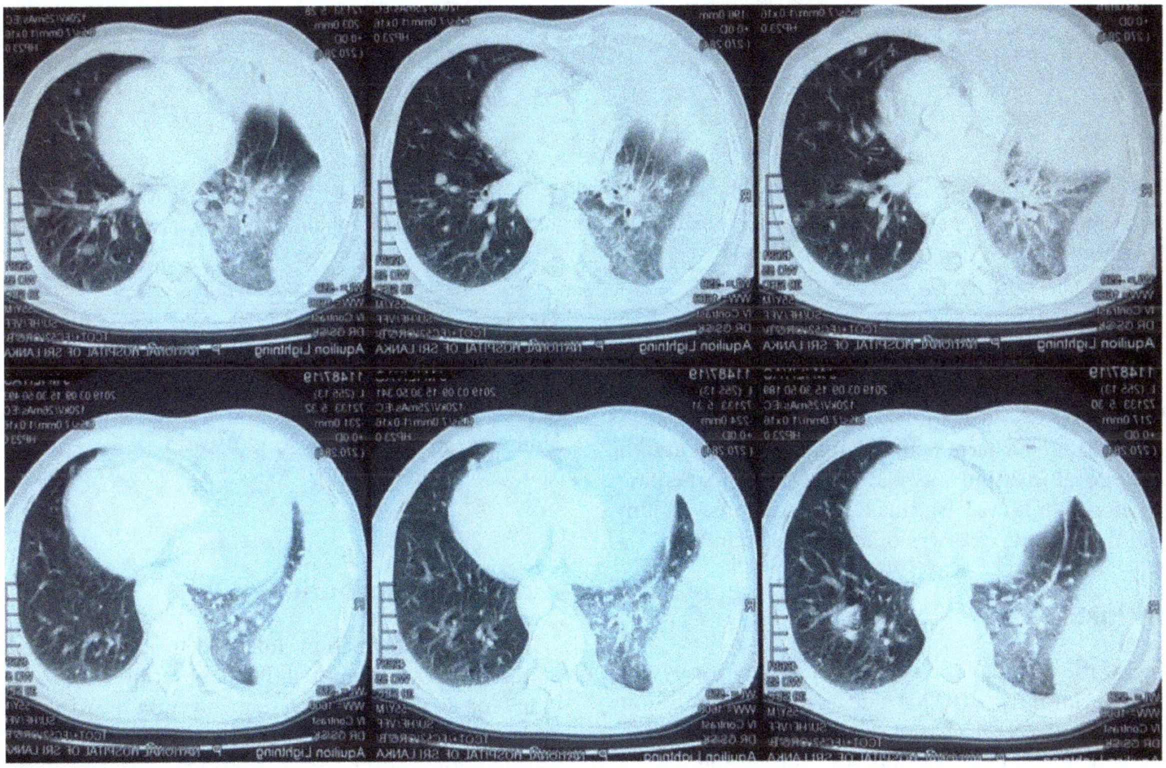

FIGURE 3: CECT chest—ill-defined enhancing malignant lesion—obliterating the right upper bronchus, right upper lobe, pulmonary artery, and pleura.

the patient also had Horner's syndrome, which is a recognized neurological manifestation of Pancoast tumors. This would have been a clue to suspect an infiltrative pathology as the cause for the LTN palsy. But ours is a case where an apical lung malignancy caused ipsilateral winging of scapula, in the absence of any other typical neurological manifestations of a Pancoast tumor, such as hoarse voice and Horner's syndrome, which are due to the involvement of recurrent laryngeal nerve and sympathetic trunk, respectively. Neither did he have any signs of compression or infiltration of the middle and lower trunks of the brachial plexus, such as pain irradiating to the upper limb or small muscle wasting of the hand [4].

The respiratory symptoms such as cough or hemoptysis are uncommon at the initial stages of apical lung neoplasms due to its peripheral location [4]. Apart from bronchial breathing heard at auscultation and cervical lymphadenopathy, a lung malignancy was not suspected as a cause for

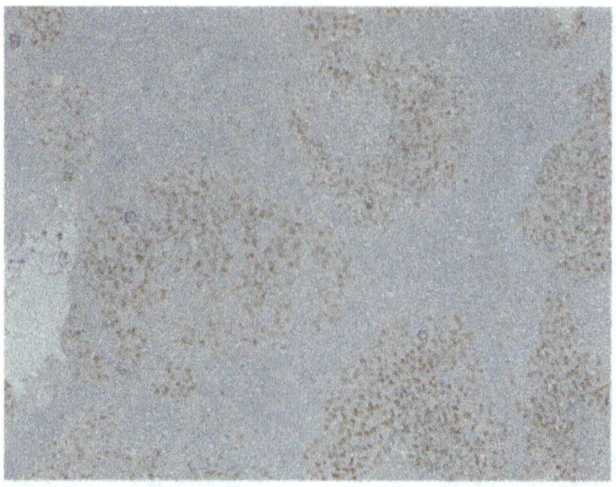

Figure 4: Immunohistochemistry of lymph node biopsy is positive for thyroid transcription factor 1 (TTF-1) confirming metastasis from an adenocarcinoma of lung.

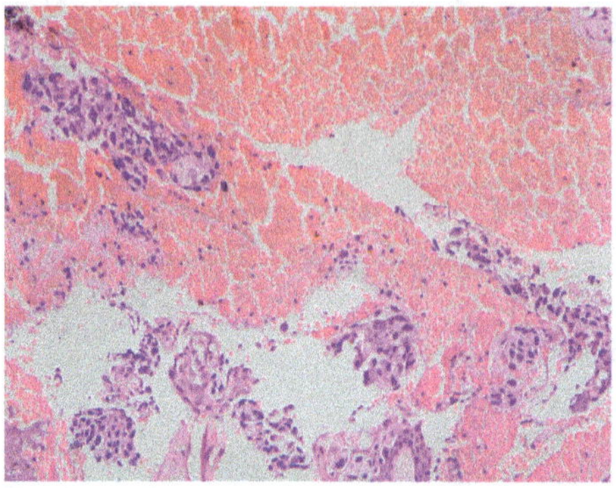

Figure 5: Histology of the biopsy taken from—endobronchial tumor at bronchoscopy—atypical cell clusters with oval and polygonal cells mixed with blood. Cells contain enlarged, hyperchromatic, pleomorphic nuclei and eosinophilic cytoplasm, and prominent nucleoli, compatible with adenocarcinoma of lung (H&E stain ×100).

winging of scapula, at the initial evaluation. Apical tumors can easily be missed on plain radiographs in the early course of the disease, as they might be hidden behind the clavicle and the first rib. CT and MR images would be useful to assess the local spread to adjacent neurovascular structures and the spine. The local invasion was classically seen in squamous cell carcinoma, followed by small cell carcinoma of lung, although the current case was of an adenocarcinoma [5].

4. Conclusion

Wingi of the scapula is commonly caused by paralysis of serratus anterior muscle (SAM), due to an injury to the long thoracic nerve (LTN) or its nerve roots.

This case highlights the value of considering a compressive lung pathology with infiltration in the differential diagnosis, when evaluating winging of the scapula.

Consent

Informed written consent for publishing the patient's details including the photos, in the journal, was obtained and is available for the perusal of the editors upon request.

Disclosure

The abstract of this case was presented as a poster presentation at XXIV World Congress of Neurology held in Dubai, United Arab of Emirates, in 2019.

Authors' Contributions

SG collected information, followed up the patient, did literature review, and drafted the manuscript. PY analyzed the lung biopsy. BS and HK were involved in the diagnosis and management of the patient and preparing the manuscript. All the authors read and approved the final manuscript.

Acknowledgments

The authors would like to acknowledge the patient who gave full support in collecting information and pictures to be published.

References

[1] R. M. Martin and D. E. Fish, "Scapular winging: anatomical review, diagnosis, and treatments," *Current Reviews in Musculoskeletal Medicine*, vol. 1, no. 1, pp. 1–11, 2007.

[2] B. W. Gooding, J. M. Geoghegan, W. A. Wallace, and P. A. Manning, "Scapular winging," *Shoulder Elbow*, vol. 6, no. 1, pp. 4–11, 2013.

[3] G. Toshkezi, J. Dejesus, J. F. Jabre, A. Hohler, and K. Davies, "Long thoracic neuropathy caused by an apical pulmonary tumor: case report," *Journal of Neurosurgery*, vol. 110, no. 4, pp. 754–757, 2009.

[4] N. Panagopoulos, V. Leivaditis, E. Koletsis et al., "Pancoast tumors: characteristics and preoperative assessment," *Journal of Thoracic Disease*, vol. 6, no. Suppl 1(Suppl 1), pp. S108–S115, 2014.

[5] M. Ghaffarpour, S. Firouzbakhsh, H. G. Omrani, and B. Mansoorian, "Neurologic manifestations as the presenting symptoms in lung cancer," *Acta Medica Iranica*, vol. 40, no. 3, pp. 198–202, 2002.

42

Cauda Canis: Variation of a Tinel's Sign for a Sciatic Nerve Tumor

Keith George[1] **Shane Burke**[1] **Knarik Arkun**[1,2] **and Ron Riesenburger**[1]

[1]*Department of Neurosurgery, Tufts Medical Center, 800 Washington Street, Boston 02111, MA, USA*
[2]*Department of Pathology, Tufts Medical Center, 800 Washington Street, Boston 02111, MA, USA*

Correspondence should be addressed to Keith George; keith.george@tufts.edu

Academic Editor: Mehmet Turgut

A patient with a prior history of intradural schwannoma and disc herniation presented with radicular pain after being hit in the thigh by a dog's tail. She was worked up and found to have a tumor of her right sciatic nerve. The tumor was resected and histology was consistent with schwannoma. The dog's tail acted as a Tinel's sign maneuver and led to timely identification of her peripheral nerve tumor. Peripheral nerve schwannomas can present in unusual forms, and Tinel's maneuver may be a useful tool in diagnosis.

1. Introduction

Radicular pain in patients undergoing neurosurgical evaluation can be attributed to a variety of causes. A majority of these causes include pathology at the spinal level, principally disc herniation, spinal stenosis, and degenerative changes leading to bone spurs [1]. However, alternative peripheral causes of radicular pain should also be considered part of the full workup. We present an interesting case and the first of its kind, where a woman was found to have a tumor of her sciatic nerve after she was hit in her thigh by a dog's tail (cauda canis translates to dog's tail in Latin) and subsequently developed radicular pain.

2. Case Presentation

A 57-year-old female, with a prior history of intradural L2 lumbar schwannoma that was resected 7 years ago, presented with right leg pain that radiated into her lateral leg, down to her ankle and big toe. A year prior to her current visit, she was found to have an L4-L5 herniated disc with right-sided radiculopathy and deferred surgical intervention, and improved with conservative measures. After some time, she was hit in the back of her right thigh by the tail of a Labrador dog, and she buckled and noticed severe electric pain shooting down her leg, akin to a Tinel's sign finding. The pain occasionally awakened her and was worse when she sat and improved with activity. She did not endorse a personal history or family history of neurofibromatosis. Physical exam was notable for 4/5 strength in her right anterior tibialis, 4/5 right extensor hallucis longus, decreased sensation to the lateral aspect of the right ankle, and positive Tinel's sign on the posterior thigh. An MRI of the right thigh showed a tumor along the right sciatic nerve, 3 cm in size (Figure 1).

A preoperative ultrasound was obtained to help localize the tumor for surgery. Ultrasound showed the center of the mass 17 cm rostral to the skin crease of the popliteal fossa, with the caudal section of the mass 16 cm from the crease and the rostral portion 18.5 cm from the crease.

During the procedure, the patient was placed prone, and an intraoperative ultrasound confirmed that the tumor was 18 cm from the popliteal fossa (Figure 2). An incision was made along the right posterior thigh, and muscle was dissected until the sciatic nerve tumor was exposed. Intraoperative electromyography (EMG) monitoring was used to delineate tumor versus intact nerve. A section of tumor was sent for pathology, and the tumor was histologically confirmed to be a schwannoma (Figures 3 and 4). Debulking was avascular, and the tumor was excised from the nerve, with minimal fascicle loss (Figure 5). The patient woke without a deficit. The patient recovered well postoperatively with no complications. She was followed up for six weeks after the surgery and was found to have an improvement in

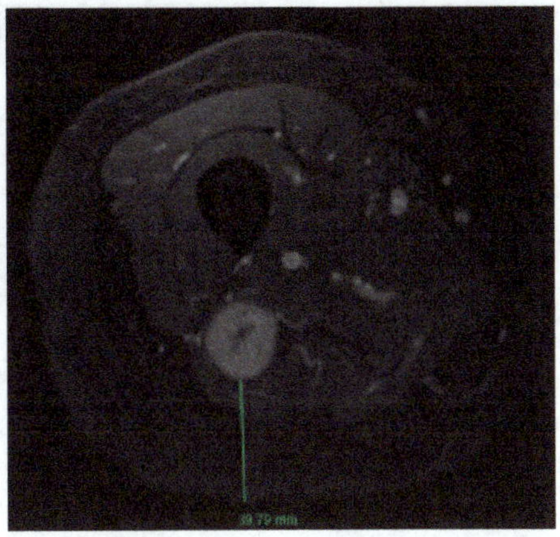

FIGURE 1: MRI axial showing right sciatic nerve tumor, 4 cm from the skin.

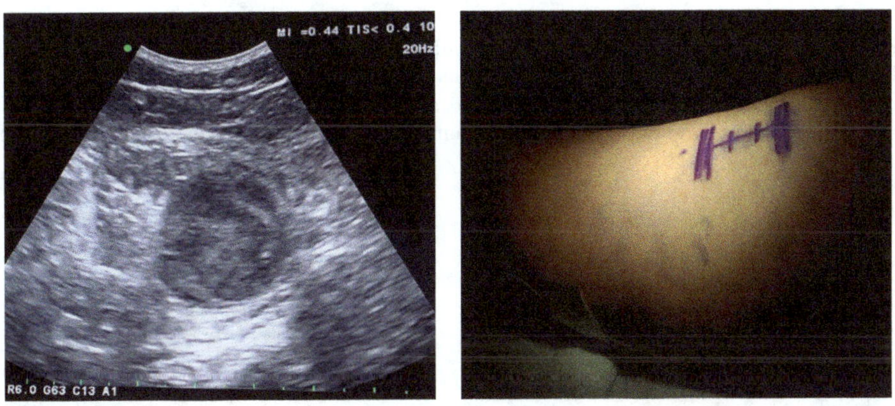

(a) (b)

FIGURE 2: (a) Intraoperative ultrasound localizing tumor. (b) Planned incision along the right posterior thigh.

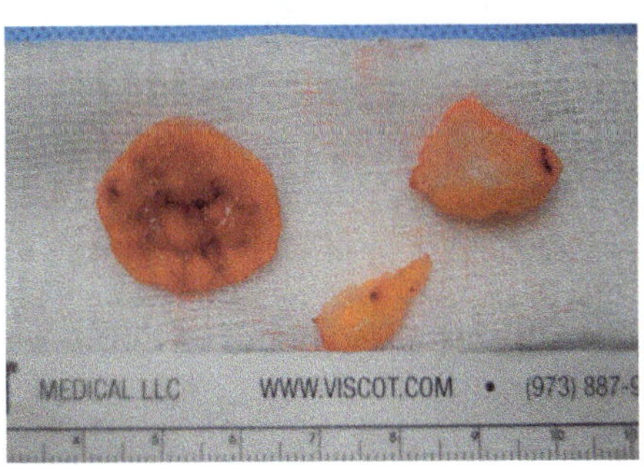

FIGURE 3: Gross specimen of schwannoma.

symptoms, with good healing of her surgical incision and 5/5 strength bilaterally in her lower extremities.

3. Discussion

This is a unique case of an underlying tumor being suspected through a patient's physical contact with a dog's tail (cauda canis sign), and the first of such a case to our knowledge. The dog's tail whipping against the posterior thigh and the resultant electric radiating pain the patient experienced can be related to a positive Tinel's sign, which was reproducible on exam. The radicular pain likely arises from the tumor impinging on the sciatic nerve. Other cases of sciatic nerve schwannomas associated with Tinel's sign have been described in the literature [2–4]. Kralick et al. describe a similar case where a patient shared similar symptoms and had difficulty sitting or lying in bed and also had a positive Tinel's sign on physical exam. Initial radiographic studies could not identify a source for the radicular pain, and as a result of the Tinel's sign, a lower extremity MRI was obtained that captured the tumor, allowing the patient to be adequately treated. In our case, the patient's presentation could have initially been attributed to a recurrence of her prior L4-L5 disc herniation. Were it not for the positive Tinel's sign as a result of the dog's tail, there could have been a delay in identifying the true cause of the patient's symptoms.

Histological analysis showed the tumor to be a schwannoma, with characteristic Antoni A and Antoni B patterns, along with the presence of Verocay bodies. Schwannomas are encapsulated nerve sheath tumors of Schwann cells. They are the most common form of peripheral nerve tumor, accounting for about 35% of all benign peripheral nerve sheath tumors [5–7]. Despite this, involvement of the sciatic nerve is still rare, typically less than 1% of cases [8].

Given her history of a prior schwannoma that was intradural, the patient could have an underlying pathology. A population-based study found that 90% of schwannomas

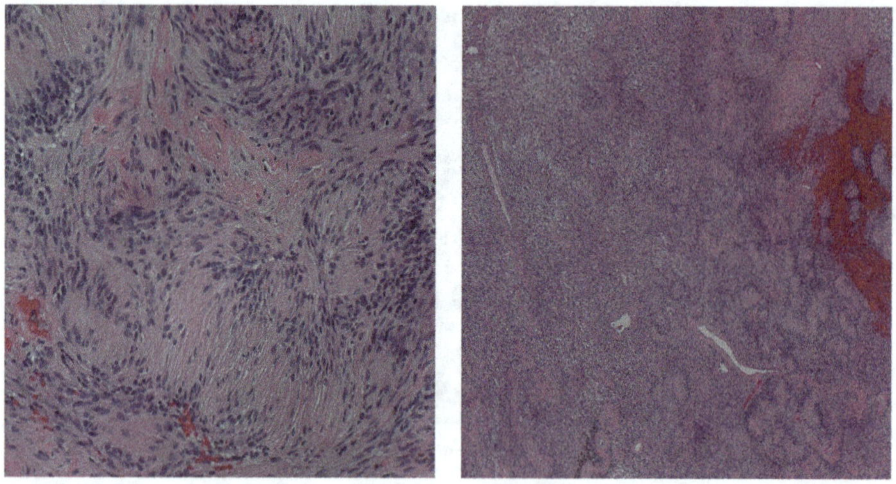

(a) (b)

FIGURE 4: (a) H&E high magnification (X200) of Antoni A area with Verocay bodies formation. (b) H&E low magnification (X40) of biphasic spindle cell lesion with cellular Antoni A areas and numerous Verocay bodies formation on the right, along with many hyalinized vessels and fresh hemorrhage, characteristic of schwannoma. Hypocellular area with looser stroma or Antoni B pattern is on the left. Pigment laden macrophages are present around vessels at the bottom of the image, representing evidence of old microbleed.

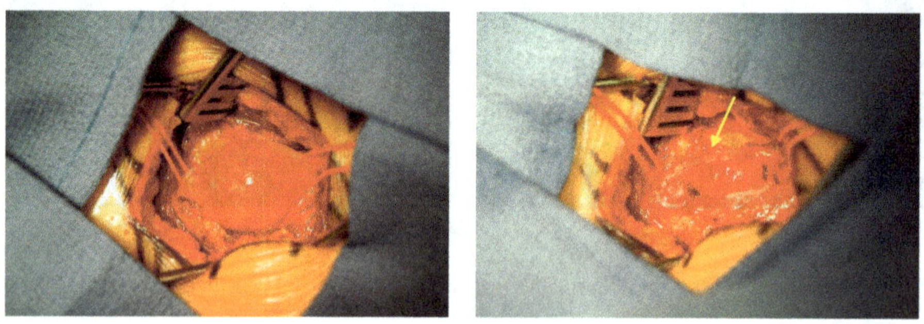

(a) (b)

FIGURE 5: (a) View of the surgical field with tumor along the sciatic nerve. (b) Tumor excised with sciatic nerve left intact (yellow arrow).

are sporadic, while 3% occurred in patients with neurofibromatosis type 2 (NF2) and 2% in patients with schwannomatosis [9]. NF2 is an autosomal dominant disease that is linked to mutations of the NF2 gene, a tumor suppressor gene, located on chromosome 22. Inactivation of this gene predisposes a patient to developing various tumors in the nervous system [10]. Patients with schwannomatosis are also susceptible to tumor spread along the nervous system, but the genes implicated in pathogenesis are distinct from the NF2 gene [11]. Differentiating between NF2 and schwannomatosis is difficult, as diagnosis is determined by clinical criteria [12]. The patient's diagnosis will depend on gene testing and follow-up MRI. If there is an absence of a vestibular tumor on MRI and no evidence of an NF2 gene mutation, this patient will qualify for a diagnosis of schwannomatosis. She will be followed up by both neurosurgery and neuro-oncology. Family testing will also be recommended.

Acknowledgments

The authors thank Walter Dent, Department of Neurosurgery, Tufts Medical Center, for acquisition of photos and other media related to the case.

References

[1] E. Patel and M. Perloff, "Radicular pain syndromes: cervical, lumbar, and spinal stenosis," *Seminars in Neurology*, vol. 38, no. 6, pp. 634–639, 2018.

[2] F. Kralick and R. Koenigsberg, "Sciatica in a patient with unusual peripheral nerve sheath tumors," *Surgical Neurology*, vol. 66, no. 6, pp. 634–637, 2006.

[3] A. Rhanim, R. El Zanati, M. Mahfoud, M. S. Berrada, and M. El Yaacoubi, "A rare cause of chronic sciatic pain: schwannoma of the sciatic nerve," *Journal of Clinical Orthopaedics and Trauma*, vol. 4, no. 2, pp. 89–92, 2013.

[4] K. Mezian, J. Vacek, L. Navrátil, L. Özçakar, and L. Navrátil, "Bilateral rectus femoris muscle rupture following statin medication," *American Journal of Physical Medicine & Rehabilitation*, vol. 96, no. 7, pp. e138–e140, 2017.

[5] A. K. Bhattacharyya, R. Perrin, and A. Guha, "Peripheral nerve tumors: management strategies and molecular insights," *Journal of Neuro-Oncology*, vol. 69, no. 1–3, pp. 335–349, 2004.

[6] O. Godkin, P. Ellanti, and G. O'Toole, "Large schwannoma of the sciatic nerve," *BMJ Case Reports*, vol. 2016, Article ID bcr2016217717, 2016.

[7] D. H. Kim, J. A. Murovic, R. L. Tiel, G. Moes, and D. G. Kline, "A series of 397 peripheral neural sheath tumors: 30-year experience at Louisiana State University health sciences center," *Journal of Neurosurgery*, vol. 102, no. 2, pp. 246–255, 2005.

[8] S. J. Omezzine, B. Zaara, M. Ben Ali, F. Abid, N. Sassi, and H. A. Hamza, "A rare cause of non discal sciatica: schwannoma of the sciatic nerve," *Orthopaedics & Traumatology: Surgery & Research*, vol. 95, no. 7, pp. 543–546, 2009.

[9] J. Antinheimo, R. Sankila, O. Carpén, E. Pukkala, M. Sainio, and J. Jääskeläinen, "Population-based analysis of sporadic and type 2 neurofibromatosis-associated meningiomas and schwannomas," *Neurology*, vol. 54, no. 1, p. 71, 2000.

[10] D. R. Evans, "Neurofibromatosis type 2 (NF2): a clinical and molecular review," *Orphanet Journal of Rare Diseases*, vol. 4, no. 1, p. 16, 2009.

[11] A. Piotrowski, J. Xie, Y. F. Liu et al., "Germline loss-of-function mutations in LZTR1 predispose to an inherited disorder of multiple schwannomas," *Nature Genetics*, vol. 46, no. 2, pp. 182–187, 2014.

[12] M. MacCollin, E. A. Chiocca, D. G. Evans et al., "Diagnostic criteria for schwannomatosis," *Neurology*, vol. 64, no. 11, pp. 1838–1845, 2005.

Permissions

All chapters in this book were first published by Hindawi Publishing Corporation; hereby published with permission under the Creative Commons Attribution License or equivalent. Every chapter published in this book has been scrutinized by our experts. Their significance has been extensively debated. The topics covered herein carry significant findings which will fuel the growth of the discipline. They may even be implemented as practical applications or may be referred to as a beginning point for another development.

The contributors of this book come from diverse backgrounds, making this book a truly international effort. This book will bring forth new frontiers with its revolutionizing research information and detailed analysis of the nascent developments around the world.

We would like to thank all the contributing authors for lending their expertise to make the book truly unique. They have played a crucial role in the development of this book. Without their invaluable contributions this book wouldn't have been possible. They have made vital efforts to compile up to date information on the varied aspects of this subject to make this book a valuable addition to the collection of many professionals and students.

This book was conceptualized with the vision of imparting up-to-date information and advanced data in this field. To ensure the same, a matchless editorial board was set up. Every individual on the board went through rigorous rounds of assessment to prove their worth. After which they invested a large part of their time researching and compiling the most relevant data for our readers.

The editorial board has been involved in producing this book since its inception. They have spent rigorous hours researching and exploring the diverse topics which have resulted in the successful publishing of this book. They have passed on their knowledge of decades through this book. To expedite this challenging task, the publisher supported the team at every step. A small team of assistant editors was also appointed to further simplify the editing procedure and attain best results for the readers.

Apart from the editorial board, the designing team has also invested a significant amount of their time in understanding the subject and creating the most relevant covers. They scrutinized every image to scout for the most suitable representation of the subject and create an appropriate cover for the book.

The publishing team has been an ardent support to the editorial, designing and production team. Their endless efforts to recruit the best for this project, has resulted in the accomplishment of this book. They are a veteran in the field of academics and their pool of knowledge is as vast as their experience in printing. Their expertise and guidance has proved useful at every step. Their uncompromising quality standards have made this book an exceptional effort. Their encouragement from time to time has been an inspiration for everyone.

The publisher and the editorial board hope that this book will prove to be a valuable piece of knowledge for researchers, students, practitioners and scholars across the globe.

List of Contributors

Ismail Ibrahim Ismail, Fathi Massoud and K. J. Alexander
Department of Neurology, Ibn Sina Hospital, Kuwait

Jasem Youssef Al-Hashel
Department of Neurology, Ibn Sina Hospital, Kuwait
Department of Medicine, Faculty of Medicine, Health Sciences Centre, Kuwait University, Kuwait

V. Montano, C. Simoncini, G. Siciliano and M. Mancuso
Department of Clinical and Experimental Medicine, Neurological Clinic, University of Pisa, Pisa, Italy

Cassi L. Calì
Department of Hand Surgery and Reconstructive Microsurgery, University of Pisa, Pisa, Italy

A. Legati
Unit of Medical Genetics and Neurogenetics, Fondazione IRCCS Istituto Neurologico "C. Besta", Milan, Italy

Nesreen Jaafar, Maria Khoueiry and Achraf Makki
Department of Neurology, American University of Beirut Medical Center, Beirut, Lebanon

Samia J. Khoury
Nehme and Therese Tohme Multiple Sclerosis Center, American University of Beirut Medical Center, Beirut, Lebanon

Catarina Falcão de Campos, Isabel Conceição, Mamede de Carvalho and Miguel Oliveira Santos
Department of Neurology, Department of Neurosciences and Mental Health, Hospital de Santa Maria, Centro Hospitalar Universitário Lisboa Norte, Lisbon, Portugal
Instituto de Medicina Molecular and Instituto de Fisiologia, Faculdade de Medicina, Universidade de Lisboa, Lisbon, Portugal

Rafael Roque
Neuropathology Unit, Department of Neurosciences and Mental Health, Hospital de Santa Maria, Centro Hospitalar Universitário Lisboa Norte, Lisbon, Portugal

The-Hao Nguyen, Van-Thanh-Cong Pham and Quynh-Trang Pham
Department of Neurosurgery, Bach Mai Hospital, Hanoi, Vietnam

Hao Nguyen Si Anh and Hoang-Long Vo
Institute for Preventive Medicine and Public Health, Hanoi Medical University, Hanoi, Vietnam

Phong Tran Nhu
Public Health Department, Nursing Faculty, Dai Nam University, Hanoi, Vietnam

Boonchai Boonyawat
Division of Genetics, Department of Pediatrics, Phramongkutklao Hospital and Phramongkutklao College of Medicine, Bangkok, Thailand

Mongkon Charoenpitakchai
Department of Pathology, Phramongkutklao Hospital and Phramongkutklao College of Medicine, Bangkok, Thailand

Piradee Suwanpakdee
Division of Neurology, Department of Pediatrics, Phramongkutklao Hospital and Phramongkutklao College of Medicine, Bangkok, Thailand

Ricky Chen
Providence Brain & Spine Institute, Providence St. Vincent Medical Center, 9135 SW Barnes Road, Suite 461, Portland, OR 97225, USA

Gurjeet Singh
Legacy Medical Group Neurology, Salmon Creek Medical Center, 2121 NE 139th St., Suite 205 Medical Office Building A, Vancouver, WA 98686, USA

J. Scott McNally
Department of Radiology and Imaging Sciences, University of Utah, 30 N 1900 E, Salt Lake City, UT 84132, USA

Cheryl A. Palmer
Department of Pathology, University of Utah, Huntsman Cancer Institute, 2000 Circle of Hope Dr., Salt Lake City, UT 84112, USA

Adam de Havenon
Department of Neurology, University of Utah, 175 N Medical Dr., Salt Lake City, UT 84132, USA

Alassane Mamadou Diop
Cheikh Anta Diop University, Dakar, Senegal
Neurology Department of the Pikine Hospital, Dakar, Senegal

Ahmadou Bamba Mbodj and Serigne Abdou Aziz Fall
Neuroscience Department of the Fann Hospital, Dakar, Senegal

Ibrahima Niang
Medical Imaging Department of the Fann Hospital, Dakar, Senegal

Nedal Bukhari
Department of Medical Oncology, King Fahad Specialist Hospital, Dammam, Saudi Arabia
Department of Internal Medicine, King Fahd University Hospital, Imam Abdulrahamn Bin Faisal University, Dammam, Saudi Arabia

Bachar Harfouch
Department of Neurosurgery, King Fahad Specialist Hospital, Dammam, Saudi Arabia

Majid Shallal Alotaibi
Department of Neurology, King Fahad Specialist Hospital, Dammam, Saudi Arabia

Hulayel Al-Harbi
Department of Medical Oncology, King Fahad Specialist Hospital, Dammam, Saudi Arabia

Omar Chamdine
Department of Pediatric Hematology Oncology and Stem Cell Transplantation, King Fahad Specialist Hospital, Dammam, Saudi Arabia

Jasmine Shimin Koh, Genevieve Lynn Yu Tan-Yu and Thirugnanam Umapathi
Department of Neurology, National Neuroscience Institute, 11 Jalan Tan Tock Seng, Singapore

James Wei Min Tung
Lee Kong Chian School of Medicine, Nanyang Technological University, 59 Nanyang Dr., Experimental Medicine Building, Singapore

Mutsumi Fujii and Miki Ohgushi
Department of Physical Medicine and Rehabilitation, Hyogo Rehabilitation Center, Kobe, Japan

Kazumi Tanigo, Hirokazu Yamamoto, Keijyu Kikugawa and Masayuki Shirakawa
Department of Rehabilitation, Hyogo Rehabilitation Center, Kobe, Japan

Takaaki Chin
Hyogo Rehabilitation Center, Kobe, Japan

Mojtaba Khazaei
Department of Neurology, Hamadan University of Medical Sciences, Hamadan, Iran

Kiana Karimi and Parinaz Sedighi
Student Research Committee, Hamadan University of Medical Sciences, Hamadan, Iran
Universal Scientific Education and Research Network (USERN), Tehran, Iran

Salman Khazaei
Research Center for Health Sciences, Hamadan University of Medical Sciences, Hamadan, Iran

Gustavo Gaitan-Quintero and Loida Camargo-Camargo
Neurology Residency Program of Sinú University, Cartagena, Colombia

Norman López-Velásquez
Universidad de La Costa, Barranquilla, Colombia

Miguel González
Duke University, Durham, NC, USA

Katerina Vraka, Dipak Ram, Siobhan West and Hui Jeen Tan
Department of Paediatric Neurology, Rotal Manchester Children's Hospital, Manchester M13 9WL, UK

Wei Yen Evelyn Chia, Praveen Kurup and Gayathri Subramanian
Department of Paediatric Intensive Care Unit, Rotal Manchester Children's Hospital, Manchester M13 9WL, UK

T. G. M. Prasadani and Kapila Panditha
Pediatric Ward, District General Hospital Avissawella, Avissawella, Colombo, Sri Lanka

D. Irugalbandara
Ophthalmology Unit, Lady Ridgeway Hospital for Children, Colombo, Sri Lanka

Fatemeh Yavari
Mashhad University of Medical Sciences, Mashhad, Iran

Sara Raji and Fatemeh Moradi
Student Research Committee, Faculty of Medicine, Mashhad University of Medical Sciences, Mashhad, Iran

Morteza Saeidi
Department of Neurology, Ghaem Hospital, Faculty of Medicine, Mashhad University of Medical Sciences, Mashhad, Iran

Ashish Chugh, Prashant Punia and Sarang Gotecha
Dr. D. Y. Patil Medical College and Hospital, Pimpri, Pune, Maharashtra, India

Yuichiro Yoneoka, Yasuhiro Seki and Katsuhiko Akiyama
Department of Neurosurgery, Uonuma Kikan Hospital, Uonuma Institute of Community Medicine, Niigata University Medical and Dental Hospital, Niigata 949-7302, Japan

Yuki Sakurai and Nobumasa Ohara
Department of Endocrine, Uonuma Kikan Hospital, Uonuma Institute of Community Medicine, Niigata University Medical and Dental Hospital, Niigata 949-7302, Japan

Go Hasegawa
Department of Pathology, Uonuma Kikan Hospital, Uonuma Institute of Community Medicine, Niigata University Medical and Dental Hospital, Niigata 949-7302, Japan

Gregory Griffin, Brittany Cunningham and Yonatan Spolter
Cleveland Clinic Akron General, Neurological Institute, Akron General Avenue, Akron, OH 44307, USA

Jonathan M. Beary
AT Still University-Missouri Campus, Neurobehavioral Sciences, 800 West Jefferson Avenue, Kirksville, MO 63501, USA

Richard Gandee
Cleveland Clinic Akron General, Neurological Institute, Akron General Avenue, Akron, OH 44307, USA
AT Still University-Missouri Campus, Neurobehavioral Sciences, 800 West Jefferson Avenue, Kirksville, MO 63501, USA

Christopher R. Newey
Cleveland Clinic Akron General, Neurological Institute, Akron General Avenue, Akron, OH 44307, USA
Cleveland Clinic, Neurological Institute, 9500 Euclid Avenue, Cleveland, OH 44195, USA

Yasunobu Nosaki, Ken Ohyama, Maki Watanabe, Takamasa Yokoi and Katsushige Iwai
Department of Neurology, Toyohashi Municipal Hospital, Toyohashi, Japan

Hedia Klaa, Thouraya Ben Younes, Hanene Benrhouma, Aida Rouissi, Ichraf Kraoua and Ilhem Ben Youssef-Turki
Department of Child and Adolescent Neurology, Research Laboratory LR18SP04, National Institute Mongi Ben Hmida of Neurology, Tunis, Tunisia
University of Tunis El Manar, Faculty of Medicine of Tunis, Tunis 1007, Tunisia

Sonia Nagi
University of Tunis El Manar, Faculty of Medicine of Tunis, Tunis 1007, Tunisia
Department of Neuroradiology, National Institute Mongi Ben Hmida of Neurology, Tunis, Tunisia

Yoshiki Esa, Yushi Watanabe, Harutoshi Fujimura, Junya Kobayashi and Yuta Kajiyama
Department of Neurology, Sakai City Medical Center, Sakai, Japan

Misako Kaido
Department of Neurology, Sakai City Medical Center, Sakai, Japan
Department of Clinical Genetics, Sakai City Medical Center, Sakai, Japan

Iwao Gohma
Department of Respiratory Medicine, Sakai City Medical Center, Sakai, Japan

Kenichi Takahashi
Department of Respiratory Medicine, Kishiwada City Hospital, Kishiwada, Japan

Janet K. Lee, Kathleen Murray and Swetha Renati
University of South Florida, Department of Neurology, Tampa, FL, USA

Mostafa Suhail Najim, Riyadh Ali Mohammed Hammamy and Sreethish Sasi
Department of Internal Medicine, Hamad Medical Corporation, Doha, Qatar

Ameet Kumar Jha
University of Central Nicaragua, Managua, Nicaragua

Prakash Baral
Department of Anatomy, Gandaki Medical College, Pokhara, Nepal

Salman Assad, Justin Nolte, Dharampreet Singh, Samrina Hanif and Paul Ferguson
Department of Neurology, Marshall University School of Medicine, Huntington, WV, USA

Nathaniel M. Robbins
Department of Neurology, Geisel Dartmouth School of Medicine, Hanover, USA

Jillian R. Ozmore
Department of Medical Genetics, Dartmouth-Hitchcock Medical Center, Lebanon, USA

Thomas L. Winder
Invitae Corporation, San Francisco, USA

Pedro Gonzalez-Alegre and Tanya M. Bardakjian
Department of Neurology, The University of Pennsylvania, Philadelphia, USA

Michael Winklehner
Institute of Neurology, Medical University of Vienna, Vienna, Austria

Claudia Stöllberger
2nd Medical Department, Krankenanstalt Rudolfstiftung, Vienna, Austria

Thomas Hummel
Krankenhaus Stockerau, Stockerau, Austria

Chanaka Amugoda
Emergency Department, Werribee Mercy Hospital, Melbourne, Australia

Noushin Chini Foroush
Medical Registrar, Austin Health, Melbourne, Australia

Hamed Akhlaghi
Emergency Physician, St. Vincent's Hospital, University of Melbourne, Melbourne, Australia

Jesus Eduardo Garcia-Berlanga, Isaac Jair Palacios, 4 Alejandro Banegas-Lagos, Augusto Rojas-Martinez and Daniel Martinez-Ramirez
Tecnologico deMonterrey, Escuela deMedicina y Ciencias de la Salud, Monterrey, Nuevo Leon, Mexico

Mariana Moscovich
Department of Neurology, Christian-Albrechts University, Kiel, Germany

Muhammet Ozer, Khadija Merchant and Zulfiya Manning
Department of Internal Medicine, Capital Health Regional Medical Center, Trenton, NJ, USA

Suleyman Yasin Goksu
Department of Internal Medicine, University of Texas Southwestern Medical School, Dallas, TX, USA

Kirti Juneja
Bharati Vidyapeeth Deemed University Medical College, Pune, Maharashtra, India

Vernard S. Fennell
Division of Endovascular Neurosurgery, Capital Health Regional Medical Center, Trenton, NJ, USA

Josef Finsterer and Sinda Zarrouk
Neurology and Neurophysiology Center, Vienna, Austria
University of Tunis El Manar, Tunis, Tunisia
Krankenanstalt Rudolfstiftung, Messerli Institute, Vienna, Austria

Mohankumar Kurukumbi and James Leiphart
Department of Neurology, Inova Fairfax Hospital, Falls Church, VA, USA

Anam Asif
VCU School of Medicine, Inova Campus, Falls Church, VA, USA

Jing Wang
Department of Neurocritical Care, Inova Fairfax Hospital, Falls Church, VA, USA

Jehad Zakaria, Pravesh Saini, Mariya Yanovskaya, John T. Tsiang, Krishnan Ravindran and Stephen Johans
Department of Neurological Surgery, Stritch School of Medicine, Loyola University Medical Center, Maywood, IL, USA

Chirag R. Patel
Department of Otolaryngology-Head and Neck Surgery, Stritch School of Medicine, Loyola University Medical Center, Maywood, IL, USA

Anand V. Germanwala
Department of Neurological Surgery, Stritch School of Medicine, Loyola University Medical Center, Maywood, IL, USA
Department of Otolaryngology-Head and Neck Surgery, Stritch School of Medicine, Loyola University Medical Center, Maywood, IL, USA

Bhupendra Shah and Roshan Chhetri
Department of Internal Medicine, B.P. Koirala Institute of Health Sciences, Dharan, Nepal

Jose Gabriel Solis, Arturo Olascoaga Lugo and Jose Malagón Rangel
Department of Internal Medicine, Hospital de Especialidades "Dr. Bernardo Sepúlveda Gutiérrez", Centro Médico Nacional Siglo XXI, Instituto Mexicano del Seguro Social, Ciudad de México, Mexico

Marco Antonio Rodríguez Florido
Department of Pathology, Hospital de Pediatría Centro Médico Nacional Siglo XXI, Instituto Mexicano del Seguro Social, Ciudad de México, Mexico

Bayron Alexander Sandoval Bonilla
Department of Neurosurgery, Hospital de Especialidades "Dr. Bernardo Sepúlveda Gutiérrez", Centro Médico Nacional Siglo XXI, Instituto Mexicano del Seguro Social, Ciudad de México, Mexico

Athanasios Astreinidis and Stephanos Finitsis
Department of Endovascular Surgery, AHEPA Hospital, Aristotle University of Thessaloniki, Panepistimioupoli, 54124 Thessaloniki, Greece

Xanthippi Mavropoulou, Elisavet Psoma and Panagiotis Prassopoulos
Department of Radiology and Medical Imaging, AHEPA University Hospital, Panepistimioupoli, 54124 Thessaloniki, Greece

Joel Leonardi, Christian Saleh, Phillip Jaszczuk, Stefanie Wilmes and Margret Hund-Georgiadis
REHAB Basel, Clinic for Neurorehabilitation and Paraplegiology, Basel, Switzerland

Kristine A. Blackham
Department of Radiology, Division of Diagnostic and Interventional Neuroradiology, University Hospital Basel, Basel, Switzerland

Sabrina Zechel
Institute of Neuropathology, University Medical Center Göttingen, Göttingen, Germany

Praveen Sripad, Jürgen Dammers and Frank Boers
Institute of Neuroscience and Medicine (INM-4), Medical Imaging Physics, Forschungszentrum Jülich GmbH, 52425 Jűlich, Germany

Jessica Rosenberg
Institute of Neuroscience and Medicine (INM-4), Medical Imaging Physics, Forschungszentrum Jülich GmbH, 52425 Jűlich, Germany
Institute of Neuroscience and Medicine (INM-11), JARA, Forschungszentrum Jűlich GmbH, 52425 Jűlich, Germany
Department of Neurology, RWTH Aachen University, Aachen, Germany

Christian P. Filss
Institute of Neuroscience and Medicine (INM-4), Medical Imaging Physics, Forschungszentrum Jülich GmbH, 52425 Jűlich, Germany
Department of Nuclear Medicine, RWTH Aachen University, Aachen, Germany

Norbert Galldiks
Institute of Neuroscience and Medicine (INM-3), Forschungszentrum Jűlich, Jűlich GmbH, 52425 Jűlich, Germany
Department of Neurology, University of Cologne, Cologne, Germany
Center of Integrated Oncology (CIO), Universities of Cologne and Bonn, Cologne, Germany

Karl-Josef Langen
Institute of Neuroscience and Medicine (INM-4), Medical Imaging Physics, Forschungszentrum Jülich GmbH, 52425 Jűlich, Germany
Department of Nuclear Medicine, RWTH Aachen University, Aachen, Germany
Center of Integrated Oncology (CIO), Universities of Cologne and Bonn, Cologne, Germany
JARA - BRAIN - Translational Medicine, Aachen, Germany

Ralf Clauss
Nuclear Medicine Department, Royal Surrey County Hospital, Guildford, Surrey GU2 7XX, UK

N. Jon Shah
Institute of Neuroscience and Medicine (INM-4), Medical Imaging Physics, Forschungszentrum Jülich GmbH, 52425 Jűlich, Germany
Institute of Neuroscience and Medicine (INM-11), JARA, Forschungszentrum Jűlich GmbH, 52425 Jűlich, Germany
Department of Neurology, RWTH Aachen University, Aachen, Germany
JARA - BRAIN - Translational Medicine, Aachen, Germany

Sigge Weisdorf and Troels W. Kjaer
Zealand University Hospital, Department of Neurology, Roskilde, Denmark
University of Copenhagen, Department of Clinical Medicine, Copenhagen, Denmark

Ivan C. Zibrandtsen
Zealand University Hospital, Department of Neurology, Roskilde, Denmark

Shania Niromi Gunasekera, Priyanka Yogananda, Harindra Karunatilaka and Bimsara Senanayake
National Hospital of Sri Lanka, Colombo, Sri Lanka

Keith George, Shane Burke and Ron Riesenburger
Department of Neurosurgery, Tufts Medical Center, 800 Washington Street, Boston 02111, MA, USA

Knarik Arkun
Department of Neurosurgery, Tufts Medical Center, 800 Washington Street, Boston 02111, MA, USA
Department of Pathology, Tufts Medical Center, 800 Washington Street, Boston 02111, MA, USA

Index

www.ingramcontent.com/pod-product-compliance
Lightning Source LLC
LaVergne TN
LVHW082229200926
848484LV00008B/2322